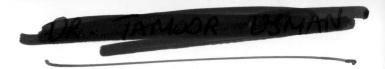

An Aid to Paediatric Surgery

*To the five women in my life, my wife
Elizabeth, and my four daughters, Kathleen,
Maureen, Madeleine and Eileen*

An Aid to Paediatric Surgery

Edited by

R A MacMahon MS FRCS FRACS

Senior Paediatric Surgeon,
Queen Victoria Children's Hospital, Monash Medical Centre

Associate Professor of Paediatric Surgery,
Monash University, Melbourne

SECOND EDITION

CHURCHILL LIVINGSTONE
MELBOURNE EDINBURGH LONDON NEW YORK AND TOKYO 1991

CHURCHILL LIVINGSTONE
Medical Division of Longman UK Limited

Distributed in Australia by Longman Cheshire Pty Limited,
Longman House, Kings Gardens, 95 Coventry Street,
South Melbourne 3205, and by associated companies,
branches and representatives throughout the world.

First edition 1984
Second edition 1991

ISBN 0-443-04185-7

National Library of Australia Cataloguing in Publication
Data

An Aid to paediatric surgery.

  2nd ed.
  Includes index.
  ISBN 0 443 04185 7.

  1. Children — Surgery. I. MacMahon, Robert A.

617.98

A Library of Congress catalog record is available for this
title

Produced by Longman Singapore Publishers (Pte) Ltd.
Printed in Singapore

Preface to the second edition

It is pleasing to have the opportunity to produce a second edition of a book. It signifies that the first edition has been successful and it gives the opportunity to incorporate second thoughts after the first edition and to include developments since the first edition. Much of the text has been rewritten and brought up-to-date, particularly in the area of special investigations where CT and MRI are replacing previous methods. Some illustrations have been dropped, new ones added and three new chapters on child abuse, sports medicine and ethics have been added to reflect the increasing interest in these areas. Fortunately, it has been possible to make all these changes without any significant change to the size of the book.

Once again I am indebted to my coauthors and to many colleagues for their helpful advice, and in particular, to Professor Arthur Clark, Professor of Paediatrics at Monash University, for many constructive suggestions. I would particularly like to express my gratitude to Mrs Laura Donnelly for all her help, particularly in typing the manuscript.

Melbourne, 1991   R. A. M

Preface to the first edition

This book is intended as an introduction to paediatric surgery for medical and paramedical students and will serve as an aid to memory for those who have already studied paediatric surgery. The aim has been to provide a basic, easy to read, easy to remember book for the student.

The book has been written in a problem-oriented rather than a didactic teaching style, highlighting the type of clinical problems encountered. It is small enough to allow an overview of the essentials of paediatric surgery, and related subjects have been kept together whenever possible, so that their relationship to each other is obvious. This will give the reader a perspective of a whole set of defects rather than presenting him with multiple short topics which, though easily read, do not facilitate unification with the whole. Where possible, we have used facts and figures which can be assimilated without difficulty, particularly in areas where there are differences of opinion or a range of figures quoted in the literature.

Emphasis has been placed on those conditions which are peculiar to paediatric surgery or which are not well understood by students. Common problems that affect both paediatric and adult patients, and which are covered extensively in adult surgical textbooks, have been put into context but have been dealt with only briefly. Contributions from Africa, Australia, India and the United States of America illustrate the similarities in the common problems faced by paediatric surgeons in different areas of the world and also highlight some of the differences.

I wish to thank the many people who have helped me in this project, particularly my coauthors and members of the Monash University Department of Paediatrics, and the many other colleagues who helped with constructive criticism. I would like also to thank Miss Janet Thompson and Miss Kay Lynch for their great patience and help with the manuscript.

Melbourne, 1984   R. A. M

Contributors

E. Thomas Boles Jr MD
Chief Pediatric Surgeon, Division of Pediatric
Surgery, Department of Surgery, Ohio State
University College of Medicine, Children's
Hospital, Columbus, Ohio, USA

W. K. Chung FRACS
Visiting Orthopaedic Surgeon, Prince of Wales
Children's Hospital, Sydney, Australia

L. J. Cussen FRCPA
Senior Lecturer in Paediatrics, Monash
University; Honorary Consultant Pathologist,
Monash Medical Centre, Melbourne, Australia

M. J. Glasson FRCS, FRACS
Director, Department of Paediatric Surgery,
Royal Alexandra Hospital for Children,
Sydney, Australia.

T. F. Lambert Dip Ed FFARCS, FFARACS
Honorary Senior Lecturer, Department of
Paediatrics, Monash University, Melbourne,
Australia

E. F. MacMahon MB ChB
Victorian Co-Ordinator, National Association
for the Prevention of Child Abuse and
Neglect, Melbourne, Australia

R. A. MacMahon MS, FRCS, FRACS
Senior Paediatric Surgeon, Queen Victoria
Children's Hospital, Monash Medical Centre;
Associate Professor of Paediatric Surgery,
Monash University, Melbourne, Australia

F. A. Nwako MCh, FRCS, FMCS, FICS, FWACS
Professor of Paediatric Surgery, University of
Nigeria, Enugu, Anambra State, Nigeria

K. C. Pringle FRACS
Paediatric Surgeon, Department of Surgery,
Wellington Medical School, University of
Otago, Wellington, New Zealand; Past
President, International Fetal Medicine
and Surgery Society

P. Upadhyaya MS, FRCS, FAMS
Professor of Paediatric Surgery, King Fahd
Hospital of the University, King Faisal
University, Al-Khobar, Kingdom of Saudi
Arabia; previously Professor of Paediatric
Surgery, All India Institute of Medical
Science, New Delhi, India

R. W. Yardley B Med Sci, PhD, FRACS
Paediatric Surgeon, Queen Victoria Children's
Hospital, Monash Medical Centre; Senior
Lecturer in Paediatric Surgery, Monash
University, Melbourne, Australia

Contents

1. The physiological differences between adults and children

T. F. Lambert

An adult in the early twenties has reached full physiological development, with considerable reserve in the various organs to cope with the stresses to which the body will be subject. These include the normal hazards of everyday life as well as those of accident or disease. Thereafter, there is a slow decline in function (ageing) over the next four decades and then a more rapid change after the age of 60. From the time of physiological maturity, excessive demand on the body systems may result in organ failure and each such insult is likely to impair function and reserve. As the individual ages, a lesser insult is needed to produce organ failure until a very minor change will have a major effect in the elderly.

THE NEWBORN INFANT

The newborn infant is in a different state. The body systems have yet to develop their full physiological function and their reserves are small. Only with growth and development will full adult function and capacity be reached. In the same way that a small stress in an old person may lead to organ failure, so it will in an infant; but because of the capacity of the small child to grow and regenerate tissue there may be little or no residual damage to the child's physiological potential. Because it is easy for a small change to produce organ failure in one system, this leads on to failure in other systems and this principle of the interdependence of body systems is much more obvious in paediatrics than in adult medicine.

Rate of change

A further major difference from adult practice is the rapidity with which children change from being fit and well to being severely ill. From being a bit miserable and snuffly a child can be moribund from meningitis within 24 hours or become dehydrated from gastroenteritis to the extent of peripheral circulatory failure within a similar length of time.

Growth as a stabilizing mechanism

There is the further difference in children that growth is a stabilizing mechanism. By utilizing energy substrates for the processes of growth, the load presented to the excretory pathways is reduced. For example, the infant kidney, although immature, can cope with the daily excretory load because of the incorporation of a large proportion of the daily intake of food into growing cells. The high utilization of energy in promoting cell growth protects the kidney to some extent and failure to thrive carries with it the likelihood of renal failure because of the spill over of protein that was previously being incorporated into, or forming, new cells.

Absolute measurements

A further requirement for the paediatric student is to adapt his or her thinking to the smaller volumes and doses that are needed in paediatrics. The rapid loss of 35 mL of blood by a newborn baby represents 10% of the blood volume and may produce circulatory failure, whereas that

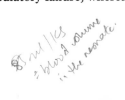

1

volume is negligible and the proportion of little significance to an adult. Further examples of these differences are given later in this and subsequent chapters but great harm can be done to the child unless the physician recognizes these differences in absolute value and proportion.

Physiological differences

Most of the comparisons that follow are between the neonate and the adult since the differences are most marked between these two groups. The underlying principles in all of the differences are those of immaturity of function and undeveloped reserve capacity.

Basal metabolic rate

Although the fetus has a rapid rate of growth, much of the regulation of energy balance occurs through the placenta. Estimates of fetal oxygen consumption suggest a rate of 4–5 mL of oxygen per kilogram per minute. Most of the energy substrate is glucose. Glycogen is laid down in the liver predominantly in the last trimester and so the very premature infant may have hardly any glycogen reserve.

The basal metabolic rate (BMR) rises rapidly after delivery and is high in the newborn period, mainly because of the rapid consumption of energy caused by cell growth and the increased requirement for heat production. Values for the neonate of 6–8 mL of oxygen per kilogram per minute are normal, with wide variation being usual. In addition, the nature of the substrate changes from glucose to free fatty acid and glycerol. In the premature infant the rate of rise in BMR may be slower and may take several days.

The BMR decreases quite rapidly over the first 18 months to 2 years and then slows gradually over the next few years until the adult value of 2–4 mL of oxygen per kilogram per minute is reached by the time of puberty. There is often a small rise in BMR at the time of puberty, presumably associated with the development of the secondary sexual characteristics.

Carbon dioxide production is increased in consequence of the increased metabolic rate and follows a similar time course of change to oxygen consumption.

Temperature regulation

The newborn infant is homeothermic and will mount an appropriate response to a thermal stress. However, the response may be short lived and inadequate because of the immaturity of the controlling and effector mechanisms and the adverse physical characteristics of the small child. The small baby is most at risk from cold stress as a result of these physiological and physical differences but it is sometimes forgotten that heat stress can be a major problem for babies and small children.

Physical factors

The physical factors that govern heat loss (conduction, convection and radiation) are the same for the child as for the adult. These are dependant upon surface area and the difference in temperature between the baby and the environment. The surface area of the newborn is 0.2 m^2 for a 3.5 kg infant (c.f. the 70 kg adult with 1.73 m^2). Because of the larger surface area to weight ratio in a baby (2–2.5 times that of an adult) loss or gain of heat is correspondingly easier in the newborn. The smaller mass means that the body heat sink is less able to protect against sudden change.

Peripheral mechanisms

The newborn is handicapped by having a thinner layer of subcutaneous tissue to insulate the core. There is poor vasomotor control of surface blood vessels so that attempts to cause vasoconstriction, and hence diminish heat loss, are inadequate and poorly sustained. The transient mottled appearance of the skin when an infant is cold is an outward manifestation of this immaturity.

Two other mechanisms that are absent or rudimentary in the newborn are shivering and sweating. An infant will not normally shiver in the first few weeks of life, so that involuntary heat production from this activity is not possible in the neonatal period. Nor is it easy to make a baby sweat: in response to a heat stress, there is marked peripheral dilatation only.

Brown adipose tissue

Most of the heat production in a resting individual comes from the processing of food. The newborn is unique in that he/she has a small reserve of brown fat from which heat can be liberated by non-shivering thermogenesis. The trigger for this is noradrenaline and the stores are found over the limb girdles and up and down the spine, but principally in the interscapular region. Once used, the brown fat stores cannot be replaced, but they serve as a protection for the baby until the BMR increases as a result of the metabolism of food.

Central controlling mechanisms

The central controlling mechanisms for homeothermic temperature control are present at birth, even in the small premature infant. The time course of the response is rapid but the efficacy of the response may be short lived and inadequate (only a few minutes in the smallest premature infant). As myelination within the central nervous system increases, so control becomes more exact, but this will not mature until after puberty. The New York skyline-like appearance of the temperature chart in a toddler with an infection is an example of the fact that the controlling negative feedback system is still not well damped and there may be rapid peak-to-peak fluctuation of 3°C over quite short periods even with a fairly mild infection. This pattern of the underdamped response is a characteristic of paediatric physiology that will be seen in the other body systems.

Voluntary control

Quite apart from these physiological differences, the infant differs from the adult in having no voluntary control over the environment or activity. On a cold day, an adult will alter the amount of heat being supplied to the room, put on warmer clothes or perform some exercise in order to achieve a state of well-being. The infant and small child are quite unable to do this and are vulnerable to extremes of temperature in an adult world. The infant left in a parked car in high summer who gets heat exhaustion is an example of this.

The neutral thermal environment

From the integration of the foregoing principles the idea has been conceived that there is an optimum zone within which a small baby can be nursed with minimum expenditure of energy on temperature regulation. This is called the neutral thermal environment. The premature infant needs a higher temperature and has a narrower range of temperature within which the least amount of metabolic energy will be consumed than does the more mature baby. Graphs of this zone for clothed and unclothed infants are available in most nurseries, but for a naked baby weighing 1 kg in a still atmosphere and 50% relative humidity, the range is from 34.4 to 35.5°C, whereas for a 3 kg infant under the same circumstances, the range is 31.5 to 34.5°C.

Two examples will serve to illustrate the clinical importance of temperature balance. First, the nursing of all sick and premature infants in incubators is a means of providing the accurate control of the thermal environment which will produce the least wastage of metabolic energy. Second, the operating theatre presents a major thermal stress for all children, but especially for the newborn, since it is normally set at a temperature that is comfortable for a gowned adult. Precautions to minimize heat loss (by leaving the infant uncovered for the shortest possible time and by using warm prep solutions) and to supply heat (by warming and humidifying inspired gases; use of a warming blanket; increasing the operating theatre temperature) are necessary to ensure that the child remains in the best possible condition.

BODY FLUIDS

The fetus and fetal tissues have an extremely high water content. Towards the latter part of gestation, around 90% of the fetus' body weight is water. After delivery the body water content falls, so that by the third or fourth day the percentage has been reduced to approximately 80% by weight. Thereafter, there is a gradual loss of body water until the age of 1–2 years, when the proportion is similar to the adult figures of 60–70% by weight (Fig. 1.1).

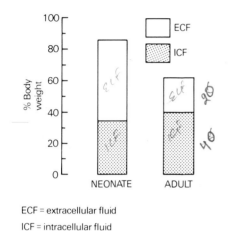

ECF = extracellular fluid

ICF = intracellular fluid

Fig. 1.1 Total body water as a percentage of body weight, showing the relative proportions of intra- and extracellular fluid.

Proportions of body water

Intracellular water changes relatively little, being 35% by weight in the newborn and rising to 40% quite quickly. Extracellular fluid is strikingly different, being about 40% in the newborn, nearly double the adult figure. This large volume of readily exchangeable water is partly present as a buffer zone to protect the child from sudden fluctuations in fluid balance, but it is also readily available to leak out quickly in disease (e.g. gastroenteritis) and water conservation is a major physiological problem for the newborn.

Principal sites of loss

Urinary system

In the newborn period the maximum concentration that can be achieved in the urine is 800 mosmol/L. This compares to the adult figure of 1400 mosmol/L. The premature infant has even less ability to concentrate urine and in particular is quite unable to conserve urinary sodium, so that the very small premature infant is likely to be both dehydrated and hyponatraemic. Any additional solute load presented to the kidney must take with it an obligatory urine volume which cannot be reduced below a figure consistent with this ability of the kidney to concentrate. The fact that the infant is growing rapidly has led to the view that the kidney is spared an excessive solute load since the nutrients are being incorporated into cells, but should growth cease, then the kidney will be presented with an immediate spill over of solute which will take with it a large volume of water. This in turn may precipitate dehydration and renal failure.

The normal values for glomerular filtration rate and for tubular function (either secretory or reabsorptive) are absolutely and proportionately lower in the neonate than in the adult. These figures are low because of the relatively poor blood supply to the infant kidney and the smaller pore size and lesser filtration pressure across the nephron. For example, glomerular filtration rate is about 38 mL/min per 1.73 m^2 in the newborn, or about one-third of the adult value. Maturation after birth is rapid so that between 1 and 2 years of life the adult value of 125 mL/min is reached.

Alimentary tract

The second conservation mechanism that is poorly developed in the newborn is the resorption of water from the alimentary tract. The alimentary tract has to obtain sufficient nutrition from the food to enable growth to take place. For this, a large surface area is required. Despite the fact that the nutrients present in breast milk are fairly simple, the mucosal surface is still comparatively smooth so that a long length of bowel is required for absorption. Despite the length of the bowel, the faeces of the newborn infant are high in water content and resorption of water from the large bowel only becomes fully mature between the ages of 1 and 2 years. When the bowel is stressed by disease its ability to absorb water is markedly reduced. So watery may the bowel actions become that they may be mistaken for urine by the unwary.

It is not uncommon for the bowel to be immature and fail to absorb the food constituents, the commonest circumstance being that of disaccharide intolerance. In this situation the sugar within the small bowel will present to the large bowel and an obligatory water loss will follow this osmotic load. Sugar intolerance is not infrequent in the postoperative period, especially after bowel surgery, and can cause even older children to become dehydrated if it goes unrecognized. Infection within the bowel is another common cause of disturbance in the small infant who may progress to pre-renal failure within 24 hours of the onset of gastroenteritis. Particularly if the fluid stools are mistaken for urine, the replacement of water and electrolytes may be inadequate or inappropriate and circulatory failure will then be added to renal failure.

The principle of the interdependence of body systems in the newborn is well demonstrated by these examples of failed water conservation. By calculating the amount of loss the difference in absolute values between adult and paediatric practice can also be made clear. Loss of 400 mL of fluid from an adult of 70 kg is insignificant and its contribution to the daily water balance of 2 or 3 L is quite small. Loss of 400 mL of fluid from a 4 kg baby represents 10% of the body weight and this degree of dehydration can produce peripheral circulatory failure.

Blood volume

The blood volume is of particular interest to the student of surgery. In the neonate this is approximately 85 mL/kg of body weight (c.f. 60–70 mL/kg in the adult). This may not seem a very large difference, but again it is the absolute values that are important.

Using the above figure, a 3.5 kg neonate will have a total blood volume of just under 300 mL. Three blood-stained gauze swabs during a surgical operation can easily total 30 mL of blood. In an adult this sort of loss is insignificant and often occurs from the skin wound at any major oper-

ation, but in the infant mentioned above 30 mL represents 10% of the infant's blood volume. If this is not replaced, then this magnitude of loss in the small baby will put him/her into, or close to, peripheral circulatory failure. The student of paediatrics has to learn to scale down his/her calculations very considerably in order to get the balance right in infant management.

CARDIOVASCULAR SYSTEM

During fetal life oxygenated blood is returned from the placenta via the umbilical vein to the right side of the heart. Here it joins venous deoxygenated blood returning from the various organ systems of the fetus. Directional flow in the inferior vena cava diverts most of the oxygenated blood coming from the placenta across the patent foramen ovale to the left atrium whence it is pumped to the head and neck, whilst most of the deoxygenated blood returning down the superior vena cava finds its way into the right ventricle and the main pulmonary artery. Approximately four-fifths of the right ventricular output

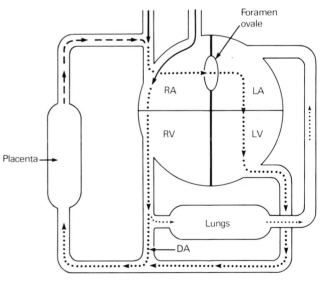

Fig. 1.2 Fetal circulation. Some streaming occurs so that most of the oxygenated blood goes to the left ventricle and most of the deoxygenated blood goes to the right ventricle. RA and LA = right and left atrium; RV and LV = right and left ventricle; DA = ductus arteriosus; Oxygenated blood — — ►; Deoxygenated blood ——►; 'Mixed' blood •••••►

is channelled away from the lungs through the patent ductus arteriosus because of the high pulmonary artery pressure in the fetus. This process allows deoxygenated blood to be returned to the placenta via the descending aorta and the umbilical arteries (Fig. 1.2).

Oxygenation

The PO_2 of the blood in the carotid artery of the fetus is between 25 and 30 mmHg. Compared with the adult arterial oxygen tension of 98 mmHg this is low but the fetal oxyhaemoglobin curve is displaced to the left of the adult curve and fetal haemoglobin is thus able to accept more oxygen for a given PO_2. The fetus also has a higher haemoglobin level of 18–21 g/100 mL (11.2–13.0 mmol/L) of blood. These two factors mean that, despite its lower PO_2, the fetus receives an adequate supply of oxygen for its metabolic needs.

Postnatally, the adult form of haemoglobin becomes the norm and the level falls rapidly over the first 3 months of life. The change in the nature of the haemoglobin and the lower viscosity of the blood help to offset the effect of the reduced oxygen carrying capacity of the blood during the period of the physiological anaemia of lactation, but the haemoglobin level does not return to more adult levels until approximately 3 years of age.

Change in the circulation at birth

The rapid change in haemodynamics following the separation of the placenta and the onset of air breathing leads to major changes in the intracardiac circulation. Since the placental return is no longer available there is a rapid fall in right atrial pressure. At the same time the pulmonary artery pressure falls by 50% over the first few breaths, thus allowing a much larger proportion of the right ventricular output to go to the lung than was possible in the fetus. This in turn allows greater flow into the left atrium and a concomitant rise in left atrial pressure. The combined outcome of these changes is to reduce, and then reverse, the flow of blood from right to left atrium thus producing functional closure of the foramen ovale. As pulmonary pressures fall and flow into the left atrium rises so there is a corresponding rise in left ventricular output and pressure. This causes reduction, and then cessation, of flow in the ductus arteriosus.

These changes take place within a few hours of delivery in a healthy newborn. The foramen ovale, although physiologically closed, may never close anatomically. Closure of the ductus arteriosus is not usually complete until 6–8 weeks of age. The lack of tight closure in the newborn accounts for the large proportion of normal right to left shunts seen in the neonate (up to 20%). When these processes have been completed the adult circulation is fully established.

Transitional circulation

Because the ductus and foramen ovale are only physiologically closed in the neonatal period it is possible for these channels to re-open and the circulation of the neonate to revert to the pattern of flow seen in the fetus. Hypoxia and acidosis lower systemic arterial and left atrial pressures and raise pulmonary and right atrial pressures. The ductus and foramen ovale now re-open and right to left shunting occurs. This is clearly a vicious circle since venous blood cannot perfuse the lung whilst these bypass channels are open. Hypoxaemia is potentiated and further acidosis occurs and this process accounts for the very high values for right to left shunts that are seen in the newborn in such conditions as respiratory distress syndrome. This reversal of the circulation can occur at any time until anatomical closure is complete. In an otherwise normal full-term infant this possibility rarely lasts beyond the neonatal period, but in the small premature infant it exists for much longer.

Heart rate

Heart rate in the fetus is rapid with an average of 140 and a range of 110 to 180 beats per minute. There is an increase in heart rate over the first month of life but it falls steadily after that over the next few years of life, not reaching adult levels until after puberty. Despite the high rate the circulation at birth is predominantly governed by inhibitory tone from the parasympathetic system. Beat-to-beat variation of heart rate can be marked and is normal in the fetus and young child. It is one of the parameters that is used in fetal monitoring to determine fetal well-being and it is one of the first indications of fetal distress. The wide fluctuation in heart rate is a further example of an underdeveloped feedback mechanism.

Myocardial contractility

Cardiac output rises during the latter part of gestation but the myocardial syncitium has a low compliance at birth and so the heart cannot respond to a fall in cardiac output by increased contractility, save at the expense of a large amount of work. This inelasticity of the myocardial fibre also limits the extent to which an infant can overcome the effects of a change in preload and all these factors add to the poor peripheral circulatory control to render the neonate particularly susceptible to blood or fluid loss. As was discussed previously, 10% of blood loss will render a neonate liable to peripheral circulatory failure. A lesser proportion of loss will have the same effect on the very small premature infant.

ECG

There is right ventricular predominance on the ECG at birth that represents the dominance of the right ventricle in fetal life. By 3 months of age the left ventricle has developed to the stage at which both ventricles are of equal size and thereafter the usual left ventricular predominance of the adult begins to be asserted. It takes several years for the adult tracing to be fully developed and interpretation of the ECG in childhood requires that the age of the child be known and taken into consideration.

RESPIRATORY SYSTEM

Functional residual capacity

The fetal lung is not an unexpanded inactive organ awaiting the first extrauterine breath, but is an actively metabolizing organ functioning like an exocrine gland producing, and being distended by, its own secretion — lung liquid. Indeed, the production and removal of lung liquid play a part in the maturation of the lung. By the time that the airways have reached the stage of alveolization and development of the terminal sacs, the lungs have sufficient capacity for postnatal survival. In humans this occurs at about 24 weeks. After delivery the lung matures rapidly but only about half of the alveoli are present at birth and therefore a premature infant has very little reserve capacity. The volume of lung liquid contained in the fetal lung close to term is almost identical to the functional residual capacity (FRC) that the infant will establish after the onset of air breathing. In the neonatal period the FRC is small compared with the total lung capacity so that alveolar instability is a particular problem for the newborn.

Breathing movement

The muscles of respiration are active in utero and become increasingly so in the latter part of gestation. This breathing movement is presumably in preparation for the onset of extrauterine respiration when the lung takes over from the placenta as the organ responsible for gas exchange. In utero, the drive to breathing movement is discontinuous and the control is rudimentary, but the fact that the vast majority of infants establish regular rhythmic respiration unaided after delivery attests to the efficiency of the process of maturation and testing of the system in utero.

Patterns of respiration

Compared to the adult, the newborn breathes at a faster rate (35–40 breaths per minute) with considerable variability within a normal range from 10–80 breaths per minute. The high rate is in response to the greater metabolic rate of the baby already discussed, whilst the variability is another manifestation of the immature feedback systems. Tidal volume (TV), on the other hand, remains constant at 7 mL/kg throughout life (with the exception of the first 24 hours when it is slightly less). The dead space also occupies a constant proportion of one-third of the TV from the time of delivery.

Rate versus volume

There are good structural reasons why the new-born utilizes an increase in rate rather than in tidal volume to provide its metabolic demand for oxygen.

In the supine infant the abdominal contents 'invade' the chest by pushing up the diaphragm. The lower ribs are much more horizontal in the newborn and the bucket-handle activity of the lowermost ribs, which is responsible for the major portion of quiet tidal respiration in the adult, is not a mechanical possibility for the infant. The rib cage is still not ossified at birth whilst the muscles of the chest wall are much weaker than the diaphragm. This means that the infant will elevate the chest wall with inspiration during a normal quiet respiration, but that if he/she tries to increase TV, then the diaphragm will tend to dissipate energy by deforming the chest wall. This produces the characteristic pattern of recession: sub-costal, substernal or intercostal depending upon the site at which it is noted. This pattern is normal in the newborn during crying and in the premature baby it is often present during quiet respiration. In the older child, as the chest wall strengthens and the respiratory muscles develop, recession is always abnormal no matter what its site. Add to these differences the narrowness of the airway and the nett result is that it is far less expensive of energy for the infant to increase respiratory rate than tidal volume.

Respiratory distress

As with other systems, the capabilities of the respiratory system at birth are adequate to the needs of an unstressed infant but the reserves are limited and the system is not fully mature. When the pulmonary system is stressed then respiratory distress will supervene. Recession now develops at rest and the respiratory rate climbs above 60 breaths per minute.

Respiratory distress may have a clearly respiratory cause or it may be a manifestation of primary failure in a different system, e.g. as a result of cardiac failure or gross abdominal distension caused by intestinal obstruction.

HEPATIC FUNCTION

In the newborn period the liver is still immature. The most common example of this is the physiological jaundice that is particularly associated with the premature infant and which is brought about by the underdevelopment of the glucuronyl tranferase system.

This is not the only enzyme system that is immature and many of the enzymes responsible for handling detoxification of drugs (e.g. cytochrome P 450) are also not at their full capacity. The liver has other functions besides excretion and detoxification. It produces a variety of proteins, particularly albumin and clotting factors, and vitamin K is given after birth to encourage pro-thrombin production. The liver acts as a store of carbohydrate in the form of glycogen and this is laid down principally in the last 6–8 weeks of gestation. Consequently, extremely premature infants will have little glycogen store and a high risk of developing hypoglycaemia rapidly. Even the full-term infant cannot withstand starvation for much longer than 6 hours without running the risk of hypoglycaemia.

Preparation for surgery

Children presenting for surgery are usually starved because of the risk of aspiration of gastric contents during anaesthesia, but the period of starvation should not be so long that the depletion of glycogen stores and lack of fluid intake combine to produce dehydration, ketosis and hypoglycaemia. The duration of preoperative fasting should not exceed the normal interval between feeds in an infant, nor 4 hours in an older child. When this is not possible then preoperative intravenous replacement should be considered.

CENTRAL NERVOUS SYSTEM

Myelination within the central nervous system and the cortical connections of the brain itself are poorly developed at birth. The several examples of the wide swings of function that have been noted thus far (heart and respiratory rate and temperature) are evidence that the negative feedback loops are not yet mature. The process of myelination is not completed until the late teens and adult control of function does not develop fully until then. The developmental milestones of childhood are related to the gradual maturation of the corticol connections within the brain.

Pain relief in children

It is commonly stated that the infant does not feel pain because of his/her lack of central myelination. Even if the infant does not appreciate pain as the equivalent adult sensation there is evidence that the baby and small child will produce a physiological response to pain. Despite this there is still a view that anaesthesia and analgesia are unnecessary for minor surgery in the neonate and that infants under 1 year of age do not need analgesia. A more rational view suggests that pain relief and anaesthesia should be provided where necessary but it is important to understand the differences in pharmacology between the infant and the older child or adult.

Principles of analgesia

Since myelination is incomplete it follows that the blood–brain barrier is less efficient, at least up to the age of 2 years. Fat-soluble drugs will permeate more freely into cells in the brain in this age group. Particularly under the age of 6 months, analgesics of the opiate group will obtain ready access to the central nervous system and may produce respiratory depression at low dosage. The effect may also be prolonged. Because the excretory pathways in the liver and kidney are immature, detoxification of the opiates will also be delayed in infancy. In the neonatal period the elimination half-life is often 2–3 times the adult value. The volume of distribution of these drugs is also larger in the neonate. The result of all these factors is that the dose of analgesia needed in the neonatal period is much smaller than that required in adult life. As an example, morphine is normally given to an adult in a dose of 0.2 mg/kg 4–6 hourly, but in the small infant 0.1 mg/kg 6–8 hourly will probably suffice. If opiates are to be given to the very young, then the practitioner must be certain that there are adequate facilities for respiratory monitoring and management of respiratory failure. Reduction in the dose, and increase in the time between doses, are general rules for the administration of any drug to the neonate or young child.

FURTHER READING

Dierdorf S F, Krishna G 1981 Anesthetic management of neonatal surgical emergencies. Anesthesia and Analgesia 60: 204–215

Llloyd-Thomas A R 1990 Pain management in paediatric patients. British Journal of Anaesthesia 64: 85–104

2. Fluid and electrolyte balance and nutrition. Pre- and postoperative care

R. A. MacMahon

In infancy and childhood, there is constant growth, well illustrated by growth percentile charts. In the physical sense this means that there is an accumulation of body constituents including fluid, major and minor electrolytes, carbohydrates, protein, fat and vitamins. It is essential to attempt to maintain growth and development, even if there is a chronic illness or disability and anything that interferes with growth has a potentially adverse effect, particularly in the young infant.

Water, carbohydrate and electrolytes are the standard constituents of simple intravenous fluids, but they are also the standard constituents of all feeding, whether by mouth, by intragastric tube, by transpyloric tube or by peripheral or central venous catheters. Other nutritional constituents, such as protein, fat and vitamins, may be given by any of these routes, but the form in which the nutrient is delivered will vary with the route. In other words, the nutritional principles are the same but the technology is different.

However, there is an order of priority for survival in the nutritional requirements. The main order of priority is water, followed by the major electrolytes, particularly sodium, the acid–base status and some carbohydrate. Hence, the initial problem, and often the only problem in the short-term illness, is to replace water and electrolyte losses that have occurred because of illness, correct any acid–base imbalance, replace any ongoing fluid and electrolyte losses that occur during treatment, and give some carbohydrate to prevent hypoglycaemia and ketosis. The body will quickly make up any deficiencies of protein, fat and other constituents when adequate normal nutrition by mouth is resumed. If complete oral nutrition will not be possible for more than one week, then other forms of nutritional support must be instituted.

All requirements and dosages in infants and children, including nutritional requirements, are quoted and prescribed per unit of size. In adult practice, it is customary to regard all adults as having the same requirements, regardless of size, even though a two-fold variation would not be uncommon. On the other hand, it should be remembered that within the childhood age range, we may be dealing with an infant weighing 1 kg or an adolescent weighing 50 kg, a 50-fold difference. The unit commonly used is weight.

BASIC CONCEPTS

Water

Water is the major constituent of the body at all ages but especially in infancy and management of water metabolism is the first step in the nutritional management of the ill patient (Table 2.1). In infancy it can be said that *weight is water*.

Water turnover is at its maximum in infancy, decreasing with growth. Compared to the older

Table 2.1 Water as a percentage of body weight

	Newborn infant	Infant at one month	Adult
Plasma	5	5	5
Interstitial fluid	35	25	15
Intracellular fluid	40	40	40
Total	80	70	60

child or adult, the infant has a larger surface area with a more permeable skin, a more rapid respiratory rate and less mature renal function, so that losses of fluid and electrolytes are large and continuous by these routes. There is also free and rapid exchange of water throughout the extracellular compartment, from plasma to interstitial fluid to lymph and there is a large enterohepatic circulation with fluids being secreted into the gut lumen and reabsorbed into the portal system. The interstitial fluid is a large component of the easily exchangeable fluid.

It follows that even mild upsets that reduce intake and/or cause excess loss by vomiting, diarrhoea, increased respiratory rate or rise in temperature will rapidly produce a degree of dehydration. Adjustments are then made between the extracellular and intracellular compartments with secondary derangement of intracellular fluid and electrolytes.

Maintenance fluid requirements

These are the requirements for growth and develoment and allow for the daily normal losses. The key rule to remember is that: *at 1 year the infant requires 100 mL/kg per day.*

The fluid requirement at various ages is shown in Table 2.2. The pattern of this table allows easy recall but such tables only give an approximate guide so that the clinical state and changes in body weight and urine output of the patient must be monitored to allow individual adjustment of the infusion rate. In particular, the increased insensible loss in prolonged periods of hot weather must be included in the estimate of fluid requirements.

The primary purpose of a fluid balance chart is to document that the patient is passing at least 1 mL/kg per hour of urine.

Electrolytes and acid-base balance

Normal levels

There is considerable variation in quoted normal levels so that the approximate levels shown in Table 2.3 are based on a '5' rule as an aid to memory. It can be seen that there is a recurrent pattern of 5 and especially 35 to 45 in the constituents that are usually clinically monitored.

Acid–base control

Acid–base control systems in the body are of three types:

1. Physicochemical buffering — an immediate effect
2. Respiratory adjustment — this occurs in minutes and develops over hours
3. Renal adjustments — these take hours to days

All processes in the body take place in an aqueous environment and H^+ and HCO_3^- are of primary importance in diagnosing and treating acid–base disturbances. The H^+ concentration is the key factor. Haemoglobin is also an important buffer system and most of the non-bicarbonate buffer of the extracellular fluid is the haemoglobin of the red cells.

Table 2.2   Approximate maintenance fluid requirements in ml /kg per day

Age	Requirements
1st days of life	75
1st months of life	150
1 year	*100*
2 years	90
4 years	80
8 years	70
16 years	60
Adult	40

Table 2.3   Normal serum levels

Na	135–145 mmol/L
K	3.5–4.5 mmol/L*
Cl	95–105 mmol/L
pH	7.35–7.45
pCO_2	35–45 mmHg
pO_2	95–105 mmHg
Standard HCO_3^-	20–25 mmol/L
Base excess	−3–+3 mmol/L

* In young infants, figures of 4.5 to 5.5 /mmol/L are more usual.

The bicarbonate buffer system is a strong system since CO_2 is produced in large amounts by the body and can be retained or excreted by the lungs.

$$H_2O + CO_2 \xrightleftharpoons[\text{anhydrase}]{\text{carbonic}} H_2CO_3 \rightleftharpoons H^+ + HCO_3^-$$

This is an extremely rapid reaction and the ionization of H_2CO_3 is almost instantaneous, so that the level of CO_2 is approximately equal to that of H_2CO_3. Ionization of HCO_3^- does not occur at body pH. In body fluids, the weak acid H_2CO_3 is in the presence of salts of the acid and so the Henderson–Hasselbalch equation shows that:

$$(H^+) = K\frac{(H_2CO_3)}{(HCO_3^-)}$$

$$\text{or pH} = pK + \log\frac{(HCO_3^-)}{(H_2CO_3^-)}$$

This K is a constant, not potassium.

This shows that blood pH is dependent on the ratio of bicarbonate to free acid and that it is directly related to HCO_3^- and inversely related to PCO_2 (as H_2CO_3).

The kidneys play a major role in control of electrolyte and acid–base disturbances and on occasions these may have opposing requirements. There is an extremely wide range of concentration of urinary constituents but there is continuous acid formation in the body and H^+ and anions are continually excreted by the kidney, so that urine is usually acid (pH 6.0–6.6). There is a limitation on the amount of H^+ that can be excreted and the minimum pH of the urine is about 4.5, so that excess H^+ can only be excreted by the simultaneous excretion of a Brönsted base, usually HPO). HCO_3^- is usually completely re-absorbed from the urine, and ammonia production from glutamine is used to conserve cation.

The tubules secrete H^+ and K^+ in significant amounts. There is a Na^+/H^+ exchange pump and a Na^+/K^+ pump. The tubular secretion of K^+ is greatly influenced by Na^+ and K^+ depletion and by changes in body H^+, while acidosis stimulates the kidneys to increase ammonia production and H^+ excretion.

It follows that clinically, there are two main methods of treatment: through respiration by bicarbonate therapy or control of respiration, or by providing appropriate fluid and electrolytes to allow renal exchange.

Key points

The major cation of the extracellular fluid is sodium (135–145 mmol/L), while the major cation of the intracellular fluid is potassium with approximately the same concentration.

The potassium concentration in extracellular fluid (3.5–4.5 mmol/L), is approximately equal to the sodium concentration of intracellular fluid.

Calcium as a cation is approximately equal in concentration in intra- and extracellular fluid but the total millimolar content is very different because of the calcium in bone.

The two major anions of the extracellar fluid are Cl^- and HCO_3^- so that if one is lost from the body there must be water loss from the extracellular space and/or its replacement by the other.

Since potassium, magnesium and phosphate are mostly intracellular ions, their concentration in serum will be greatly influenced by the method of collection of the specimen. Haemolysis of red cells and tissue damage will give falsely high values. This is often seen in the serum potassium concentration in pyloric stenosis, because one of the standard methods of collecting such samples in infants is by heel prick and heel squeezing to extract sufficient sample.

WATER, ELECTROLYTE AND ACID–BASE DISTURBANCES

The effect of these disturbances depends on:

- The nutritional state of the patient at the onset
- The type of fluid lost
- The amount and rapidity of the loss
- Other major abnormalities
- Attempts at treatment

Dehydration

Dehydration will occur from either inadequate intake or excess loss, or both. Because of the high metabolic rate, large surface area and relatively great needs of the infant, reduction in intake by itself can quickly result in dehydration without abnormal losses being present. If abnormal losses are present, the degree of dehydration will progress relative to the severity of the loss and the reduction in intake.

In the infant, weight is water so that acute weight loss is acute loss of water, mostly from the extracellular compartment. The signs of dehydration are basically the signs of reduced extracellular fluid and include loss of body weight, decreased urine output, decrease of fontanelle tension, sunken eyes and decreased elasticity of the skin.

Major electrolyte loss accompanies water loss so that electrolyte replacement, particularly of sodium and anion, must accompany the water replacement. Carbohydrate is also added to replacement fluid to combat hypoglycaemia.

Chronic weight loss represents loss of all body constituents as well as water and electrolytes.

Loss of weight is the best guide to dehydration in the acute situation, but a recent weight may not be available for comparison. In such situations, an approximate guide to the level of dehydration is shown in Table 2.4. It should be noted that the per cent dehydration is a percentage of body weight, not of body water, as this latter figure is usually only available in special metabolic clinical units.

The first problem to be faced when dealing with an infant or child with dehydration is to decide the method of providing fluid and electrolytes. If the disease is short term and self-limiting, e.g. mild diarrhoea of infancy or appendicitis in a healthy older child, it is usually possible to maintain fluid and electrolyte balance by giving fluids by mouth until full oral intake is re-established. This is the usual situation in Group 1 patients in Table 2.4 with 0–5% dehydration. However, if there is continued vomiting or other interference with intake then intravenous therapy may be required.

In the second group with 5–10% dehydration, hospital admission and intravenous therapy will often be required.

The third group with 10–15% dehydration will have a markedly decreased circulating blood volume and the infant or child may be in a state of shock. Shocked patients require restoration of a circulating blood volume as fast as possible but in infants the volume required to do this will be very small compared with adults. Continuous monitoring is required during this phase of treatment. When the patient is stabilized, reassessment of fluid and electrolyte requirements can be made.

Clinical example 1 shows a method of estimating fluid requirements in a dehydrated infant.

Clinical example 1

An infant aged 3 months has been vomiting intermittently for 2 days and refusing to feed. Two days ago the infant weighed 5 kg. Weight loss and clinical examination indicate 5% dehydration. What will be the fluid requirements in the next 24 hours?

$$\text{Maintenance requirements} = 5 \times 150 = 750 \text{ mL}$$

$$\text{Fluid to replace dehydration} = \frac{5}{100} \times 5000 = 250 \text{ mL}$$

$$\text{Total} = 1000 \text{ mL}$$

Plus any ongoing losses.

Table 2.4 Degrees of dehydration as a percentage loss of body weight

	Group 1 0–5%	Group 2 5–10%	Group 3 10–15%
History	Reduced intake and/or excess loss	More severe reduction of intake and/or excess loss	Markedly reduced intake and/or excess loss
Signs	None or only mild signs of dehydration	Signs of dehydration	Signs of dehydration and shock

In such an infant without major dehydration and without major ongoing losses once feeding is ceased, a reasonable rate of rehydration would be to give the same hourly rate over 24 hours. (But see fluid replacement in burns, Ch. 14.)

Types of dehydration and electrolyte replacement

Dehydration is also classified according to the serum sodium concentration into three types:

1. Isonatraemic: serum sodium concentration is 130–150 mmol/L
2. Hypernatraemic: serum sodium concentration is more than 150 mmol/L
3. Hyponatraemic: serum sodium concentration is less than 130 mmol/L

Mild degrees of dehydration are of the isonatraemic type because the adaptive mechanisms of the body, particularly the kidney, maintain the solute concentration close to the normal range.

Loss of fluid from the body is always in excess of the loss of electrolyte, except in special situations such as cardiopulmonary bypass, so that in replacing the usual type of clinical loss, either an isotonic (0.9%) or hypotonic saline solution will be used.

Remember that the term 'normal' saline solution is used clinically to mean isotonic saline solution. A commonly used intravenous solution, 4% dextrose in N/5 normal saline, will supply basic maintenance requirements of sodium and chloride, but is inappropriate for the replacement of dehydration electrolyte losses. A more concentrated solution, such as N/2 normal, will be more appropriate, always including dextrose to supply some calories and avoid hypoglycaemia.

Even if there is hypernatraemic dehydration, there is loss of sodium from the body so that an electrolyte-containing solution is still necessary for replacement. In this type of dehydration the osmotic effects lead to a shift of fluid from the intracellular to the extracellular compartment, masking the clinical signs of dehydration so that its severity is often underestimated. In addition, in this type of dehydration sodium has entered the cell in exchange for H^+. Sodium recrosses the blood–brain barrier slowly so that too rapid rehydration may lead to intracellular overhydration with convulsions and neuronal damage.

Rate of rehydration

The mildly dehydrated patient without major ongoing losses can be rehydrated at a steady hourly rate over 24 hours. The moderately dehydrated patient should be given 50% of the replacement fluid over the first 8 hours and the other 50% over the next 18 hours, with hourly replacement of any ongoing losses. If the patient is shocked, then the rehydration fluid must be given at as fast a rate as possible with continuous monitoring. When the shock is controlled, repeated re-assessment is necessary to determine the continuing therapy.

Oral rehydration therapy

Oral rehydration therapy (ORT) is now an established method of treating the dehydration of diarrhoea in adults and children, even those with severe dehydration short of shock. The World Health Organization (WHO) has developed a standard solution for use in this situation and its components in *millimoles per litre* are:

$$Na^+ = 90$$
$$K^+ = 20$$
$$Cl^- = 80$$
$$citrate = 10$$
$$glucose = 101$$

This represents slightly less than 3 g (2.79 g) of powder per 100 mL.

The WHO solution can be used to orally rehydrate an infant or child who is dehydrated. For maintenance therapy, especially in infants, a more dilute solution is used and half-strength ORT or one of the various commercial solutions are suitable for this purpose. Chronic diarrhoea with fluid and electrolyte loss is common after some surgical procedures, such as massive gut resections, and oral rehydration fluids are required if repeated admissions for intravenous therapy are to be avoided.

Acid–base disturbances

Patients with dehydration will have some electrolyte and acid–base disturbances but if these are mild, compensation will take place and physiological levels will be maintained. In moderate and severe dehydration correction of electrolyte and acid–base disturbances are a fundamental part of patient management.

The four clinical acid–base problems are:

1. Metabolic alkalosis
2. Respiratory alkalosis
3. Metabolic acidosis
4. Respiratory acidosis

The pH level indicates the end result of the pathological forces at work and the body's attempt to modify them. It is only when the buffering powers of the body are overcome that a significant change in pH occurs, either on the acidic or basic side. Remember that a change in pH from 7.4 to 7.1 represents a doubling of hydrogen ion concentration.

Measurement of the serum electrolytes and acid–base status with, if necessary, measurement of oxygen concentration, will give a good indication of the overall state of the body fluid and electrolyte composition. Comparison of the urine and serum concentrations of the major constituents, particularly of sodium, urea and the osmolality, will give a good indication of the state of hydration. Examples of the main types of acid–base problems are shown in Table 2.5.

Clinical example 2

An infant aged 6 weeks commenced occasional vomiting after feeds 5 days ago. The vomiting has become more frequent and forceful and the vomitus contains milk and gastric fluid but no bile. The infant fed hungrily till the day of examination but now is becoming somewhat lethargic. On examination there is a palpable pyloric tumour. The history and findings are diagnostic of hypertrophic pyloric stenosis. Examination also shows dehydration of approximately 5% of body weight. The electrolyte and acid–base levels are listed under metabolic alkalosis in Table 2.5.

Management.

1. Cessation of oral feeds. This will markedly reduce the vomiting and excess loss.
2. Correction of dehydration. See clinical example 1. This will indicate the volume and rate of fluid infusion.
3. Correction of electrolyte and acid–base disturbance. Loss of gastric juice leads to a marked loss of H^+ and Cl^- with some loss of Na^+ and K^+. As this is only a partial intestinal obstruction and feeding has continued, some

Table 2.5 Examples of electrolyte and acid–base values

	Metabolic alkalosis (pyloric stenosis)	Respiratory alkalosis (respirator hyperventilation)	Metabolic acidosis (obstructive uropathy)	Respiratory acidosis (diaphragmatic hernia)
Na (mmol/L)	133	136	130	138
K (mmol/L)	3.8	4.0	6.0	5.0
Cl (mmol/L)	86	100	100	95
pH	7.48	7.52	7.28	7.27
PCO_2 (mmHg)	46	25	30	64
Standard HCO_3^- (mmol/L)	32	24	14	24
Actual HCO_3^- (mmol/L)	34	20	14	30
Base excess (mmol/L)	+9	0	−12	0
PO_2 (mmHg)	95	105	95	70

food and fluid passes from stomach to duodenum. The dehydration is hyponatraemic.

The loss of H^+ will cause an immediate adjustment in the bicarbonate system.

$$H_2O + CO_2 \rightleftharpoons H_2CO_3 \rightleftharpoons H^+ + HCO_3^-$$

This equation is pushed to the right with an increase in plasma bicarbonate and a rise in pH. The bicarbonate takes the place of the Cl^- lost by vomiting.

The respiratory compensation for metabolic alkalosis is the production of a degree of respiratory acidosis by depression of the respiratory centre causing a rise in the level of CO_2. However, CO_2 is a potent stimulator of the respiratory centre and any degree of hypoxia produced by the respiratory depression will also stimulate the centre, so that the respiratory compensation for metabolic alkalosis is variable.

The renal compensation involves conservation of H^+ and excretion of HCO_3^- with K^+ and some Na^+, but as the body stores of Na^+ and K^+ fall, the kidney will commence conserving sodium ion rather than hydrogen ion and the urine becomes acid, the so-called paradoxical aciduria of metabolic alkalosis.

Treatment. Isotonic or at least 0.5 isotonic sodium chloride will be needed as the replacement fluid because of the large loss of sodium and chloride. As there is also potassium depletion, potassium should be added to the replacement fluid in concentrations between 20 and 30 mmol/L for mild to moderate alkalosis and between 30 and 40 mmol/L for moderate to severe alkalosis, provided that there is good renal function and urine flow is established. Glucose is added to this solution in a concentration of 50 g/L (278 mmol/L).

While ammonium chloride and arginine or lysine hydrochloride may be used as acid salts in the correction of alkalosis, their use in this condition is not necessary.

There is no necessity for emergency surgery in pyloric stenosis and if enough fluid, sodium, potassium and chloride are infused to allow the kidney to conserve H^+ and excrete bicarbonate, then even severe degrees of metabolic alkalosis will return to normal electrolyte and acid–base levels within 2–3 days.

While the operation for pyloric stenosis can be performed under local anaesthesia, it is now usual to perform it under general anaesthesia. This carries a risk of respiratory alkalosis with ventilation and this would complicate any uncorrected metabolic alkalosis, making resumption of spontaneous respiration difficult. For these reasons, the metabolic alkalosis should be completely corrected before surgical correction is carried out.

Clinical example 3

A male infant aged 2 months has a 3 day history of fever, lethargy, occasional vomiting and a few loose stolls. A good urinary stream has never been seen and he has had poor weight gains since birth. On examination he is febrile and dehydrated and has lost 7% of his weight since being weighed one week ago. Bladder and both kidneys are palpable and enlarged. Investigations confirm a urinary tract infection and obstructive uropathy due to posterior urethral valves. Electrolyte and acid–base studies are listed under metabolic acidosis in Table 2.5. Metabolic acidosis is very quickly accompanied by a compensatory hyperventilation leading to fall in PCO_2. This gives a component of respiratory alkalosis that helps minimize the change in hydrogen ion concentration.

Management.

1. Establishment of adequate urinary drainage (Ch. 19)
2. Treatment of urinary tract infection
3. Fluid management — see clinical example 1
4. Electrolytes and acid–base correction

Metabolic acidosis results from the inability of the kidney to excrete acids produced in metabolism/catabolism. Control of the urinary tract infection, establishment of free urinary drainage and provision of non-protein calories with adequate fluids will allow excretion of acid radicals.

Release of the back pressure effect on the kidney will produce a diuresis of poorly concentrated urine so that strict attention must be paid to the fluid balance and serum osmolality and electrolyte concentrations.

An immediate effect on the degree of acidosis can be obtained by infusing base such as sodium bicarbonate. An estimate of the amount of bicarbonate to infuse in the first instance can be obtained by the use of the formula:

$$\text{Number of mmol HCO}_3 = \frac{\text{BE} \times \text{Wt in kg}}{3}$$

where BE is the base excess and the 3 indicates that administered HCO_3 is distributed to approximately 30% of body weight.

As ever, clinical estimates and formulae can only be used as an approximate guide and repeated reassessment clinically and by electrolyte and acid–base measurements are necessary for ongoing management.

Clinical example 4

A 3 day old infant has developed acute on chronic respiratory distress over 24 hours. Breath sounds are diminished in the left chest. On chest X-ray, there is an obvious left diaphragmatic hernia with mediastinal shift to the right. The acid–base findings are those listed under respiratory acidosis in Table 2.5.

Management.

1. Correction of acid–base abnormality
2. Correction of anatomical abnormality

The immediate buffer for excess CO_2 is the physiochemical system:

$$CO_2 + H_2O \rightleftharpoons H_2CO_3 \rightleftharpoons H^+ + HCO_3^-$$

The excess CO_2 is retained as HCO_3^-, some of which is buffered by haemoglobin and some by intracellular buffers, but there is also a rise in concentration in the free interstitial fluid and this is an important component in the neonatal infant with a large extracelluular fluid volume.

The compensation for a continued elevation of CO_2 is mainly renal. The kidney excretes hydrogen ion as titratable acid or as ammonium and the bicarbonate has to be excreted with cation. Associated hypoxia may produce a degree of metabolic acidosis.

Treatment of the respiratory acidosis in this condition is adequate ventilation followed by operative reduction of the hernia.

NUTRITION

As pointed out earlier, growth and development are a continuous facet of the infant and child and it is essential to try to maintain these even during illness or surgery. It should be remembered that there is a steady obligatory loss of nitrogen and electrolytes in the urine so that if these are not replaced, the body tissues are being broken down and excreted. If the patient will be unable to eat in a normal fashion after surgery, e.g. an infant with a massive gut resection, or if there are excess demands, e.g. a child with burns, then specialized feeding by whatever route is necessary should be commenced as soon as possible and certainly before there has been a major loss of body tissue.

The basis of infant nutrition is breast milk which is the 'gold' standard. All the basic nutritional requirements are estimated from the composition of breast milk. The healthy infant who is demand feeding from the breast and is happy and thriving is deemed to be receiving optimal nutrition even though no consideration is given to the individual constituents.

For the sick infant, who may need to be fed a specialized diet or in a specialized manner, a knowledge of the individual constituents is fundamental to successful feeding. Under these circumstances the constituents of breast milk are taken as the basis for feeding.

For the older child, the constituents of a broad-based diet leading to optimal growth and development in normal children, is taken as the basis for the requirement of the individual constituents.

Methods of feeding

Feeding may be by the following methods:

- Breast
- Bottle
- Table
- Intragastric tube via mouth or nose
- Gastrostomy
- Transgastric duodenal or jejunal tube
- Jejunal tube by separate abdominal incision
- Intravenous

The nutritional principles are similar in each case but the form of the food varies with the

Table 2.6 Comparative values of some nutritional requirements according to age (per kg/day).

	Infant	Child	Adult
Fluid (ml)	150	80	40
Calories	100	80	40
Kilojoules	400	320	160
Sodium (mmol)	3	2	1
Potassium (mmol)	2	1.6	0.8
Calcium (mmol)	1.4	0.7	0.1
Phosphorus (mmol)	1.4	0.7	0.15
Magnesium (mmol)	0.3	0.2	0.08
Carbohydrate (g)	To supply the caloric content		
Fat (g)	To supply the caloric content and essential fatty acids		
Protein (g)	2.5	1.6	0.8

method, e.g. intravenous protein is supplied as a sterile solution of amino acids.

In the same way that the fluid requirements vary markedly with age, the nutritional requirements also vary. Some comparative requirement figures are shown in Table 2.6. However, as stated previously, water, sodium and some carbohydrate are all that are required in the short term to tide a patient over an acute illness.

PRE- AND POSTOPERATIVE CARE

Preoperative and postoperative care will vary depending on whether the child is being admitted for elective surgery or whether the admission is an emergency, but management of fluids, electrolytes and nutrition are an integral part of this care.

Elective surgery

Adequate preparation for surgery includes an explanation to the child of the reason for admission to hospital and, if he/she is old enough to understand, an explanation of the type of surgery that will be performed. This should be done before admission to hospital. For elective surgery the child should be in good general health and if this is not the case, e.g. anaemia, upper respiratory tract infection, or local sepsis, the operation should be postponed. Food and fluid is withheld

for several hours before operation, preferably for the time of the usual interval between feeds for the particular patient.

Infants and children should be kept in hospital for as short a time as possible so that much elective surgery is done on a day-stay basis in which the child is admitted in the morning, the operation is performed during the day and once recovery from anaesthesia is complete the child then returns home that some day. During this time the parents are encouraged to stay with the child so that there is minimal disruption to the family unit.

Appropriate management during elective operations means that the anaesthesia and surgery have gone smoothly, temperature has been maintained, blood and fluid loss have been measured and replaced and there has been a rapid recovery from the anaesthetic. In these circumstances, postoperative care only requires continued monitoring of the vital signs and airway until it is certain that the child has completely recovered from any respiratory depression caused either by drugs used in premedication before anaesthesia or by the anaesthetic itself; and of observation of the area of the wound for such things as haemorrhage, e.g. following circumcision.

For the day-stay patient, the effect of anaesthesia and surgery will have worn off within a few hours so that the patient may then drink and can be discharged from hospital. For the patient with major surgery and a long anaesthetic, it may be 24 to 48 hours before oral intake can commence. Intravenous fluids will be required during this time. For the patient with major bowel surgery, oral intake should be withheld until there is evidence of return to normality of gastrointestinal function, demonstrated by a reduction of nasogastric aspirate to normal levels and passage of flatus and/or faecal material per anus or ostomy.

Emergency surgery

The aim of preoperative care in this situation is to attempt to return any disordered metabolism to normal before surgery; and of postoperative care to maintain this normality. The infant group is the one most at risk because of their poor ability to maintain bodily homeostasis.

Preoperative care

Transport. Special arrangements must be made to transport sick infants to a referral hospital for surgery. These requirements include a portable incubator so that the infant's temperature can be controlled and access and observation is facilitated without cumbersome wrappings. An oxygen and suction supply must be available in a form suitable for such an incubator.

Depending on the clinical condition, there are special requirements during transport. If an infant has an intestinal obstruction, then a nasogastric tube should be in place and should be allowed free drainage and be aspirated regularly to decrease the risk of vomiting and inhalational pneumonia. If the infant has a major respiratory problem, e.g. diaphragmatic hernia, then an endotracheal tube may be necessary. Ordinarily the time taken to insert an intravenous catheter will merely delay transport but on occasions this may also be necessary. Problems such as a tension pneumothorax would need to be aspirated or drained before attempted transfer. This is particularly necessary if the infant will be transported by air.

Preparation for surgery. The aim of preparation for surgery is to achieve a clinical condition such that the anaesthesia and operation constitute as small a risk to the patient as possible. This includes maintenance of body temperature, care of the airway and oxygenation, the treatment of shock, correction of fluid, acid–base and electrolyte imbalance and correction of major metabolic disturbances such as hypoglycaemia or hypocalcaemia.

Correction of chronic anaemia and malnutrition are not possible preoperatively in the emergency situation.

This emergency treatment in preparation for surgery can be thought of as a system of tubes. These are:

1. Endotracheal tube to maintain the airway
2. Intragastric tube to decompress the stomach
3. Intravenous catheter for fluid and blood infusion
4. Indwelling urinary catheter to monitor urine flow
5. Central venous catheter to monitor central venous pressure

Correction of shock will depend on the cause of shock, whether it is due to blood loss, fluid loss, loss from burns, septic shock or the shock of adrenal insufficiency. Loss of more then 10% of the body weight as dehydration or loss of more than 10% of the circulating blood volume, especially with continuing loss, may produce shock. Treatment of the shock will depend on the cause — see Group 3 dehydration above. Because of possible delay in cross-matching blood, such shock may be treated by emergency intravenous infusion of stable plasma protein solution (SPPS), which is a solution of 50 g of plasma proteins per litre, of which 86% is albumin and 14% is globulin. Alternatively, an albumin solution may be used. This consists of 200 g of human plasma protein (95% albumin) per litre. This is a far more concentrated solution than SPPS and should be accompanied by crystalloid infusion. It should not be used if SPPS is available. The concentrations of such solutions may vary between countries.

These solutions are infused at the rate of 10% of estimated blood volume as fast as possible and then a clinical reassessment is made.

In acute emergency situations, e.g. midgut volvulus, all that is possible before surgery is stabilization of the patient by treating shock, stabilizing the control of respiration and the commencement of the correction of major fluid, electrolyte and acid–base imbalances.

Postoperative care

Postoperative care is critical in the management of the infant or child who has had major emergency surgery. There may be continuing problems of anaemia or malnutrition and fluid, electrolyte and acid–base status may not have been completely corrected before surgery. A long anaesthetic and loss of blood, fluid and electrolytes at surgery with possible errors in the estimation of this loss, lead to a complicated clinical picture.

Monitoring of vital signs, particularly the airway, pulse and colour, as well as the temperature and blood pressure, is a fundamental part of postoperative care. Unrecognized respiratory depression, or internal bleeding, and fluid or electrolyte imbalance are the main dangers. The pulse rate may vary markedly, but a steadily rising pulse rate is a dangerous sign. It must be remembered that in neonates, severe infection may produce a fall, rather than a rise in temperature. Repeated clinical examination, accurate fluid balance and repeated electrolyte and acid–base estimations may be necessary to control the patient adequately.

If there is any possibility of postoperative respiratory difficulty the patient should be placed on a respirator electively until the respiratory condition is stable. This will be controlled by blood-gas monitoring.

Pain management is an integral part of postoperative care (see Ch. 1).

Postoperative water intoxication. This is a problem that may occur in the postoperative period, particularly following major abdominal procedures. It is a particular risk to infants and small children because of the difficulty of monitoring fluid loss during long operations and of collecting timed urine output after surgery, particularly if there is oliguria and a urinary catheter is not in place.

This syndrome is due, in part, to inappropriate fluid replacement during surgery and in part to antidiuretic hormone (ADH) secretion. The fluid lost from the bowel and abdominal cavity during surgery is extracellular fluid and should be replaced by at least N/2 saline or preferably Hartmann's (lactated Ringer's) solution. More dilute solutions tend to produce water intoxication. The inappropriate ADH secretion is a physiological response to the trauma of major surgery and the kidney produces only a small amount of concentrated urine. The features of this syndrome are oliguria, normal or high urinary osmolality with continuing sodium excretion, hyponatraemia and low plasma osmolality. The patient is well hydrated and there is a gain in weight. The differential diagnosis is hyponatraenic dehydration in which there is a loss of weight and signs of dehydration. If this syndrome is not recognized, convulsions may occur from cerebral oedema.

The key to adequate postoperative care is adequate monitoring and repeated clinical assessment.

FURTHER READING

Breaux C W, Hood J S, Georgeson K E 1989 The significance of alkalosis and hypochloremia in hypertrophic pyloric stenosis. Journal of Pediatric Surgery 24: 1250–1252

Finberg L, Harper P A, Harrison H E, Sack R B 1982 Oral rehydration for diarrhoea. Journal of Paediatrics 101: 497–499

3. An approach to lumps and swellings

R. A. MacMahon

Lumps and swellings are common but children often present with unusual lumps or a common type of lump in an unusual situation or with unusual features. Most such lumps can be diagnosed and the management planned after an adequate history and physical examination without the need for further investigation.

If the child is obviously afraid, in pain, or in fear of separation from parents, then the general approach to the examination of children is of great importance. Thus, when approaching an infant or young child, a parent should be comforting the child by sitting the child on the parents' knees or by the parent holding the child's hand.

It is important to be gentle, sympathetic and efficient in asking the right questions, applying the right physical examination techniques and being confident when all the signs have been elicited, that nothing has been missed. Every attempt should be made to avoid hurting or frightening the patient and this can be achieved with practice and commitment, even with the most tender of swellings.

In order to avoid missing things by oversight, it is essential to have a system or check list and in older children this may be applied seriatim. In younger children and less cooperative patients it is imperative that we adapt the physical examination technique to that which the child will tolerate. Thus, unpleasant things, e.g. eliciting a gagging reflex or looking in the auditory canal, should be left until last and the sequence of examination adapted to the child's activity and tolerance. This, however, does not mean that a system is unnecessary; on the contrary, a system

is then even more essential to avoid omissions and it is the sequence which is varied.

It can be difficult to remember immediately all the characteristics of a lump which need to be considered and this is one of the situations in which a mnemonic is helpful. One possible mnemonic is *Surgeons Can Find The Lumps*.

Surgeons Can Find The Lumps	
S Site	**C** Colour
Size	Contour
Sinus	Consistency
Surface	Cough impulse
F Fixation	**T** Temperature
Fluctuation	Tenderness
Filling–emptying	Transillumination
Flow–bruit	Thrill/pulsation
L Local features	
Lobulation	
Lymph drainage	
Lumps elsewhere	

In the above system accurate definition of the site will be found to be one of the most valuable and one of the most frequently neglected aspects of physical examination, i.e. determine not only that the mass is in the medial part of the arm, but check whether it is deep to the skin, to the deep fascia, or to the muscle, and whether it is anterior or posterior to the intermuscular septum and the neurovascular bundle. Similarly, in the abdomen, is a mass in the anterior abdominal wall, in the posterior abdominal wall or between anterior and posterior walls? If it is within the abdominal cavity, is it fixed or does it move with respiration and is it part of, or superficial or deep to, adjacent viscera such as kidney, liver, or mesentery?

In some cases a few key characteristics will indicate that some of the items on the check list do not apply, e.g. a lump at the side of the knee, covered by normal skin, attached to bone and bony hard will not need examination for a cough impulse, fluctuation, transillumination or filling–emptying.

On the other hand, the importance of applying a systematic examination is well illustrated by a soft, cystic, fluctuant lump over the posterior fontanelle and which also has a cough impulse, indicating an encephalocele and not a simple scalp cyst.

Not infrequently the practitioner will be confronted with a lump either not seen before or at least not immediately possible to diagnose. After an adequate examination it should at least be possible to apply a simple pathological classification and this will give an immediate indication of the treatment requirements and prognosis of such a lump. Again a simple mnemonic is useful: *Causes That Very Inconveniently Produce Noxious Disease.*

Causes That Very Incoveniently Produce Noxious Disease	
Congenital	Parasitic
Traumatic	Neoplastic
Vascular	Degenerative
Inflammatory	

If the question of neoplasia arises, then the subgroups must be considered:

Neoplasia — benign
          \ malignant —— primary
                       \ secondary

The skin and subcutaneous tissues are the common sites for lumps and swellings and the common swellings are of the lymph nodes, haemangioma, lymphangioma, pyogenic granuloma and pilomatricoma. Sebaceous naevus is a lesion that it is important to recognize because of its propensity to undergo neoplastic change and possible associated abnormalities.

ENLARGED LYMPH NODES

These are extremely common especially in the neck, where they are commonly found in the anterior triangle along the anterior border of the sternomastoid muscle. They usually have no associated symptoms but are visible or palpable. Non-complicated nodes are smooth, firm, rounded, somewhat mobile swellings in the subcutaneous tissue or beneath the cervical fascia, 0.5–1 cm in diameter. Enlarged neck nodes are presumably related to mild chronic or recurrent infection in the oropharynx, while enlarged nodes at other sites are usually related to infection in areas which they drain.

Surgical intervention is used as an excisional biopsy if:

1. The gland is more than 2 cm in diameter and has been present for more than 2 months
2. There is generalized lymphadenopathy
3. The spleen is also enlarged
4. There are signs in other organs and a cause is not obvious on other investigations

Specific cervical lymphadenitis

There are three main groups:

1. Acute inflammatory lymphadenitis
2. Anonymous mycobacterial infection (*Mycobacterium avium-intracellulare-scrofulaceum* — MAIS)
3. *Mycobacterium tuberculosis* infection

Acute lymphadenitis

These lymph nodes are enlarged and tender with periadenitis and are usually related to an infected lesion in the skin or oropharynx.

Staphylococcal and streptococcal infections constitute over 75% of acute infections. In addition to appropriate local and antibiotic therapy, surgical drainage may be required if suppuration has occurred as indicated by central softening, reddening of the overlying skin, or by the persistence of a very hard centre to a node which is not responding to medical treatment. Antibiotic-modified lymphadenitis leaving a suppurating node which flares up days or weeks later has now become the commonest surgical lesion of cervical nodes in childhood.

Atypical mycobacterial lymphadenitis

This is now more common than tuberculosis in Western countries. There is a mass in the side of the neck, with local signs of chronicity, matting of node groups, collar-stud abscesses or bluish-edged sinuses. These features are indistinguishable from infection with *M. tuberculosis*. The patient's general health, however, is unaffected, there is a lack of contact with open tuberculous patients and though the Mantoux test is positive, the specific atypical mycobacterial skin tests should be strongly positive and diagnostic. A-typical mycobacterial lymphadenitis is unresponsive to chemotherapy and operation may be indicated to prevent skin breakdown or to remove groups of chronically infected lymph nodes.

Tuberculous cervical lymphadenitis

This is now rare in developed countries but is still common in developing tropical countries. Full investigation is required to assess the extent of the disease and to search for open cases amongst the patient's contacts. Bacterial diagnosis is made by Mantoux skin test along with stain and culture of sputum and gastric aspirate, as well as any material evacuated from the nodes. The patient, and other susceptible children, should be excluded from contact with patients with open tuberculosis and prolonged antituberculous chemotherapy should be given if the patient is a young child, e.g. under 5 years, who has been recently infected. Operative evacuation of caseous material or removal of caseous nodes is indicated to prevent skin breakdown, discharging wounds and later scarring. The frequently favourable prognosis in cervical tuberculous lymph node infection before specific chemotherapy was available probably indicates misdiagnosis of atypical mycobacterial infections.

Lymph node neoplasia

Lymph nodes may be enlarged in leukaemia, lymphoma or in the reticuloses (See Ch. 4).

Lymph node metastases of neoplasms

These are firm to hard in consistency and non-tender. Malignant disease should be considered in the investigation of all such patients. Full history and examination at the first visit will usually indicate a primary site but if not, blood film and X-ray of chest and abdomen should be taken. If no other suggestion of malignancy is found, observation of firm, non-tender nodes for periods of up to 8 weeks may be desirable before biopsy is undertaken.

Biopsy material should be examined by experienced paediatric pathologists whenever possible, and ideally should include material for touch preparations, culture and fresh specimens for light and electron microscopy and cytogenetic and cytological studies. In the lymphomata, detected T and B cell markers have significant prognostic value.

In children under 5 years of age leukaemia and neuroblastoma are the common causes of cervical node metastases and in the 7–15 year group, leukaemia and lymphoma predominate. The so-called lateral aberrant thyroid is a lymph node metastasis from papillary or follicular carcinoma of the thyroid gland which may lie dormant for many years but can still be treated with excellent results.

HAEMANGIOMA

A subcutaneous mass, which is ill-defined, partially empties on pressure and has a blue or red patch in the overlying skin, is a haemangiomatous mass.

The term haemangioma describes a developmental malformation which consists of proliferating blood vessels. Haemangiomata most usually occur in the skin and subcutaneous tissue but can be situated in any organ. The clinical features and natural history vary according to the predominant component vessel. A capillary haemangioma which is situated entirely within the dermis (naevus vinosis or port-wine stain) produces a flat or slightly elevated reddish lesion which remains unchanged throughout life. In the face, such a haemangioma may constitute a significant cosmetic problem and is treated by the application of appropriate cosmetics or laser coagulation. Surgical treatment is only occasionally helpful.

Cavernous haemangiomata consist of proliferated venous channels and are more common than capillary haemangiomata. Many lesions contain a mixture of cavernous and capillary elements. At birth, there is either no lesion or a small pink spot on the skin. Over ensuing months, there is an increase in size with elevation. The phase of rapid growth may last for upwards of 12 months and subsequently there is gradual regression (presumably due to thrombosis and sclerosis of vessels). Most lesions disappear completely without any treatment (Fig. 3.1) by 5 years of age.

The majority of patients with cavernous or mixed haemangiomata require no active treatment but need to be maintained under medical supervision until the lesions either spontaneously disappear or a decision is made about treatment. There are some exceptions to this general rule. Cavernous haemangiomata of the lip do not regress and usually require surgical excision. Subglottic haemangioma causes airways obstruction and the recommended treatment is irradiation from an implanted radioactive gold grain, protected by tracheotomy.

LYMPHANGIOMA

This is a soft, multicystic, ill defined fluctuant mass that, if very superficial, is brilliantly trans-

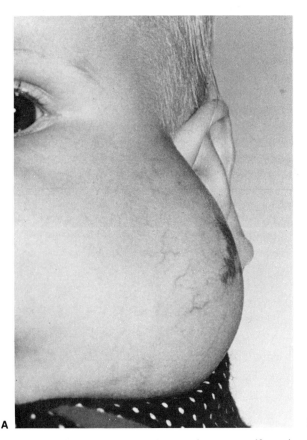
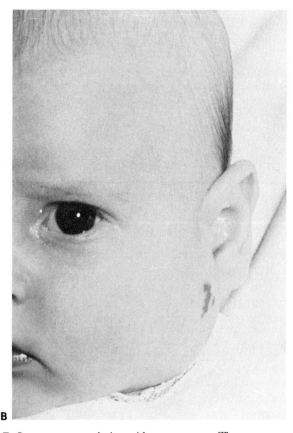

A   **B**

Fig. 3.1 A: Infant with large haemangiomatous malformation. **B**: Spontaneous resolution without treatment. The haemangioma had completely disappeared by childhood.

illuminable. In the neck, if the separate loculi are large and obvious, it is called a cystic hygroma. It arises as a result of an abnormality of development of the lymphatic system with failure of coalescence of primitive lymphatics.

It is a benign, congenital hamartoma which can occur in any area where there are lymph vessels. The neck is one of the commonest sites and one of the most difficult for operative removal. Lymphangioma develops before the organization of fetal fascial planes and thus takes the place of fascia, epimysium, epineurium and vascular adventitia in the region. As the fascia of the neck, mediastinum and axilla are one continuum, each of these areas should be checked when a lymphangioma presents in one of them. Like the vessels from which they are derived, cervical lymphangioma does not traverse the midline.

The history is usually of a soft, lax, non-tender swelling, rarely evident at birth, becoming bigger during infancy or early childhood. The mass varies in size from day to day and enlarges rapidly during intercurrent infection, subsequently returning towards its previous size.

The physical signs of lymphangioma are those of a soft, cystic mass, reducible in part or not at all. Though one or more borders may be well-defined where the loculi are larger, other edges taper imperceptibly into the surrounding tissue. The depth of the lesion varies, at times involving skin and subcutaneous fat, sometimes only deeper fascial planes. The overlying skin may show coarser texture, thicker skin folds or peau d'orange. Transillumination is diagnostic if the lesion is sufficiently accessible. The fluid, if aspirated, has the characteristics of lymph with minimal haemorrhage.

A less common infiltrative form can occur within the oropharynx as an isolated lesion involving the tongue. This topic is also discussed in Chapter 16 (see Fig. 16.8).

Unlike haemangioma, lymphangioma does not regress completely and usually requires surgical excision. Repeated aspiration or the injection of sclerosants always fail to eradicate the lesion and make operative resection more hazardous. They should not be used. Radiotherapy has no place in the treatment of resectable lymphangioma as the dosage required to cure the lesion will also destroy surrounding vessels, impair growth, induce premature senility and there is a significant risk of malignancy in the area of irradiation and scatter.

Surgical excision of lymphangioma should be considered a major undertaking even under the most ideal circumstances. The younger the child the smaller the scars and the better the compensatory growth of adjacent skin and fascia subsequently. Thus, if anaesthetic and nursing, as well as surgical facilities, are ideal, a lymphangioma should be excised in infancy after the age of 3 months. Unlike cancer surgery, this benign lesion is excised without a margin of normal tissue and thus lymphatic vessels will be unroofed and incompletely excised where they abut on vital structures. However, provided all macroscopically abnormal lymphatics are removed along with their fibrovascular pedicle and provided suction drainage of the cavity is meticulous and maintained for several days, the recurrence rate is only 10%.

PYOGENIC GRANULOMA

Pyogenic granuloma is a common, red, raised, usually single lesion, which commences as a tiny spot and may grow up to 2 cm in diameter. It is most often found on the face, extremities or mucous membranes. It is not familial, there is no predilection for sex, it may occur at any age and there may be a history of recent injury or possible insect bite to the site of the lesion. It grows rapidly over weeks or months to its final size and then frequently remains unchanged, although involution may occur. The surface is usually smooth, but it bleeds easily in response to mild trauma and it may become ulcerated. Satellite lesions are common and the main lesion may recur following treatment, but there is no tendency to neoplastic change. It is treated by the use of diathermy or simple excision. The main differential diagnosis is granulation tissue following local injury.

PILOMATRICOMA

Pilomatricoma is a hamartoma of hair follicles, found mostly in children and young adults and more often in girls than boys. While it is not hereditary, cases have been reported in more than one member of a family. It is usually a single lesion, occurring almost always on the face, neck or upper arm. Pilomatricoma is usually a hard, white or yellow, irregular nodule, from a few millimetres up to 2 cm in greatest dimension and is situated in the dermis, with normal or slightly discoloured overlying epidermis. Complications are infrequent. It may occasionally become inflamed and malignant neoplastic change has been reported but is extremely rare. The treatment is simple excision of the lesion and there is no tendency to recurrence.

SEBACEOUS NAEVUS

Sebaceous naevus is a fairly common, smooth, raised, round, oval or elongated salmon-pink or yellow lesion found usually on the scalp or face. It is present at birth but becomes larger, more yellow and more irregular at puberty. It is not familial and there is no predilection for sex. It is a hamartoma and may be associated with malformations of the central nervous system, seizures or intellectual handicap. There is a definite propensity to neoplastic change, usually in the form of basal cell carcinoma, in from 5 to 10% of patients. The treatment is simple excision.

LATERAL NECK LUMPS

The neck is a common site for lumps, including the common lumps.

Neck lumps are conveniently classified as lateral or midline.

Sternomastoid tumour

This is a firm smooth ovoid mass, 2–3 cm in diameter, attached to the sternomastoid muscle. It is not neoplastic but is a localized fibrotic nodule within the muscle. It may be present at birth but is usually found in the first few weeks of life. Untreated, the tumour gradually resolves over several months but there is progressive fibrosis and shortening of the muscle producing torticollis (wry neck) with flexion of the head to the same side and rotation of the head to the opposite side. The infant then lies continually on the opposite parieto-occipital area when lying on his/her back, because of the rotation, with gradual deformation of the head, involving flattening of the parieto-occipital area on the side opposite to the tumour (plagiocephaly) and of the frontal area on the same side (facial hemiatrophy).

There are variations in the method of presentation. There may be an anterior nodule attached to the sternal head only; a fusiform dilation of the muscle belly; or fibrosis and shortening of the muscle without an obvious nodule.

Treatment consists of physiotherapy, either postural or active, to stretch the sternomastoid muscle, though there is debate about its efficacy. Postural physiotherapy involves holding the infant so that the head falls away from the affected side; positioning cots and infant seats so that the infant looks to that side; and by encouraging the prone position for sleep with the face turned to the side of the tumour. Active physiotherapy involves firm but gentle rotation of the head so that the chin approaches the top of the shoulder of the affected side. These movements need to be done several times at each session and there should be several sessions per day. Most cases respond to this treatment within 6 months.

If there is persistent shortening of the muscle, particularly if plagiocephaly and facial hemiatrophy are developing, the sternomastoid should be divided surgically and physiotherapy continued vigorously. Gradual resolution of the plagiocephaly and hemiatrophy occurs but if they are marked, they may not completely resolve.

The torticollis may occur during childhood, usually at the time of a growth spurt, either from a previously unrecognized fibrosis of the muscle, or from residual fibrosis in a previously treated sternomastoid tumour. Division of the muscle is required, with continuing physiotherapy.

Other causes of torticollis, such as vertebral anomalies, neuromuscular problems or a vertical squint, need to be excluded.

Branchial cyst

A branchial cyst appears as a smooth, unilocular, fluctuant, mildly transilluminable swelling beneath the anterior border of the sternomastoid muscle. It is a remnant of the 2nd branchial cleft (see Ch. 16). It may become inflamed but there are no other associated features. The characteristics are sufficient for diagnosis and further investigations are not necessary. Treatment is by excision.

Thyroid gland

The clinical features of thyroid lumps are well covered in standard surgical texts.

MIDLINE NECK LUMPS

Midline lymph nodes are much less commonly enlarged than lateral lymph nodes but have the same characteristics.

Submental lymph node

This node, situated just behind the symphysis of the mandible, may cause diagnostic problems when it is the only enlarged lymph node in the region, unless the infection in its lymph shed is recognized, i.e. infections of the lower incisor teeth, adjacent gum or median segment of the lower lip. Adequate physical examination should give the diagnosis.

Dermoid cyst

This is usually either immediately beneath the jaw or suprasternal, is subcutaneous or subfascial and is smooth, firm, rounded and unilocular. Because this is an inclusion dermoid, formed by skin and skin appendages, it is full of keratin and so is not transilluminable, though it is usually too small and too deeply situated to be certain of this.

Note: Dermoid cysts occur along lines of fusion and the commonest site is at the lateral end of an eyebrow, the external angular dermoid. Those situated over skull sutures, such as at the base of the nose or in the midline of the skull, may have a dumbbell type of intracranial extension.

Such cysts should be distinguished from epidermoid cysts and from teratomatous dermoid cysts. The epidermoid cyst is composed of epidermis without skin appendages and is usually seen at the umbilicus. Teratomatous dermoid cysts are usually seen as the sacrococcygeal teratoma of infancy or in the ovary in older children.

Surgical excision is the treatment of all such cysts.

Thyroglossal cyst

This is a unilocular cyst in the midline, usually superficial or subfascial and attached to the hyoid bone. It develops as a sequestration of tissue from the thyroglossal duct, which runs from the foramen caecum at the base of the tongue to the site of the thyroid gland.

These congenital cysts are not usually noted until months or years after birth. There may be a thyroglossal fistula in the midline between the submental triangle and suprasternal notch as part of the congenital malformation, or a fistula may arise following discharge or incision of the cyst.

Clinical signs are those of a unilocular cyst in the midline, except at the level of the thyroid cartilage which may displace a thyroglossal cyst to one or other side. They may show positive translucency if sufficiently accessible. Movement upwards on swallowing is a feature of cysts below the hyoid or on protrusion of the tongue with those above. Cysts close to the hyoid, whether thyroglossal or dermoid, tend to move with hyoid movements.

Rarely, the thyroid tissue associated with a thyroglossal cyst is the only thyroid tissue present so that examination of a thyroglossal cyst or fistula should always include inspection and palpation of the back of the tongue and identification of a thyroid gland in the normal position. If the gland cannot be identified clinically with certainty, a thyroid scan should be performed.

Treatment

A thyroglossal cyst or fistula requires the same treatment, which is complete excision of the cyst or fistula, the central segment of the hyoid body and all remnants of thyroglossal duct from foramen caecum to thyroid gland, if recurrence is to be avoided. Adequate excision is more likely to be achieved if carried out before infection, incision or rupture of the cyst. The skin incision must be in the line of the skin creases to achieve a satisfactory cosmetic result and the shorter the neck at the time of operation, the smaller the incision which will allow adequate resection. Thus, in units where surgery, anaesthesia and nursing are optimal, thyroglossal cysts are removed in infancy or early childhood.

FURTHER READING

Clain A 1980 Hamilton Bailey's demonstration of physical signs in clinical surgery, 17th edn. Bristol Wright, Bristol

4. Tumours in childhood

E. Thomas Boles Jr

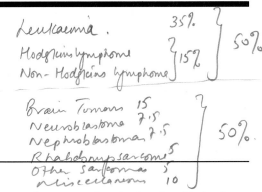

Although much less common than tumours in adults, tumours in the childhood age group are significant causes of morbidity and mortality. In the Western world malignant tumours account for more deaths in children over 3 years of age than any other cause excepting accidental injuries. Unfortunately, knowledge of tumours in adults has little applicability to children. The usual location of primary tumours, the cell types, the biological behaviour, response to therapy, and prognosis are all quite different in children as compared with adults. The therapy of childhood malignancies has undergone profound changes in recent years with a consequent marked improvement in prognosis. This improvement primarily has been the result of chemotherapy, and combination therapy including appropriate surgery and radiation therapy make management of these children complex. Hence, children having or suspected of having a malignancy are best served by referral to a multidisciplinary paediatric oncology unit.

The purpose of this chapter is to discuss primarily the tumours which arise within the abdominal cavity. The commonest childhood malignancy, leukaemia, is covered in medical texts and will not be discussed here. Other tumours will be mentioned briefly.

CLINICAL MANIFESTATIONS

Unlike the case with adults, no convenient list of 'cardinal manifestations of cancer' has been developed for children. However, the most common and significant finding is the development of a mass. An intra-abdominal mass or a superficial mass anywhere on the body should lead to prompt investigation.

Another constellation of manifestations is systemic symptoms, including failure to thrive, irritability, anorexia and fever. Evidence of pain is unusual in infants with tumours, but becomes a significant symptom in the older child. Loss of function and other neurological manifestations are also helpful. Weakness or paresis, loss of urinary or bowel control and loss of ability to stand erect or walk, all fall under this category.

Age of the patient

Age is an important factor in the types of tumours and their prognosis. In the newborn period, true neoplasms must be distinguished from benign developmental lesions. Thus, congenital hydronephrosis or multicystic kidney commonly are present in the newborn, and must be distinguished from renal or retroperitoneal tumours. Although nephroblastoma (Wilms' tumour) is rare in this age group, mesoblastic nephroma (a benign renal tumour) mimics the Wilms' tumour from a diagnostic point of view. Other tumours arising in the newborn or very young infant are ovarian cystic lesions and a form of neuroblastoma which frequently is metastatic at diagnosis but curiously has an excellent prognosis, the so-called stage IV-S type. Sacrococcygeal tumours are most often quite obvious lesions of the newborn, and fortunately in this age group are almost invariably benign.

During infancy (up to 2 years of age) nephroblastomas, the more common forms of neuroblastoma, and hepatoblastomas are all relatively common and reach their peak incidences during this time. After 3 years of age solid malignant lesions tend to become less common, and this is true of the three above-noted neoplasms. Rhabdomyosarcomas, however, are most frequent between 2 and 6 years of age. These tumours arise with roughly equal frequencies in the pelvis, the head and neck area, and the muscles of the extremities and trunk. Ovarian tumours, particularly teratomas, either cystic or solid, arise in the school age child for the most part. Lymphomas also generally occur for the most part in children over 3 years of age.

Associated manifestations

A variety of associated manifestations provide diagnostic clues in some of the affected children. Commonly a child over 1 year of age with neuroblastoma will be ill with such non-specific symptoms as fever, failure to thrive or even loss of weight. The same sort of manifestations also are seen in association with lymphomas, but not in children with Wilms' tumours and only rarely in association with hepatomas. Superficial nodules involving the skin and subcutaneous tissues are occasionally seen in infants with stage IV-S neuroblastoma. The 'panda bear' sign, or periorbital ecchymosis, is a sign of metastatic neuroblastoma, usually seen in children over 1 year of age. A small proportion of children with Wilms' tumour will have aniridia or hemihypertrophy.

Physical examination

On physical examination the most significant finding is a mass. Particularly with abdominal tumours, the characteristics of this mass are frequently of great diagnostic value. Location is an important factor. Wilms' tumours almost invariably are on one side of the midline. On the other hand, retroperitoneal neuroblastomas frequently extend from one side of the midline to the other. Liver tumours are upper abdominal masses which move with respiration, and enlarged spleens have the same characteristic. Tumours arising from the ovary, uterus, or bladder are either pelvic or, more commonly, lower abdominal in location.

The distinction between a solid and a cystic lesion is clearly important, and often can be made by transillumination, particularly in infancy. Most Wilms' tumours are round or ovoid in shape, and the majority of tumours arising from the liver or ovary share this characteristic. On the other hand, neuroblastomas and lymphomas are commonly irregular. Many ovarian or mesenteric lesions are moveable, but Wilms' tumours, neuroblastomas, and other retroperitoneal lesions characteristically are fixed. Tenderness is an uncommon feature that may be seen with torsion of ovarian lesions such as teratomas.

The general appearance on physical examination of these children correlates with specific tumours in many instances. The baby or young child with a Wilms' tumour usually is outwardly completely well. Those with neuroblastoma, however, most often are clearly ill. Hypertension is found in approximately a quarter of the children with Wilms' tumours, and in a somewhat lesser percentage in those with neuroblastoma.

LABORATORY INVESTIGATIONS

Overall at the present time laboratory studies are not particularly helpful in the initial evaluation. A full blood examination will be found to be normal in the majority of these patients, although anaemia often is associated in children with neuroblastoma or lymphoma. The routine urinalysis also usually is normal, although a urinary tract infection may herald an obstructing lesion in the urinary tract.

Increasingly, the production of specific metabolites by certain tumours has led to the identification of tumour markers. Many of these biochemical tests are sophisticated and time consuming, limiting their initial diagnostic value. This problem surely will eventually be solved. In all cases these tumour markers are helpful in following the patients and in many instances are of considerable prognostic value. An example is the production by neuroblastoma of products of catecholamine metabolism, particularly vanillylmandelic acid (VMA) and homovanillic acid

Table 4.1 Some biochemical markers of tumours

Tumour	Marker
Neuroblastoma	Vanillylmandelic acid
Phaeochromocytoma	Vanillylmandelic acid
Carcinoid tumour	5-hydroxyindole acetic acid
Medullary carcinoma of the thyroid	Calcitonin
Islet cell tumour	Insulin
Yolk sac tumour*	α-fetoprotein
Granulosa cell tumour	Oestrogen
Hepatoblastoma	α-fetoprotein

* Yolk sac tumour = archenteronoma = endodermal sinus tumour = embryonal carcinoma

(HVA). These compounds are excreted in the urine, and may be reported either as the total amount excreted in 24 hours or as the ratio to urinary creatinine. The excretion of both of these substances is markedly increased in nearly all patients with neuroblastoma. Alpha fetoprotein characteristically is elevated in patients with endodermal sinus tumours and often with hepatoblastoma. Elevation of the serum alpha fetoprotein level in a patient with a teratoma, such as a sacrococcygeal or ovarian lesion, is strong presumptive evidence that the tumour is malignant and that the malignant component is an endodermal sinus tumour (Table 4.1).

In an infant or child with a presumptive diagnosis of neuroblastoma or lymphoma, a bone marrow examination is a routine part of the evaluation. This study obviously is important in the staging of the tumour and in the subsequent chemotherapeutic management.

DIAGNOSTIC IMAGING STUDIES

The increasing availability and sophistication of imaging techniques in the past decade has dramatically improved the evaluation of abdominal masses. These studies should follow promptly the initial clinical evaluation, and should be done in a logical sequence. Plain abdominal and chest radiographs are obtained first. By displacement of the intestinal tract, the position and size of the mass often are clearly shown. Areas of calcification within the mass may be seen with neuroblastoma, teratoma and hepatoblastoma. The outline of the kidneys often is clearly demonstrated. A chest X-ray is essential for the possibility of metastatic lesions; and, of course, a mediastinal mass or widening of the mediastinal shadow is often a characteristic of both Hodgkin's and non-Hodgkin's lymphomas.

Ultrasonography

Ultrasonography (US) is almost always the next appropriate study. This study will distinguish between cystic and solid tumours, and subsequent evaluation is determined by this finding. The kidneys are particularly well seen with this technique. A kidney of normal size and architecture is evident or the finding of a cystic or a large solid mass replacing the kidney may indicate lesions such as multicystic kidney, hydronephrotic kidney, or a Wilms' tumour. This study also is extraordinarily helpful in delineation of the pelvic viscera. With a full bladder the uterus and ovaries can be seen, and the study is frequently diagnostic in showing an ovarian cyst or an ovarian teratoma, either cystic or solid. The usefulness of this study in examination of the mid portion of the abdomen is more limited because of the gas-filled loops of intestine, but mesenteric cysts or intestinal duplications often can be clearly shown. The liver also is well displayed by this technique, and such lesions as solid tumours or cystic lymphangiomas are clearly seen. Ultrasonography demonstrates the inferior vena cava well, and has essentially replaced the inferior vena cavagram for this purpose. This study can determine whether the cava is open, obstructed, filled with tumour or displaced.

In some instances, as with clearly seen ovarian lesions, no further diagnostic studies are required. However, in the majority of instances the finding of a solid or a cystic lesion will dictate additional studies. If a cystic lesion is found in a renal fossa, then further investigations will follow those outlined in Chapter 19.

Computerized axial tomography

If the ultrasound demonstrates a solid intra-abdominal mass, in most instances the next study should be an enhanced computerized tomography (CT) scan. It is important that the patient be prepared for such a study with adequate filling of the gastrointestinal tract with barium solution, and that intravenous dye be injected to outline the collecting structures of the kidneys. With most solid intra-abdominal masses, the enhanced CT scan will accurately indicate the organ of origin, the size of the lesion, and its anatomic relationships. It can almost invariably distinguish between renal tumours and extrarenal retro-peritoneal tumours such as neuroblastoma or lymphomas. With a retroperitoneal neuroblastoma, the relationship of the tumour to the aorta and its major intra-abdominal branches can often be precisely determined. Local invasion of adjacent viscera as well as the extent of local spread often are seen. Renal function and the presence or absence of distortion of the collecting systems can be noted. Calcification is well displayed.

In the liver, metastatic lesions, e.g. neuroblastoma, often can clearly be seen. With primary hepatic lesions, the size, the presence or absence of necrosis with haemorrhage or calcification, and the extent usually are readily apparent. In pelvic lesions the extent of the lesion and often the presence or absence of involvement of adjacent structures, such as the rectum, can be noted. The study is also valuable in infants with sacrococcygeal teratomas, inasmuch as any intrapelvic extension of the tumour is clearly outlined.

Magnetic resonance imaging

Magnetic resonance imaging (MRI) is the most recently introduced technique for imaging, and has been demonstrated to be particularly useful in children with lesions involving the central nervous system, both brain and spinal column. It has also proved to be very useful in defining lesions of the musculoskeletal system and of the bone marrow. Its precise role in evaluation of abdominal lesions in children has not, thus far, been clearly defined. MRI of solid lesions of the kidney (e.g. Wilms' tumour) is comparable in sensitivity to CT. In a Wilms' MRI will also demonstrate tumour thrombosis in the inferior vena cava.

For the demonstration of pulmonary metastases, CT remains the procedure of choice. With neuroblastomas, again MRI appears to have accuracy comparable to CT in terms of diagnosis and defining the extent of the tumour. It also permits accurate evaluation of extension into the spinal column or superior extension into the mediastinum. Clearly evaluation of posterior extension into the spinal column is a major advantage and can replace myelography for this purpose. With respect to hepatic masses, MRI has accuracy similar to CT in the evaluation of solid tumours, and may be superior to either CT or angiography in terms of predicting resectability.

Technical considerations are of great importance in determining the value of MRI. The lack of radiation exposure to the patient is a clear advantage, but the exact relative places of CT and MRI in the evaluation of paediatric abdominal masses await further experience.

BIOPSY

Biopsy is always required, and in most cases this will be an open surgical procedure. Increasingly, needle biopsies are finding a place. Because the type of biopsy and location of the incision often influence later therapy, patients should be referred to a major paediatric cancer centre before biopsy whenever possible.

STAGING OF TUMOURS

The staging of tumours is used to decide the methods of treatment and to give an idea of prognosis. The staging of all tumours varies but, in general, stage I is that in which the tumour is limited to one organ or localized tissue; stage II is a tumour that has already spread locally; stage III is a tumour that has spread within the general area of the tumour but not beyond the confines of the immediately contiguous structures; and stage IV is a tumour in which there are haematogenous or distant metastases. More precise staging criteria for specific tumours have been determined by international agreements.

The treatment of tumours is by surgery, irradiation and chemotherapy and may involve one or all of these, depending on the type of tumour, the age of the patient, and the stage of the tumour.

If a tumour can be completely surgically excised this usually indicates a good prognosis. If it cannot be completely surgically excised then radiotherapy or chemotherapy will be necessary. All these methods of treatment have their drawbacks. The area involved in radiotherapy suffers from growth disorders and long-term cosmetic problems and there is also an increased risk of malignancy in the areas within the irradiated field, e.g. thyroid carcinoma following irradiation of a neck lymphoma. There is also an increased risk of neoplasia following the use of chemotherapy, particularly if alkylating agents are used in conjunction with radiotherapy. The commonest secondary tumours are myeloid leukaemia, thyroid carcinoma and bone sarcoma. They usually occur within 10 years of treatment and mostly from 3–7 years after treatment.

SPECIFIC ABDOMINAL TUMOURS

WILMS' TUMOUR (NEPHROBLASTOMA)

Probably the most common of all abdominal tumours in childhood, this embryonal renal tumour occurs for the most part in infancy and early childhood, rarely in the school age child. The tumour most often grows in a concentric fashion, pushing aside rather than invading adjacent renal parenchyma and collecting structures. However, this produces the appearance of intrarenal distortion of architecture on investigation (Fig. 4.1). Characteristically, a well-developed capsule develops. Local invasion into local structures (retroperitoneum, liver) is uncommon. The tumour rarely outgrows its blood supply, so that haemorrhage, necrosis and calcification are infrequent.

Distant spread occurs both through lymphatic channels and the bloodstream. Lymph node spread to the renal hilar, para-aortic, and paracaval areas may occur. The most common distant metastatic lesions are blood borne pulmonary metastases; metastatic lesions to the bone and liver are infrequent. At diagnosis most children have localized disease confined to the kidney or with regional lymph node involvement.

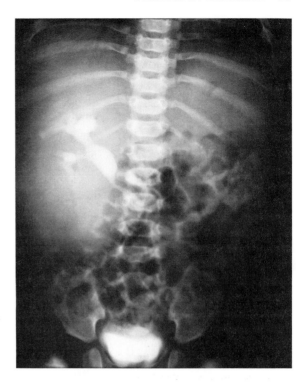

Fig. 4.1 IVP showing a large soft tissue mass in the right side of the abdomen and marked distortion of the right renal collecting system, typical of a Wilms' tumour.

Diagnosis

The infant or child is usually asymptomatic, the diagnosis first being suspected in an otherwise healthy child as a consequence of the inadvertent palpation of an abdominal mass. The mass is often large, filling much of one side of the abdomen. It is usually firm, fairly well fixed in position, and smoothly contoured. Hypertension is associated with the tumour in 20–25% of the children.

The diagnosis is often strongly suspected on clinical grounds alone. Using the format of imaging studies described previously, plain films of the abdomen outline the position and size of the mass. The ultrasound study shows that the mass arises from a kidney and is solid. This study also defines the status of the inferior vena cava. The definitive study is the enhanced CT scan, showing an intrarenal mass with distortion of the collecting system (Fig. 4.2A). This study also evaluates the status of the opposite kidney, an

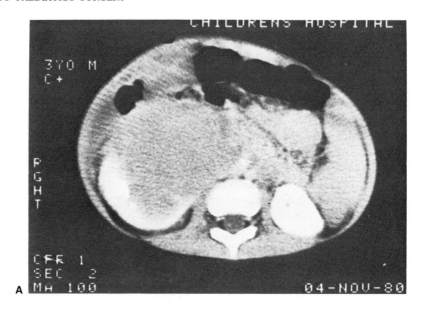

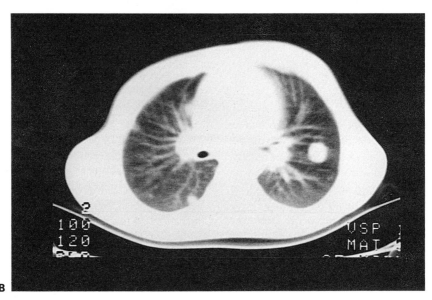

Fig. 4.2 A: Abdominal CT scan with enhancement showing a large right intrarenal tumour (Wilms'). Left kidney normal. **B**: Chest CT scan with bilateral pulmonary metastases in child with Wilms' tumour.

important consideration since bilateral tumours occur in about 5% of the cases. The CT scan is essential for evaluation of pulmonary metastases (Fig. 4.2B).

Treatment

Multimodal treatment plans include surgery, radiotherapy, and chemotherapy. Surgical removal of the involved kidney is performed by a transperitoneal approach with early ligation of the renal vein and artery. Precise and gentle dissection is essential to avoid rupture of the tumour capsule and consequent spillage. In localized tumours in which all tumour can be grossly removed and in which regional lymph node spread has not occurred, radiotherapy is not required. However, in more advanced cases in which regional lymph node spread has occurred or in which all of the primary tumour cannot be removed, radiotherapy is necessary.

Chemotherapy is essential postoperatively in all cases and is largely responsible for the truly remarkable improvement in results which has occurred in the last two decades. The chemotherapeutic agents commonly employed include actinomycin D, vincristine, and adriamycin. Combination drug therapy has proved superior to single drug therapy.

Prognosis

The prognosis of children with Wilms' tumours has improved dramatically since the addition of chemotherapy to the management program. With current therapy, previously significant prognostic factors such as age, regional lymph node metastases, and tumour weight no longer are relevant. The only significant factors now are cell type and stage at diagnosis. In a recently completed multi-institutional study on Wilms' tumour, done in the United States (Third National Wilms' Tumour Study), 89.3% of the tumours (1465 patients) were classified as having favourable histological types. The remainder of the tumours (10.7% of the patients) were classified as unfavourable. The 4 year survival for the entire group was 89.1%. For those with stage I disease and favourable histology (607 patients) the 4 year survival was 96.5%. For high-risk patients (stage IV at diagnosis and all those with unfavourable histology) the 4 year survival was 73.0%.

NEUROBLASTOMA

This tumour arises from the adrenal medulla or from the sympathetic ganglia extending in their perivertebral locations from neck to the pelvis. Overall, this tumour is somewhat more common than Wilms' tumour with approximately 70% of the cases arising within the abdomen. Most of the remaining are mediastinal. The biological behaviour of these tumours is aggressive both locally and with respect to metastases. Most of these tumours either do not have a capsule or the capsule is poorly defined. The tumours com-

monly spread locally to encase the inferior vena cava, aorta and celiac vessels. They cross the midline, invade the mesenteries, and even extend superiorly under the diaphragm and into the mediastinum. Posterior spread through intervertebral foramina and into the spinal column produces dumbbell lesions. Early spread to regional lymph nodes is common, and at times spread to such distant nodes as those in the supraclavicular fossa is apparent at diagnosis. Distant metastases also are found early in the course of the disease with involvement of liver (early infancy), bone (older children), bone marrow, skin and meninges. Inexplicably, pulmonary metastases are rare.

In approximately two-thirds of the cases distant metastases are present at diagnosis, and in no more than 5% is the tumour confined to the organ of origin.

Clinical features

As with the pathology, the clinical manifestations are in marked contrast to those seen in Wilms' tumour. However, age distribution of children with this tumour is similar to that in Wilms' tumour, with 50% occurring in the first 2 years and about 75% within the first 5 years of life.

These infants and children are almost always symptomatic and systemic symptoms are common. Anorexia, irritability and fever are often prominent. Abdominal pain, gastrointestinal symptoms and symptoms secondary to pressure on the bladder are not unusual. Bone pain or loss of function of the legs secondary to bony metastases are also at times apparent, particularly in early childhood. Posterior extension through an intervertebral foramen and into the spinal canal (dumbbell tumours) results in pain and loss of function.

An abdominal mass is the most common finding. The mass is usually upper abdominal, hard, fixed, often irregular and frequently crosses the midline. In those arising at or inferior to the aortic bifurcation, pelvic and/or lower abdominal masses present.

Hypertension occurs in a significant number of these children, with an incidence of between 10 and 20%.

Investigations

Anaemia is a common finding, probably as a consequence of bone marrow replacement. As a corollary, bone marrow examination is essential, since bone marrow spread is present in more than half of these children at diagnosis and such spread obviously is a major determinant of therapy. Urine determinations of VMA and HVA are helpful in some for diagnosis and in essentially all for following the course of the disease.

With respect to imaging techniques, radiographs of the abdomen commonly show a large abdominal mass, sometimes with fine calcifica-

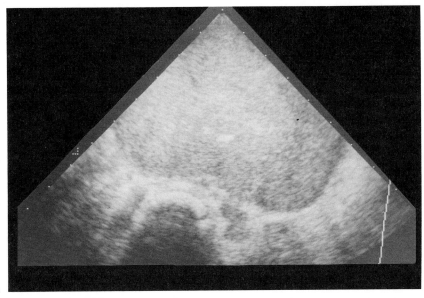

A

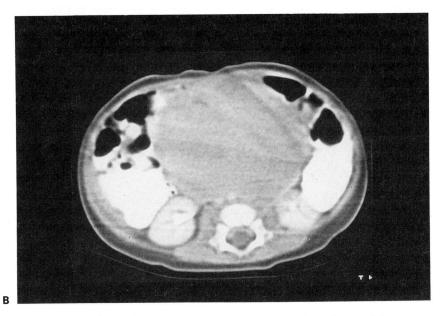

B

Fig. 4.3 A: Ultrasound of the abdomen (transverse) showing a large, solid tumour crossing the midline (neuroblastoma). **B**: Abdominal CT (same patient) with huge, centrally positioned neuroblastoma. Normal kidneys.

tions. Ultrasonography defines the mass more accurately, indicates that it is solid, and usually clearly separates it from the kidneys (Fig. 4.3A). The status of the inferior vena cava is also determined by this study. At the present time in most centres the definitive imaging study is an enhanced CT scan. This usually accurately outlines the tumour in terms of position and extent, and frequently permits the relationship of the tumour to major blood vessels, particularly the celiac axis, aorta and vena cava, to be assessed. The study also shows the kidneys, which are frequently displaced but not involved by the tumour (Fig. 4.3B). MRI, as noted previously, has similar attributes in terms of accuracy to the CT scan, and has the additional advantage of clearly showing invasion of the tumour into the spinal canal if this is present. Bony metastases are looked for either by X-rays of the skeletal system or by nuclear scans.

Treatment

As might be predicted in a tumour so aggressive and with such a high incidence of metastases at diagnosis, treatment generally has been unsatisfactory and disappointing. Tumours which are localized to the organ of origin and which can be completely resected surgically are uniformly cured by surgery alone. Somewhat more extensive but still localized tumours which can be grossly removed also have an excellent prognosis with surgery alone. Tumours in the latter category may have microscopic residual or may have lymph nodes positive for tumour attached to the surgical specimen. Approximately 18% of neuroblastomas fall into this localized category, and a prospective study of 101 such patients showed a 2 year disease-free survival of 89%.

With more advanced but still localized tumours (stage III) or with metastatic tumours (stage IV) curability remains low, although there are some indications that both more aggressive schedules of chemotherapy and more aggressive surgery may increase long-term survival or even cure. Multidrug chemotherapy does result in marked reduction in the size of the primary tumours in about 70% of such patients. Delayed surgery with an attempt to remove all or most of the primary lesion has been a technique used commonly after several courses of chemotherapy. Although such surgical procedures may be difficult, particularly when aorta, vena cava, superior mesenteric artery and celiac axis are involved, frequently all or nearly all of the primary tumour can be safely removed.

Prognosis

Unfortunately, the overall survival of patients with metastatic disease at diagnosis or with extensive intra-abdominal disease has not changed significantly in the past 15 or 20 years. In a recent cooperative group study on patients with stage IV disease at diagnosis who were treated with chemotherapy followed by delayed surgery, survival rates were 26% at 2 years and 16% at 3 years following diagnosis. Another study by the same group, however, suggests that tumour excision together with chemotherapy may improve ultimate survival.

Age continues to be an important, perhaps the single most important, prognostic factor. Infants less than 1 year of age invariably fare better than do older children. A schema for classifying patients into favourable or unfavourable groups on the basis of age and histology has been proposed by Shimada and appears to have true significance. More recently, the N-myc gene has been identified in neuroblastoma cell lines, and a correlation between the amplification of the N-myc oncogene and prognosis has been repeatedly demonstrated. Invasiveness of the neuroblastoma and a poor prognosis correlate with amplification of the N-myc oncogene, a good prognosis with lack of such amplification. Interestingly, in a recent study of infants with either stage IV-S or localized neuroblastoma, both of which have excellent prognosis, the tumours lacked N-myc gene amplification.

Stage IV-S neuroblastoma is a form of the disease seen almost exclusively in infants under 1 year of age. The primary tumour is often small, but metastases to liver, skin, or bone marrow are present. Liver metastases often are massive. Cure rate with this unique form of metastatic neuroblastoma with little or no treatment approximates 75%.

LIVER TUMOURS

Primary tumours of the liver are uncommon. Approximately 70 to 75% of these tumours are malignant, the rest benign. Children with primary liver tumours frequently are asymptomatic and present because of an upper abdominal mass. Pain, gastrointestinal symptoms, and systemic symptoms usually are absent. In most instances the diagnostic plan outlined previously will provide the necessary information for diagnosis and management. Serum alpha fetoprotein levels should be obtained in such patients. Ultrasonography distinguishes cystic from solid tumours (Fig. 4.4). A CT scan of the upper abdomen has been the most helpful study in the past decade with accurate demonstration of tumour size and position. Hepatic artery angiography has been thought to be an essential diagnostic study when a major resection is planned, but unfortunately neither the angiographic or CT findings are accurate in predicting surgical resectability. MRI is comparable to CT in most parameters, and may provide useful information concerning resectability, by delineating the relationship of portal lobules to the tumour tissue.

Benign tumours

The most common benign tumour of the liver is the haemangioma. These usually are single lesions, asymptomatic and require no treatment in most instances. In the rare instance of associated congestive heart failure, surgical resection may be appropriate if medical management of the heart failure is unsuccessful. Haemangioendotheliomas may be asymptomatic and require no management, but in most cases present with a very large hepatic mass and congestive heart failure. Severe thrombocytopenia secondary to sequestration of platelets produces a bleeding diathesis in about half of such patients. These tumours or malformations characteristically regress spontaneously within a year, and obviously, therefore, no treatment is required except for the complications. With congestive heart failure, again medical management should be the first line of therapy. If this is unsuccessful, a trial of steroid therapy or a brief course of low dose radiotherapy should be attempted. If these fail, hepatic artery ligation has been reported to be successful. In other benign tumours, such as adenomas and hamartomas, appropriate surgical resection is usually all that is required.

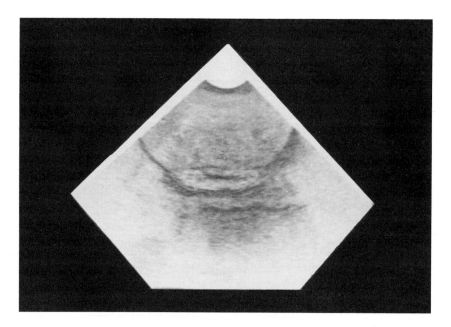

Fig. 4.4 Abdominal ultrasound (right longitudinal) outlining a large, solid tumour of the right lobe of the liver (hepatoblastoma). Compression of underlying right kidney.

Malignant tumours

The most common primary malignant tumour is the hepatoblastoma, making up about two-thirds of this group. Most of the remaining are hepatocellular carcinomas, and there are a few sarcomas such as the rhabdomyosarcoma. The outlook for children with a primary malignant tumour depends to a great extent on whether or not complete surgical resection can be accomplished. If this is possible and chemotherapy is added, the cure rate is high, approximating 80%. However, in only about one-third of these children is complete surgical resection possible. In the remaining two-thirds, even with intensive chemotherapy, the prognosis has, to date, been dismal. Studies are underway to determine whether or not the use of intense chemotherapy in some of these unresectable tumours may shrink the tumour sufficiently so that complete surgical resection can be accomplished. Because of the striking relationship between resectability and curability, an aggressive surgical approach is essential.

RHABDOMYOSARCOMA

Overall, rhabdomyosarcoma occurs in children with a frequency which approximates that of Wilms' tumour and neuroblastoma. The largest number of these tumours occur in the head and neck area, including the orbit. Most of the rest occur either in the pelvis or in the muscles of the extremity or trunk. In childhood there are two histological types: alveolar and embryonal. These make up almost all of the tumours. The embryonal type predominates in primary lesions of the genitourinary tract and, to a somewhat lesser extent, in those arising in the head and neck region. The alveolar type makes up almost half of those occurring in the extremity and somewhat more than a third of those arising in the trunk.

These histology patterns are very significant in terms of prognosis, those with the embryonal type having a considerably better outlook than those with the alveolar pattern.

In those tumours involving the genitourinary organs, symptoms usually arise as a consequence of urinary tract obstruction, a suprapubic mass,

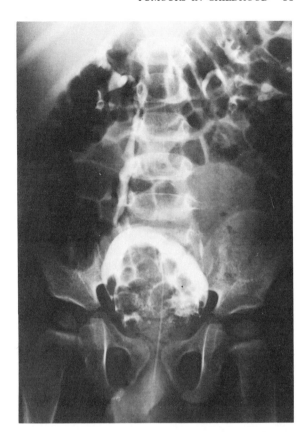

Fig. 4.5 Large intravesical rhabdomyosarcoma of the botryoid type seen on IVP. Surprisingly, the upper collecting systems are not dilated.

or vaginal bleeding. A high proportion of these tumours are botryoid, embryonal tumours which take on a polypoid appearance (Fig. 4.5). These botryoid tumours may be seen in the bladder on cystoscopy or may protrude from the vaginal introitus. Most of these pelvic tumours can be readily diagnosed by biopsy, frequently through an endoscope. Treatment is combined chemotherapy, radiotherapy and surgery. Many of these tumours have proved to be very responsive to chemotherapy, and this has become the primary mode in some studies. Radiotherapy is given when chemotherapy fails to completely eradicate the tumour, and radical surgical excision has been used when combined chemotherapy–radiotherapy has failed.

Generally, the results with this approach have been satisfactory. This has been particularly true in vaginal lesions, although vaginectomy and hysterectomy have been required in a considerable number of cases.

Chemotherapy has not been as effective in bladder and prostate lesions, and in about 20% of the cases an anterior exenteration has been required because of failure of the chemotherapy-radiotherapy programme. The overall cure rate in the genitourinary group of tumours is approximately 75%.

With respect to head and neck lesions, those arising in superficial areas for which complete surgical excision is practical, as in the scalp, face and parotid gland, have an excellent prognosis following such excision and adjuvant chemotherapy. However, deep-seated lesions occurring in such areas as the nasopharynx, inner ear or pterygoid fossa, have been found to have a much poorer prognosis despite intensive radiation therapy and chemotherapy. Complete surgical excision of such deep-seated lesions rarely can be done. Of all the sites, the orbit is the most favourable. Orbital exenteration is now rarely required, and the cure rate with combined chemotherapy and radiotherapy is in the neighbourhood of 90%. Early diagnosis is the rule with such lesions. Cataracts are a common complication secondary to the radiation therapy.

With extremity lesions, the results at present are not as favourable. The incidence of alveolar pathology is much higher than with either genitourinary or head and neck primaries, and this probably largely accounts for the poorer results. Every attempt should be made to surgically remove the primary by wide local excision. This is followed by radiotherapy to the primary and by chemotherapy. Overall, survival of children with primary extremity lesions is at present slightly less than 50%.

OVARIAN TUMOURS

Ovarian neoplasms and cysts are uncommon lesions in childhood but increase rather markedly in incidence with age. Approximately half of these occur during adolescence, and twice as many occur in the years between 5 and 10 as in the first 5 years of life. The most common cause of presentation is pain. This usually is from torsion of an ovarian mass, but can be due to bleeding into the mass or to perforation. Quite often the clinical presentation in such girls mimics acute appendicitis. The second most common presentation is that of a lower abdominal mass. Quite infrequently precocious feminization from oestrogen production is the initial manifestation.

The diagnostic approach to girls with ovarian masses is ordinarily straightforward. In all postmenarcheal girls a pregnancy test is essential to rule out an intrauterine or tubal pregnancy. Ultrasonography is particularly helpful since a relatively high proportion of ovarian lesions are non-neoplastic and cystic. For solid lesions, CT imaging is helpful not only in assessment of the ovarian lesion but in demonstrating the status of the liver, para-aortic nodes, the kidneys, and the possibility of ascites. Blood for human chorionic gonadotrophin and alpha fetoprotein determination should be routinely drawn in all patients with demonstrable solid tumours.

Approximately 25% of symptomatic ovarian masses will be non-neoplastic. Most of these cystic lesions occur in the adolescent years, and most do not require surgical therapy. However, laparotomy is indicated for large cysts (over 5 cm in diameter), those responsible for pain secondary to torsion, and those which do not decrease in size over a period of 2 or 3 months' observation. At surgery, every effort should be made to remove the cysts totally or subtotally without sacrificing the ovary.

The true neoplasms consist of:—

- Epithelial tumours
- Stromal tumours
- Germ cell tumour

Epithelial tumours predominate in the adult, but are quite infrequent in children. Stromal tumours (granulosa cell and theca) also are quite infrequent but of particular interest because of their production of oestrogen and the clinical picture of precocious feminization. These tumours are ordinarily solid and encapsulated. Relatively conservative surgical management is appropriate with removal of the tumour and the ipsilateral fallopian tube. Prognosis is excellent.

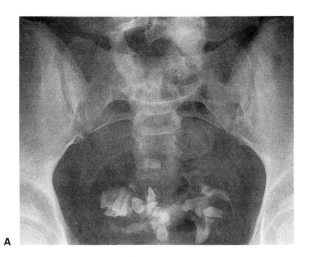

A

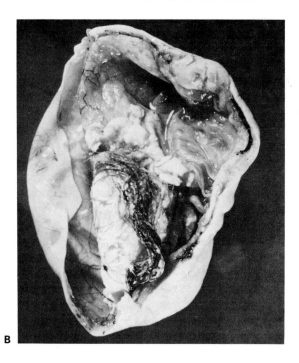

B

Fig. 4.6 A: Abdominal X-ray of a girl with a large pelvic and lower abdominal mass showing calcifications typical of a benign ovarian teratoma. **B**: Benign teratoma (opened) of ovary showing cystic and solid components.

By far the most common ovarian neoplasms in childhood are germ cell tumours, making up approximately two-thirds of the entire group. Teratomas, dysgerminomas and endodermal sinus tumours are the most frequent.

Teratomas are the single most common neoplasm in this age group and usually present clinically because of torsion or because of a mass. In many instances the diagnosis becomes clear on finding areas of calcification within the mass on a plain X-ray of the abdomen (Fig. 4.6A). The majority of these are benign, cystic teratomas (dermoid cysts) and are satisfactorily managed by unilateral salphingo-oophorectomy (Fig. 4.6B). A small proportion (10%) of these teratomas are immature because of the presence in any component of poorly differentiated embryonal tissue. A histological grading classification of these tumours from 0 to 3 has been proposed correlating with the proportion of the embryonal tissue. Management of these immature lesions is an unsettled issue, but clearly more extensive surgical procedures are indicated if the tumour has spread beyond the involved ovary.

Dysgerminoma is the most common form of ovarian malignancy in childhood. It is indistin-

guishable histologically from testicular seminoma. Most of these are seen in adolescent girls, and most of the affected patients present because of an abdominal mass or discomfort. Most are well-encapsulated tumours replacing one ovary; but both ovaries have been reported to be involved in up to one-fifth of the patients. Therefore, bisection with biopsy of the opposite ovary is indicated. These tumours spread primarily to the regional lymph nodes and are highly sensitive to radiotherapy. The combination of surgical removal and postoperative radiation results in very high cure rates. Chemotherapy also has been reported to be effective in children with intraperitoneal dissemination, and therefore should be used in the presence of distant metastatic lesions or local recurrence.

Endodermal sinus tumours are highly malignant and aggressive. The tumours produce alpha fetoprotein, and hence this tumour marker is an important diagnostic aid and is also very helpful in follow-up management. Prior to chemotherapy the outlook in children with this tumour was extremely poor. Aggressive chemotherapy is now the mainstay of management following surgical removal, and reported results have dramatically improved with approximately 80% long-term survival.

MEDIASTINAL TUMOURS

These tumours form a diverse and most interesting group. As with abdominal tumours, there are important differences between children and adults. The location is usually posterior mediastinal in children and anterior in adults, and the predominant tumour types are neuroblastoma or lymphoma in children and thymoma or teratoma in adults. Finally, about half of these mediastinal tumours are malignant in children, but only about 20–30% are malignant in adults.

Clinical features

These are often caused by encroachment of the tumour on the tracheobronchial tree, spinal cord or superior vena cava. Cough, wheezing and dyspnoea result in the first group. When a posterior mediastinal tumour grows through the intervertebral foramen and into the extradural space of the vertebral column, pain or neurological deficits result. Rapidly growing tumours in the superior mediastinum often produce the superior vena caval syndrome. However, significant specific symptoms occur only in about 50% of cases. In the rest, the tumour is found because a chest X-ray is taken on a routine basis or for the evaluation of systemic symptoms.

Investigations

Because the various tumours arise characteristically from one of the mediastinal compartments (anterior, middle or visceral and posterior or paravertebral), lateral as well as posteroanterior X-rays are essential. CT scan defines the relationships of the mass with great accuracy. MRI in all posterior lesions is important to define the possibility of posterior extension into the spinal cord. Oesophograms are useful in lesions of the middle or posterior compartments. Bronchograms are rarely needed, although the outline of the air-filled trachea is often of considerable value. Evaluation of the skeletal system for me-

tastases is particularly important in posterior lesions. Bone marrow examination is essential for neuroblastomas and lymphomas, and, of course, urinary catecholamine excretion levels are important in neurogenic tumours.

Anterior compartment

The thymus in early infancy is normally quite large and may present a diagnostic problem in a symptomatic baby, but the radiological picture is usually diagnostic. Thymomas are very rare in children and when present behave like lymphomas. Teratomas also arise in this compartment. These usually are benign and cystic. They may produce pulmonary symptoms by compression but are more often asymptomatic. Treatment is surgical excision.

Middle (visceral) compartment

Under 2 years of age these lesions are usually congenital, cystic and benign. Bronchogenic cysts, usually close to the carina, often produce respiratory symptoms. Neuroenteric duplications of the oesophagus are usually associated with anomalies in the thoracic or low cervical vertebrae. They may end blindly in the chest and cause respiratory symptoms or occasionally extend below the diaphragm and communicate with the duodenum or proximal jejunum. Some are lined with gastric mucosa and may, therefore, be responsible for intestinal bleeding. These various lesions should be managed by surgical excision.

In children over 2 years of age the tumours in this compartment are usually lymphomas, either Hodgkin's or non-Hodgkin's. In most instances, mediastinal involvement by Hodgkin's disease is found on the basis of a chest X-ray in the evaluation of a patient with cervical lymphadenopathy. Only rarely is Hodgkin's disease in the mediastinum responsible for symptoms. The treatment depends on the stage of Hodgkin's disease in most centres, and the overall results with extended field radiotherapy or with a combination of radiotherapy and chemotherapy are extremely good.

Non-Hodgkin's lymphoma, on the other hand,

is most often a fast growing lesion which is large at diagnosis and responsible for symptoms including respiratory distress and the superior vena cava syndrome. These tumours are frequently wide spread at diagnosis, often with involvement of the bone marrow. Although highly responsive to radiotherapy, curability has been extremely rare until the advent of chemotherapy. However, with radiotherapy and intensive multidrug chemotherapy, 80% survival at 12 to 48 months has been reported.

Posterior (paravertebral) compartment

The lesions in this compartment are almost all neurogenic and most are malignant (neuroblastoma or ganglioneuroblastoma). About 20–25% of all neuroblastomas are mediastinal. An occasional benign ganglioneuroma is seen in older children.

In about one-third of cases a 'dumbbell' configuration of the tumour results from posterior extension through intervertebral foramina and into the vertebral canal. Compression of the cord then produces loss of function in the infant and pain in the older child as the earliest clinical manifestations. In the infant regression of motor function with loss of ability to sit or crawl, or urinary dribbling, may be noted. The pain in older children is accompanied by neurological abnormalities including paresis, abnormal deep tendon reflexes and impaired sphincter function.

Imaging studies are usually diagnostic. Radiographs show the lesion and indicate its posterior position. Spreading of the ribs at the site of the lesion is often seen and sometimes actual destruction of the ribs. CT scans are again most helpful, and MRI demonstrates quite clearly any posterior extension.

Treatment of mediastinal neuroblastoma or ganglioneuroblastoma consists of surgical resection and radiation therapy. With extension into the spinal canal, laminectomy with decompression and resection is the first step. This is followed by radiotherapy to the tumour bed and then thoracotomy and removal of the mediastinal tumour.

The overall results with mediastinal neuroblastoma are much better than with abdominal lesions. The reasons for this difference are not clear, although more of the tumours in the mediastinum show some degree of differentiation (ganglioneuroblastoma) than do those in the abdomen. The cure rate is approximately 60%. As is the case elsewhere, the prognosis is distinctly better for those under 1 year of age than for older children. The cure rate is not adversely affected by spinal column extension. Most of those with dumbbell lesions recover from their neurological deficits entirely or in a large part. However, spinal deformities develop in most children with dumbbell lesions; and this long-term complication of therapy frequently is a major problem requiring additional surgical procedures for stabilization and correction of curvatures.

SACROCOCCYGEAL TERATOMA

In most instances the diagnosis is obvious at birth because of a large mass extending down and out from the sacral area. Occasionally the mass is so large as to present problems in delivery of the baby. (Fig. 4.7). About three-quarters of these infants are girls. Differential diagnosis from a myelomeningocele must be made, but the more proximal location and the associated neurological deficits of the latter usually permit this distinction.

These tumours in the newborn period are almost invariably benign and are ordinarily successfully managed by excision with in-continuity removal of the coccyx by a posterior approach. In some, however, intrapelvic extension is of such a degree as to require a combined abdominal and posterior approach. The diagnosis of such anterior extension is made preoperatively on the basis of a rectal examination, ultrasonography and CT imaging.

A small percentage of these tumours are diagnosed later in infancy or early childhood after palpation of a mass which often was not obvious and was not apparent in the newborn period. Tumours in infants 6 months or older are malignant and carry a poor prognosis. Radical surgical excision should be followed by chemotherapy, but experience to date on the most appropriate agents to use or results with such combined therapy is meager.

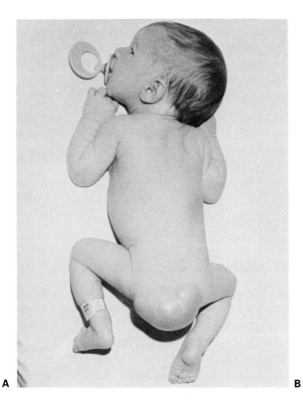
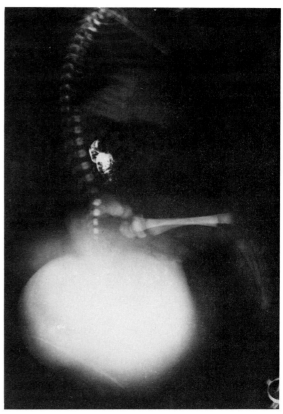

A   B

Fig. 4.7   A: Newborn with large mass arising in the sacrococcygeal area typical of a sacrococcygeal teratoma. **B**: Lateral X-ray of newborn with a large sacrococcygeal teratoma. Areas of calcification are visible within the mass.

TESTICULAR TUMOURS

An enlarged, painless testicular mass requires careful evaluation for the possibility of a testicular neoplasm. The major consideration in differential diagnosis is a hydrocele. Transillumination is a very useful technique in distinguishing a cystic hydrocele from a solid neoplasm but occasionally tumour is associated with a hydrocele.

As with ovarian tumours, testicular neoplasms may be divided into germ cell and non-germinal tumours. In children, the former make up about three-quarters of the total and almost all occur in the first 5 years of life. The usual tumour is an embryonal cell carcinoma (endodermal sinus tumour), which is managed by radical orchidectomy followed by chemotherapy. Retroperitoneal node dissection is probably not necessary. Serum for alpha fetoprotein determination should be drawn preoperatively and followed subsequently as a tumour marker. Teratomas occur but are much less common.

Rhabdomyosarcoma may occur as a para-testicular tumour, presenting as a painless, solid mass. This also is managed by radical orchidectomy but this should be followed by a retroperitoneal node dissection. Chemotherapy is always given, as well as radiotherapy, if the retroperitoneal nodes are involved or there is local extension.

INTRACRANIAL TUMOURS

These are relatively common childhood tumours. Two-thirds arise below the tentorium and one-third above. The commonest of the infratentorial tumours are astrocytoma and medulloblastoma, while the commonest supratentorial tumour is astrocytoma. Craniopharyngioma and tumours of the pineal gland also occur above the tentorium while ependymoma occurs in both sites.

Clinical features

The clinical features will depend on the state of closure of the sutures and fontanelles. The child in whom the sutures and fontanelles have closed will present with headache, vomiting and visual disturbance and sometimes with peripheral signs, as in the adult patient. If the sutures are still open, the child will present with an enlarging head and minimal peripheral signs. However, involvement of the cerebellum by a subtentorial tumour may cause ataxia and nystagmus and involvement of the brain stem may cause cranial nerve palsies.

Investigations

The CT scan is the method of choice for diagnosis and localization of tumours of the CNS, but the increasing availability of nuclear magnetic resonance, positron emission tomography and other rapidly evolving techniques makes consultation with imaging specialists mandatory.

X-ray of the skull may show separation of sutures, and occasionally calcification within the tumour. Cerebral angiography may occasionally be useful for the diagnosis of vascular tumours. A lumbar puncture should not be attempted in a child with closed sutures and clinical features of raised intracranial pressure.

Treatment

Treatment may be curative or palliative. The type of treatment will depend on the anatomical site of the tumour and on its histological type, e.g. a well-differentiated cerebellar astrocytoma is best treated by surgical excision alone, while this is obviously impractical for a glioma of the brainstem. Cerebellar medulloblastoma, a highly malignant tumour, metastasizes within the subarachnoid space and is best treated by chemotherapy and craniospinal radiation. On the other hand, craniopharyngioma grows very slowly and even partial removal may result in complete relief of symptoms for many years.

FURTHER READING

Boechat M I, Kangarloo H 1989 MR imaging of the abdomen in children. American Journal of Roentgenology 152: 1245–1250

D'Angio G J, Breslow N, Beckwith J B, et al 1989 Treatment of Wilms' tumour. Results of the Third National Wilms' Tumour Study. Cancer 64: 349–360

Grosfeld J L, Weber T R, Weetman R M 1983 Rhabdomyosarcoma in childhood: analysis of survival in 98 cases. Journal of Pediatric Surgery 18: 141–146

Hartman G E, Shochat S J 1989 Abdominal mass lesions in the newborn: diagnosis and treatment. Clinics in Perinatology 16: 123–135

Hays D M, Raney R B Jr, Lawrence W Jr, et al 1982 Primary chemotherapy in the treatment of children with bladder-prostate tumours in the intergroup rhabdomyosarcoma study (IRS-II). Journal of Pediatric Surgery 17: 812–820

Mahaffey S M, Ryckman F C, Martin L W 1988 Clinical aspects of abdominal masses in children. Seminars in Roentgenology 23: 161–174

Matthay K K, Sather H N, Seeger R C, et al 1989 Excellent outcome of stage II neuroblastoma is independent of residual disease and radiation therapy. Journal of Clinical Oncology 7: 236–244

Shimada H, Chattern N, Newton W et al 1984 Histopathological prognostic factors in neuroblastic tumors: Definition of subtypes of ganglioneuroblastoma and an age-linked classification of neuroblastomas. Journal of the National Cancer Institute 73: 405–416

5. Abdominal pain — acute and recurrent

R. W. Yardley

Children frequently have episodes of abdominal pain and as many as 20% will have episodes of pain severe enough to induce absence from school or attendance to the family doctor. These episodes of pain fall into two main groups: acute abdominal pain and recurrent abdominal pain.

If the illness is an isolated episode it is labelled acute abdominal pain or if it consists of recurrent episodes of pain which may recur over many months or years, it is referred to as recurrent abdominal pain (N.B. not chronic abdominal pain).

ACUTE ABDOMINAL PAIN IN CHILDHOOD

The child with acute abdominal pain represents a different diagnostic challenge to the adult with abdominal pain. The child can have any of the conditions that occur in adult life, e.g. cholecystitis, duodenal ulcer or pancreatitis, but for all practical purposes the diagnostic decision lies between acute appendicitis (AA) and non-specific abdominal pain (NSAP).

While the astute physician must always be alert for the unusual case, the beginner tends to diagnose rare conditions, perhaps remembering clearly the features of the only case they have seen of a particular condition and regarding the details of that particular case as typical. Unfortunately also, patients do not always present with so-called classical patterns of symptoms and signs.

Analysis of clinical information

Obtaining an accurate history and precise physical findings is the major way to make a diagnosis. There are few helpful special investigations.

It is important to have a strategy when confronted with a cluster of symptoms. The first thing to do is to make some judgement as to which of the symptoms is the one most likely to provide an anatomical diagnosis, and analyse this first. In other words, in which cavity of the body is the pathological process — in the abdomen, the chest or elsewhere. After making an anatomical diagnosis concentrate on symptoms which indicate the pathological process involved, e.g. fever is strongly indicative of an inflammatory process.

Consider the example of a child who presents with central abdominal pain associated with bright red rectal bleeding and obvious pallor. The symptom to analyse first is the rectal bleeding as in this case the abdominal pain is likely to be secondary to gastrointestinal hurry associated with the blood within the gut. The passage of blood rectally focuses our attention on a shorter list of diagnoses than if we examined all causes of abdominal pain. However, analysis of abdominal pain will usually provide the most direct route to a diagnosis when it is a prominent symptom. Associated symptoms such as vomiting and anorexia are less specific in indicating the cause of the illness. These symptoms may often be present in extra-abdominal conditions in children (e.g. meningitis, pneumonia). There are usually features in the physical examination which will point in the right direction if the site of the pathology cannot be ascertained from the history, e.g. abdominal tenderness is absent, in the presence of guarding, in the child who has referred pain to the abdomen from basal pneumonia.

The analysis of an abdominal pain symptom must include its onset and duration, the site at

49

onset, any shift of the pain site with time, the character of the pain, whether constant or colicky, and any aggravating or relieving factors. The speed of onset of the pain gives a clue to the pathological process involved. Very rapid onset may suggest vascular occlusion or volvulus, while gradual onset over hours suggests an inflammatory process. If vomiting is the predominant symptom associated with colicky pains and absence of bowel actions or flatus, then bowel obstruction should be considered (see Ch. 8).

Analysis of the pain

Site at onset

The abdomen is often divided into regions for didactic purposes. The schemas need not concern us here but it is a generalization of some value that if the site of pain is asymmetrical or localized at some distance from the umbilicus then it is more likely to be of significance. The viscera do not have a precise somatotopic cerebral representation and pain due to pathology within an organ is referred to the abdominal wall with the same segmental innervation. The appendix receives its segmental innervation from T10 and as a consequence pain arising from pathology in this organ is referred to the region of the umbilicus. As the pathological process spreads to involve the parietal peritoneum the site of the pain is accurately localized. When organs are inflammed or distended tenderness is usually experienced at the site of palpation.

Duration and severity of the pain

The severity of pain is very subjective and must often be assessed by recourse to the observations made by the child's parents. In the pre-school age child, parental observations are often the only information that is available while in the older child one must keep in mind that the child will frequently minimize his/her symptoms if the possibility of hospital admission or operation is raised early in the interview. Careful observation of the child's facial expression and general affect helps to decide the veracity of the story. The pain may be judged severe if it interferes with the

child's normal activities, wakes him/her from sleep, causes crying or induces a posture or activity calculated to relieve the pain, e.g. lying in bed with the legs drawn up suggests peritonitis or colic due to intussusception. The duration of the pain is also of some importance as it is usual for the pains of major pathology to last longer than 6 to 8 hours. If the child is seen early in the illness and no decision as to the cause of the pain can be made, a period of watchful waiting can be undertaken without undue risk.

Shift of site of the pain

Shift in the site of the pain during the illness usually implies involvement of the parietal peritoneum. In appendicitis the initial pain is often referred to the region of the umbilicus and as the inflammatory process involves the parietal peritoneum the pain is experienced in both the right iliac fossa and the periumbilical region. The right iliac fossa pain then dominates the clinical picture. Shift of pain, although characteristic of appendicitis (~65%), also occurs in children with NSAP (~15%). Continued periumbilical pain, particularly if colicky, is found in obstructive appendicitis. This variant is often associated with perforation and early operation is advisable.

The character of the pain

Colicky pain is more characteristic of obstruction within hollow tubular organs, e.g. ureter, bile ducts and bowel. It is also present with functional disorders of the bowel motility and in children with constipation. Constant pain, particularly if of prolonged duration, is more indicative of an inflammatory process.

Aggravating and relieving factors

The child with severe abdominal pain will resist movement and the pain may be aggravated on walking or hopping if appendicitis is present. If pain is relieved by opening of the bowels, this suggests some form of bowel disturbance and the character of the stool is important in deciding the nature of the problem. Loose watery bowel actions often tinged with blood are characteristic of enteritis, hard stools of constipation.

Appendicitis or NSAP

In surveys of admissions to hospital of children with abdominal pain it has been found that about 55–60% are for NSAP, 30% are for AA and 10–15% have a large variety of conditions including urinary tract infection, constipation, and traumatic lesions. Patients who attend their family doctor are more likely to have NSAP than AA in the proportion of 20:1.

What is NSAP? It is not a diagnosis in the conventional sense but is a useful umbrella term to cover those patients in whom no specific pathology is identified and the illness subsides spontaneously without specific therapy. The symptoms in this group of patients often mimic those with appendicitis closely enough to cause genuine confusion, but easy recourse to surgery results in a high rate of removal of a normal appendix. Careful history taking and physical examination should ensure that the removal rate of normal appendices is only 10%. The frequency of symptoms in patients with appendicitis compared with those with NSAP are shown in Table 5.1.

It will be noted from this list that most of the symptoms are more regularly present in AA. A symptom like anorexia seems at first sight to be of no discriminatory value, but in a child who has a normal appetite, then AA is very unlikely, though it is not excluded.

The incidence of physical findings in these two conditions is shown in Table 5.2.

Table 5.1 Relative frequency of symptoms in AA and NSAP

Symptom	AA	NSAP
Central pain at on set	70%	25%
Shift of pain to right iliac fossa	65%	15%
Aggravation by movement	75%	25%
Anorexia	98%	85%
Diarrhoea	18%	9%
Headache	14%	30%

Table 5.2 Relative frequency of signs in AA and NSAP

Sign	AA	NSAP
Local tenderness	100%	50% (usually more diffuse)
Guarding	90%	5%–10%
Rebound tenderness	75%	5%

In a situation where acute appendicitis is suspected but cannot be distinguished from NSAP on the basis of history, it may be thought prudent to operate. If an operation to remove the appendix is performed on all such children with right iliac fossa pain as soon as they present to hospital then 50% will have a normal appendix removed. The added information that is required to make a more accurate diagnosis is to be found in the physical signs (Table 5.2). A period of observation of 6–8 hours, if no decision is made on presentation, is also useful. In the child with AA the symptoms and signs progress while in the child with NSAP they remain the same or improve. While there is no deterioration in the patient's condition then a watch and wait policy has been demonstrated to be safe.

Various presentations of appendicitis

The typical case

The majority of patients will present with periumbilical pain followed by vomiting or nausea and a shift of pain to the right iliac fossa over 6–8 hours. Physical examination reveals localized tenderness at McBurney's point and often guarding of the muscles in the same region.

Other patterns

The pain may begin in the right iliac fossa from the outset and consequently there is no shift of pain. The point of maximal tenderness may not be at McBurney's point. The site of tenderness is related to the situation of the distal portion of the appendix where the inflammatory changes begin. Therefore, the site of maximal tenderness may be in the pelvis (detected on rectal examination), the right loin in a child with a retrocolic appendix or more towards the umbilicus in a child with a pre- or post-ileal appendix. In the case of a retrocolic appendix, tenderness may be masked by the overlying gas or confusion may occur with pyelonephritis as there may be erythrocytes and neutrophil polymorphonuclear cells in the urine sample (as a result of extension of the inflammatory process to the ureter). There are usually no other urinary symptoms, however, and a period of observation will usually resolve the dilemma.

The child under 4 years

The incidence of AA is much lower in this group than in older children but it is still an important common cause of severe abdominal pain, and since other causes of severe abdominal pain are rare the possibility of AA should always be considered. In the inarticulate toddler the complaint of abdominal pain is often not obtained and the provisional diagnosis is made on the associated symptoms of vomiting and perhaps diarrhoea. Gastroenteritis is the usual working diagnosis. It is usually only when generalized peritonitis supervenes that the thought of AA is entertained by the family doctor. The inability of the child to accurately convey their symptoms and the difficulty in examining a restless, crying and irritable child combine to delay the diagnosis.

The clinical presentation is irritability, particularly when disturbed, a high fever, vomiting and anorexia. Examination shows a child lying quietly when not disturbed, with a listless expression and a distended abdomen. If the child has a persistent umbilical hernia there may be signs of inflammation over the umbilical skin. Assessment of guarding is difficult in the younger patient who almost never has the board-like rigidity that is found in the older child or adult patient with peritonitis. Nevertheless, there is increased reflex abdominal tone (guarding) and this is best assessed during sleeping episodes which are frequent in these sick patients. Differential tenderness and guarding between the right and left iliac fossae is generally present and confirms the diagnosis. Light percussion of the abdomen is also useful in assessment of the site of maximum tenderness.

The obese child

The child who is excessively obese presents a particular problem. In these patients it is easy to miss guarding of the abdominal muscles due to the softness of the thick layer of subcutaneous fat. If the possibility of this error is borne in mind then it should be minimized.

Not appendicitis

A common presentation of children which is the cause of great concern is one in which the child presents with diffuse tenderness, which although most marked in the right iliac fossa, is present in all other areas to a varying and often fluctuating extent. Despite other findings that might support the diagnosis of appendicitis, if guarding is not present then the illness is unlikely to be due to appendicitis, the proviso being that the child has normal spinal cord reflexes at the abdominal level (which may not be the case in the child with spina bifida, or cerebral palsy). It is often suggested that the removal of a normal appendix is not attended by any adverse effects but morbidity rates of up to 15% are regularly recorded and deaths have also been recorded. The incidence of postoperative bowel obstruction seems to be similar in both patients with and without appendicitis. It therefore is necessary to attempt to make an accurate diagnosis before proceeding to surgery.

Management of acute abdominal pain

Rational management of any condition depends upon the diagnosis of the particular condition and an assessment of the degree of severity. The child with AA must be assessed for the level of hydration, spread of infection and level of pain. If significant dehydration is present intravenous Hartmann's solution should be given prior to surgery to restore extracellular volume before the induction of anaesthesia. Rectal administration of metronidazole is given for the purpose of wound infection prophylaxis in the case of localized infection. In the presence of spreading peritoneal infection gentamicin and amoxicillin should be administered in addition to the metronidazole.

(Other combinations may be used according to availability and known patient drug sensitivity.) Pain control should be instituted as soon as practicable; the patient should not be left to suffer because of a mistaken notion that the diagnosis will be masked.

Paracetamol suppositories can provide early relief of pain and may reduce any associated fever. Postoperatively, narcotic analgesia is usually required and is best given as a continuous intravenous infusion.

RECURRENT ABDOMINAL PAIN

It is difficult to have strict criteria for the diagnosis of recurrent abdominal pain (RAP) but John Apley has suggested the following, which are widely accepted:

1. The pains should have recurred over a period at least longer than 3 months (not necessarily every day).
2. The pain attacks should have occurred on at least three occasions before the diagnosis can be made.
3. The pains need to be severe enough to interfere with the child's normal activity, even if only for a short time.

Prevalence

The prevalence of RAP in the childhood population is not known with any accuracy but estimates are between 5% and 15% of children in the age range 5–15 years. The presentation is usually in the 5–10 year old group and pain syndromes outside this age should heighten suspicion of an organic cause. There appears to be a slight female predominance.

Classification of RAP

Traditionally, RAP was classified into organic and psychogenic groups but with so few patients in the organic group (much less than 10%) and few positive criteria for psychological disorder in the so-called psychogenic group, a new classification has emerged. This classifies the majority as dysfunctional with two smaller groups of organic and psychogenic. Evidence has been produced that the orderly motility of the bowel is disturbed in many of these patients and the other signs of autonomic instability are present (such as increased sweating, abnormal pallor and altered pupillary reflexes). There is no specific explanation as yet for these observations or whether they are intrinsic to the patient or represent some response to an as yet undefined environmental stimulus. It seems, however, that the majority of these patients have normal health as adults.

Many children experience episodes of abdominal pain which recur and which cause anxiety in their parents because of the fear of acute appendicitis. These attacks of pain do not represent 'grumbling appendicitis' which does not exist as a pathological entity and therefore appendicectomy is not required as treatment. The clinical problem is similar to that of acute abdominal pain in that the majority of patients have benign self-limiting conditions which require only symptomatic relief. A few will have specific conditions requiring accurate diagnosis and management. It is important at the outset to establish a sound idea of the site of the pain, the severity and duration of the attacks, as well as the frequency of the attacks. A thorough physical examination is also required, including measurement of blood pressure, urinalysis and sometimes stool culture. The majority of other investigations should only be instigated if there is a clinical suspicion of a particular condition. A limited list classification of the possible entities is outlined in Table 5.3 and is by no means exhaustive. The point to emphasize is that the majority of the conditions are of a functional nature and that should be the focus of attention in the discussions with the parents.

The diagnostic approach

The common occurrence of RAP in childhood should be kept in mind, but at the same time other possibilities must be considered. The presence of an abdominal mass, hypertension or haematuria would direct inquiries to an organic cause. The persistence of pain in the same site and particularly if severe, that wakes the child

Table 5.3 Short list of possible causes of recurrent abdominal pain

1. Dysfunctional	80%
2. Psychogenic	10%
3. Organic	10%

4. Alimentary tract disorders
   (a) Peptic ulcers
   (b) Gallstones
   (c) Inflammatory bowel disease.
       Crohn's disease
       Ulcerative colitis
       Amoebiasis
   (d) Pancreatitis
       Steroids and other drugs
       Familial hyperlipidaemias
       Common channel syndrome
       Pancreas divisum
   (e) Malrotation of the midgut
   (f) Recurrent intussusception
   (g) Chronic constipation — all forms
   (h) Uropathies
       Vesicoureteric obstruction
       Pelviureteric obstruction
       Vesicoureteric reflux
       Urinary tract infection
   (i) Others

from sleep, would also point towards an organic condition. It is unusual, however, for the child with urinary tract infection to have no other urinary symptoms or the child with Crohn's disease to have only abdominal pain without weight loss, change in bowel habit, fever, anaemia, anorexia or mouth ulcers. It is the very absence of any other specific symptoms or signs which gives us the confidence to make a diagnosis of dysfunctional RAP.

The typical case

The child is generally in the early years of school. The attack of pain is often severe at the outset and of sudden onset although its description by the child or his/her parents is often vague. The pain may be accompanied by vomiting which is seldom bile-stained but is frequently associated with circumoral pallor, cold, sweating palms and may be relieved by defaecation. The episode may last only a few seconds or as long as 3 to 4 hours. The child's general health is not altered. The attacks may be accompanied by headache and

many commentators suggest that RAP represents a stress response in the child similar to casual headaches in the adult. There is seldom any identifiable precipitating factor. Physical examination in these children is unremarkable (by definition as it were). Apart from a low-grade fever and the features previously alluded to there should be no abnormal findings. If the child has a loaded rectum and colon on physical examination then a diagnosis of constipation can be made and steps taken to improve evacuation of the bowel, either by dietary, pharmacological or mechanical means.

Management

It is often a difficult matter to manage a situation in which there is a great deal of psychological uncertainty such as RAP. The uncertainty is not just present in the patient and parents, but also the doctor. Sufficient time must be given to listen to the parents complaints and to take them seriously. A short history taking and a perfunctory physical examination followed by some glib information about functional disturbance is likely to be dismissed by the parents as an insult. Reassurance is the mainstay of therapy in this condition and can only be given and received against a background of confidence. This must be established by a sympathetic hearing of the symptoms and the reassurance of having seen similar cases. An ability to help the parents understand that the symptoms are not imaginary any more than a headache is imaginary often helps them to understand the concept of dysfunctional pain. Their own experience with headache will also give them confidence to understand that although pain may at times be severe it does not necessarily have a serious cause requiring extensive investigation. Always leave the way open to review the problem again and to institute a series of 'tests' if things deteriorate. Reassurance may have to be repeated in the form of further explanation regarding the nature of the child's illness. The teacher may need to be informed of the problem to prevent unnecessary urgent calls to parents during school hours to take the child home every time an attack occurs. During an acute attack pain relief may be required and paracetamol is usually sufficient. In the majority of cases it must be said that the pain will usually subside before any benefit ensues.

If real doubt exists about the possibility of an underlying cause, then an abdominal ultrasound is non-invasive and a useful screening test of the solid organs. Supine and erect plain X-rays will show the bowel gas pattern, the presence of faecal loading of the large bowel and areas of pathological calcification (e.g. appendicular faecolith).

Normal results on these investigations add weight when reassuring the parents and the child.

FURTHER READING

Edwards F H, Davies R S 1984 Use of a Bayesian algorithm in the computer-assisted diagnosis of appendicitis. Surgery, Gynecology and Obstetrics 158: 219–222

Hoffmann J, Rasmussen O Ø 1989 Aids in the diagnosis of acute appendicitis British Journal of Surgery 76: 774–779

Jones P F 1976 Active observation in the management of acute abdominal pain in childhood. British Medical Journal 2: 551–553

6. Constipation, diarrhoea, enuresis and related problems

M. J. Glasson

Children frequently have symptoms of disturbed passage of faeces and urine, such as constipation, diarrhoea or wetting while retention of urine also occurs but is uncommon. The underlying cause of these symptoms sometimes requires surgical treatment.

DEFINITIONS

Constipation is usually defined as the infrequent and difficult passage of hard stools, though in special conditions, e.g. infant Hirschsprung's disease, the infrequent passage of soft stool is regarded as constipation.

Encopresis is the term given to soiling occurring in the absence of a gross organic cause and associated with psychological factors. There may be passage of stool in abnormal places at abnormal times.

Diarrhoea is the frequent passage of very soft or fluid stools which may or may not contain blood or mucus.

Wetting refers to the involuntary passage of urine after the age at which voluntary control would be expected.

Enuresis is the term given to wetting which does not have a recognizable organic cause.

Retention of urine refers to the inability to completely empty the bladder and is rare as an acute phenomenon in childhood. Chronic retention of urine frequently masquerades as wetting because of overflow of urine from the chronically distended bladder.

NORMAL BOWEL FUNCTION

The act of defaecation is a complex one, involving nerves, muscles, training and habit. The nerves concerned include those to the voluntary muscles of the external sphincters and those to the involuntary muscle of the intestine and internal sphincter.

Intestinal content is propelled as the result of coordinated alternate contraction and relaxation of bowel musculature (peristalsis). It is attributed to a series of coordinated local nervous reflexes in response to chemical and mechanical stimulation from luminal content. The autonomic nervous system exerts a controlling influence; parasympathetic nerves cause contraction whilst sympathetic stimulation inhibits colonic motility. Absence of ganglion cells in the rectum and lower colon (Hirschsprung's disease) results in failure of relaxation of the affected segment and constipation.

Normal bowel control is dependent upon normal function of the external and internal sphincter muscles, especially that part of the levator ani complex which is often described as the puborectalis muscle. Normally, the rectum and anal canal are empty. When stools enter and distend the rectum (often as a result of mass movement of the colon after meals), reflex relaxation of the internal sphincter muscle occurs and there is desire to defaecate. The stool passes into the anal canal and defaecation ensues when the external anal sphincters are voluntarily relaxed. There is great variation in the frequency of defaecation in infancy and childhood. Nerve pathways responsible for voluntary control of defaecation are not present at birth and they do not usually mature until the age of approximately 2½ years.

Infants open their bowels automatically, but

with growth and development they are subjected to social pressures and are conditioned to go to the toilet to pass faeces. If the social pressure and methods of training are restrictive or coercive they may interfere with the development of a regular bowel pattern. Hence the problems of stool retention and consequent constipation and soiling may be seen in so-called normal children, as well as in those with some obvious anatomical abnormality of muscles and nerves such as exists in spina bifida.

If motions are not passed at regular intervals, the absorption of water, which occurs in the large intestine, continues and the faeces tend to become hard and more difficult to pass.

CONSTIPATION

Table 6.1 outlines a classification of the causes of constipation. Careful analysis of the clinical features of children who present with constipation usually enables the clinician to make an accurate diagnosis of the cause.

History

The age of the child and the presence or absence of other symptoms are of great importance. When constipation is an isolated symptom, the length

Table 6.1   A classification of constipation

1. **Constipation occuring in an acute illness**
   Secondary to
   (a) Fever
   (b) Dehydration
   Mechanical acute intestinal obstruction
   Hypertrophic pyloric stenosis

2. **Chronic constipation**
   'Surgical' causes
   (a) Congenital anal stenosis
   (b) Treated imperforate anus
   (c) Hirschsprung's disease
   'Medical' causes (these are rare)
   (a) Hypothyroidism
   (b) Renal tubular acidosis
   (c) Lead poisoning
   (d) Coeliac disease
   Neurological
   (a) Myelomeningocele
   (b) Other spinal lesions (e.g. trauma)
   (c) Cerebral palsy
   Functional

of history is important: sometimes the onset of constipation can be dated to a minor illness associated with fever or dehydration or to a change in diet or environment (perhaps at holiday time).

It is helpful to ascertain the frequency of bowel actions, the nature and size of the stool and information concerning pain and bleeding with defaecation. Older children who do not use the toilet for defaecation or occasionally pass enormous stools which obstruct the plumbing are unlikely to have organic disease. Painful defaecation associated with hard stools and small amounts of bright blood on the stool suggests a complicating anal fissure.

Constipation occurring in acute illnesses is likely to be overshadowed by other symptoms notably vomiting. In the immediate postnatal period, constipation is manifested as failure to pass meconium with many (but not all) causes of neonatal intestinal obstruction; there is always vomiting (usually bile-stained) and very often abdominal distension (see Ch. 8). At a slightly older age when there is non bile-stained vomiting, co-existing constipation provides a clue to the diagnosis of hypertrophic pyloric stenosis.

Although feeding with cow's milk may produce firm stools, the onset of constipation and pain and difficulty with defaecation coincidental with the cessation of breast-feeding and the introduction of solid foods may be due to an unrecognized anorectal anomaly with stenosis. History taking in toddlers and older children who are constipated should specifically seek other symptoms such as vomiting, blood and mucus per rectum, soiling, encopresis and failure to thrive if such symptoms are not volunteered.

Physical examination

An assessment is first made of the general condition and appearance of the child. Acutely unwell patients requiring prompt treatment should thus be identified. Failure to thrive will be identified from measurement of height and weight using percentile charts. Associated disorders such as cerebral palsy or spina bifida with hydrocephalus should be readily identifiable. In an otherwise well child with chronic constipation, careful examination of the vertebral column may reveal clues (e.g. midline tuft of hair, palpable sacral deficiency) suggestive of an occult spinal anomaly. When there is mechanical intestinal obstruction, there is likely to be distension, tenderness and increased bowel sounds on abdominal examination. The classical findings in infants with hypertrophic pyloric stenosis are visible gastric peristalsis and a pyloric tumour palpable in the right hypochondrium. Although older children with chronic constipation may have faecal masses palpable along the line of the colon (especially in the left iliac fossa), it is possible for there to be a large amount of faecal retention in the colon with few abnormal physical signs on abdominal examination apart from mild fullness.

It is vital to carefully inspect the anus, noting especially its position and size. The congenitally narrow anus may be normally sited or may be situated in an anterior ectopic position on the perineum or (in girls) on the vulva. Faecal staining from soiling or encopresis may be obvious to inspection or be suggested by a perianal rash. Gentle separation of the anus with two fingers will reveal an anal fissure.

Rectal examination is a distressing experience for children and in some clinical situations (e.g. the acute abdomen) may not assist the overall assessment. It usually will be helpful with well patients who present with constipation. In early infancy, the examination is best undertaken with the fifth finger. Explosive passage of flatus and stool following withdrawal of the gloved finger in a neonate with abdominal distension and vomiting is highly suggestive of Hirschsprung's disease. With anorectal stenosis, attempts at rectal examination are unsuccessful. Older children with a large faecal mass in the rectum extending to the anal verge are likely to have functional constipation.

Investigation

With some of the conditions listed in Table 6.1 (e.g. hypertrophic pyloric stenosis, congenital anal stenosis, myelomeningocele) a confident diagnosis can be made clinically and no investigations are required before instituting treatment. With others (e.g. mechanical acute intestinal obstruction, Hirschsprung's disease) tests will be required to confirm the diagnosis. When functional constipation is suspected investigation may be deferred pending the outcome of management for that condition (see below) unless the symptoms date from early infancy.

The following tests may be useful.

Plain abdominal X-ray

This must be obtained when there is an acute illness with vomiting and abdominal distension. With intestinal obstruction there will be dilated loops of bowel and fluid levels (see Fig. 8.6).

In a well child with abdominal pain and some disturbance of bowel habit, abdominal X-ray confirms constipation and provides a guide to its severity.

Contrast enema

This is indicated when there is a possibility of low small bowel or large bowel obstruction or when there is suspicion of Hirschsprung's disease. Barium sulphate is the usual agent; water soluble material may be chosen in very early infancy.

With Hirschsprung's disease, there may be a narrow distal segment and a 24 hour film will demonstrate retention of barium. When colonic dilatation extends down to the anus the diagnosis is likely to be functional constipation rather than Hirschsprung's disease.

Anomanometry

Anorectal manometry (Fig. 6.1) is a functional test which will show a characteristic abnormal pattern in Hirschsprung's disease. The pressure in the lumen of the normal anal canal changes in a biphasic manner when the rectum is acutely distended. The initial rise in pressure is mediated by a local intramural reflex. Subsequent fall to a level below the resting pressure is due to a spinal inhibition reflex whose efferent arc involves a synapse at the ganglion cells in the bowel wall. Normal anomanometric studies exclude Hirschsprung's disease but abnormal pressure studies are not necessarily diagnostic.

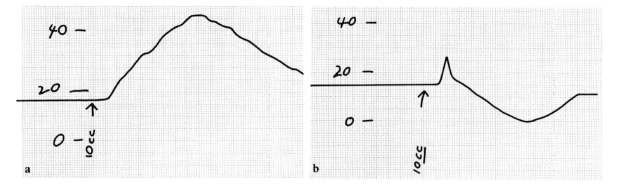

Fig. 6.1 Anomanometry **A**: In a patient with Hirschsprung's disease. **B**: In a normal child.

Rectal biopsy

This is required to confirm a diagnosis of Hirschsprung's disease by demonstrating absence of ganglion cells. The collection of a suction biopsy is a simple procedure; for the specimen to be adequate it must contain submucosa and the histological sections should be examined by a paediatric pathologist. Full thickness biopsy requires general anaesthesia and enables the pathologist to examine the intermuscular plexus as well as the submucosa.

Management

The management of constipation occurring in acute illnesses (Table 6.1) is dealt with elsewhere.

'Surgical' causes

Congenital anal stenosis. Some cases may respond to intermittent passage of an anal dilator but usually a simple anoplasty is undertaken on diagnosis to enlarge the anal orifice. Girls with an ectopically sited anus at or close to the vulva may require no particular treatment provided the anal orifice is of adequate calibre. Transplantation of the anus to a more normal position can be undertaken using the Pena technique with good cosmetic and functional results, but necessitates preliminary colostomy.

Treated imperforate anus. Imperforate anus is a common cause of neonatal intestinal obstruction (see Ch. 8). Numerous anatomical variations of the malformation have been described but, for practical purposes, there are two distinct groups:

1. Low level types — bowel terminates close to perineal skin or by fistulous opening in an ectopic site.
2. Intermediate and high level types — bowel terminates well above perineum at or above the puborectalis muscle complex.

Low level imperforate anus. Because the bowel ends at or close to the surface, immediate treatment consists of anoplasty to create an anus in the normal site. With the anoplasty technique of Hendren, intermittent anal dilatation may not be necessary postoperatively to prevent anal stenosis. The prognosis for continence is excellent but many of these children are predisposed to constipation throughout childhood and require the management necessary for chronic functional constipation (see below).

Intermediate and high level imperforate anus. The external anal sphincter muscles may be absent in these children and continence after rectoplasty relies upon the levator ani. For this reason, most authorities prefer to perform a colostomy in the newborn period and to defer definitive rectoplasty until the age of 6 to 12 months. With the Pena technique, the rectum can then be accurately placed within the sphincter muscle complex. Subsequent continence is not guaranteed, partly because of deficient development and innervation of the puborectalis muscle.

Chronic constipation and soiling following treatment of high level anorectal agenesis is best managed by regular colonic irrigation via the perineal anus. Revision rectoplasty can be considered if muscle stimulation of the perineum under general anaesthesia suggests that there was inaccurate placement of the rectum at the original surgery.

Hirschsprung's disease. In Hirschsprung's disease ganglion cells are absent from the bowel wall for a variable distance upwards from the anus. The peristaltic wave from above does not continue into the aganglionic segment which remains contracted. The normal proximal bowel becomes dilated and hypertrophied. Most cases of Hirschsprung's disease are diagnosed in the neonatal period because of symptoms of acute intestinal obstruction. Chronic constipation is the method of presentation of those children not diagnosed in the first months of life. Intestinal obstruction does not commonly occur in older children with Hirschsprung's disease but a careful history will usually reveal that the disturbance of bowel habit originated in the neonatal period with delayed passage of meconium, bile-stained vomiting or even diarrhoea at that time. Soiling, though not a feature of chronic constipation due to Hirschsprung's disease, may occur.

Definitive treatment of Hirschsprung's disease involves resection of the aganglionic segment and restoration of intestinal continuity according to one of a number of described techniques (i.e., Duhamel, Soave, Rehbein, Swenson). Many surgeons prefer to perform a decompressing colostomy at the time of diagnosis (regardless of age) and to delay definitive operation for some months. Following subsequent closure of colostomy, the prognosis is good; some patients (especially those with long segment aganglionosis) have ongoing difficulty with bowel habit and require prolonged medical surveillance.

'Medical' causes

The management of constipation in such patients is essentially the treatment of the causative illness (Table 6.1).

Neurological constipation. Constipation is the rule in neurological disorders and depending upon the type of neurological problem it may be due to various combinations of inability to learn defaecation patterns, deficient sensation, poor motility and disordered reflexes.

The constipation in these patients has a pathological basis and will be a long-term problem so

that the management regimen must fit into the continuing general management of the patient. The management will also vary with the type of underlying problem, the age of the patient and the degree of cooperation.

The aim of management is to achieve regular bowel actions. The use of laxatives must be on an individual basis. Some children never need them and for some they are essential. Others may need them for short periods only at different stages of development.

The type of laxative that suits one person will be found quite unsuitable for another and too much laxative will produce soiling between bowel actions and sometimes colic, whereas too little will not produce an emptying of the rectum and colon.

In the infant, a dose that gives regular evacuation without too much soiling and without colic is the ideal. Sometimes, in the infant, manual expression, of the type used to express the bladder, will be sufficient to empty the rectum.

When the child is old enough for conscious cooperation, a programme of regular training and the evacuation of the rectum should be commenced. In the spina bifida patient, as the faeces are usually firm and as the sphincters may form little or no obstruction to the passage of faeces, straining by contraction of the abdominal muscles with suprapubic pressure with the hands will often empty the bowel. This will need to be done on a regular basis two to three times per day. An occasional dose of laxative may still be necessary for such a child and even without laxative, occasional soiling is still a problem. A larger dose of laxative at the weekend may give a regular emptying without interfering with the week's schooling. Alternatively, the parents may be taught the technique of removal of faeces via the anus, using a gloved finger, well lubricated. As an alternative, suppositories of various types can be inserted via the anus to achieve emptying. Some children do well with regular enemas utilizing the tube and technique described by Shandling.

The great problem for children attending school is the offensive odour of even minimal soiling or a small pellet of faeces that may escape from the rectum. Their classmates strongly object to this and this situation may interfere with their continuance at a normal school. For this reason, vigorous efforts must be made to achieve the best possible bowel control, particularly for children who will be attending normal school and for those about to commence adult employment. But no matter what method of bowel management is used, minimal soiling will often occur and various products are now available which, when used appropriately, will dissipate any offensive odour.

Functional constipation. This is the type of constipation which has no other features to suggest an underlying or associated cause and which, on examination, shows faecal masses down to the anus. Further investigation is non-contributory.

This is the most common cause of chronic constipation and occurs more often in boys than in girls. There is no abnormality of intestinal function in the newborn period and the history of constipation often dates from specific postnatal events such as a febrile episode, dietary change or an event of psychological significance such as early or coercive toilet training or separation from a parent. Persistent soiling (encopresis) is a very common feature. The child is usually well nourished and may have a large faecal mass palpable in the abdomen. Occasionally, there is some abdominal discomfort and distension; the anus may be soiled and digital examination reveals hard or 'putty like' stools just inside the anal verge and distending the anal canal.

The first step in management is to explain to the parents and to the child, if appropriate, the underlying problem and the proposed course of management. Large faecal masses distending the rectum and lower colon when the child is first seen should be evacuated utilizing enemas, washouts and possibly manual disimpaction. Subsequently, enemas and suppositories should be avoided, if possible, because they serve to focus attention upon the anus and may provoke adverse secondary psychological effects.

Once the bowel is empty of hard faecal masses, the mainstay of treatment is the use of oral faecal softening or bowel stimulating agents in appropriate dosage to produce regular soft bowel actions. The parents are instructed in the technique of palpation of the lower abdominal faecal mass so that the dose of medication can be ad-

justed to need. Agents which are commonly used include Senokot, Coloxyl, Milk of Magnesia, Duphalac and liquid paraffin. Liquid paraffin is effective but should not be used before the age of 12 months because of the risk of inhalational lipoid pneumonia. Severely constipated children may require a dose of liquid paraffin of up to 3 mL/kg per day initially, but over a period of weeks it is usually possible to reduce the amount and eventually reach the situation where the child merely requires a small dose intermittently when the stools become hard or when there is a period of more than 2 days without a bowel action.

If the terminal bowel has become overstretched by chronic constipation, then occasional enemas or suppositories may be required to complete the emptying process until the bowel regains adequate functions. A positive habit training programme should be a part of the laxative programme.

Rarely, psychiatric referral is necessary. The underlying psychodynamic problem occasionally revolves around a disturbed relationship with one or both parents where the child is expressing anger and hostility in a negative manner by refusing to open the bowels normally.

DIARRHOEA

Table 6.2 lists important causes of diarrhoea. Acute diarrhoea has sudden onset and may quickly cause the child to become very ill with dehydration and hypovolaemia. Diarrhoea which persists for more than 2 weeks can be described as chronic. A detailed study of the clinical features provides a clue to the diagnosis and makes it possible to institute effective management.

History

It is important to obtain detailed information about the stools, including the time of onset of diarrhoea and the frequency, consistency, colour and content of the bowel actions. The passage of blood and/or mucus in the stool is suggestive of a surgical cause, but could be due to bacterial enteritis. Sudden onset associated with fever is suggestive of a viral infection.

Diarrhoea is a common symptom at all ages

Table 6.2 Important causes of diarrhoea

Acute diarrhoea
In the neonatal period
'Surgical' causes
1. Necrotizing enterocolitis
2. Hirschsprung's disease
3. Abnormalities of intestinal rotation and fixation
'Medical' causes
1. Gastroenteritis
2. Carbohydrate intolerance
3. Congenital adrenal hyperplasia

Infants and children
'Surgical' causes
1. Acute appendicitis
2. Intussusception
3. Hirschsprung's disease
4. Intestinal malrotation
5. Short gut syndrome and other postoperative phenomena
'Medical' causes
1. Gastroenteritis
   (a) Viral
   (b) Bacterial
   (c) Parasitic, e.g. *Giardia lamblia*
2. Antibiotic therapy
3. Carbohydrate intolerance

Chronic diarrhoea
1. Intestinal malabsorption
   (a) *Giardia lamblia*
   (b) Cystic fibrosis
   (b) Coeliac disease
2. Ulcerative colitis
3. Crohn's disease
4. Ganglioneuroma
5. Spurious diarrhoea

and the most common cause is gastroenteritis, but in early infancy (especially the neonatal period), a surgical diagnosis should be considered.

The presence or absence of other symptoms (especially abdominal pain and vomiting) are vital aspects of the history. Pain (usually periumbilical or in the right iliac fossa) invariably is a feature of acute appendicitis but is uncommon in gastroenteritis. Detailed analysis of the duration and frequency of vomiting is important: bile-stained vomitus must always arouse suspicion of a surgical lesion; the vomitus of gastroenteritis consists of gastric content only.

History taking should also include specific enquiry concerning whether or not the child has been passing urine in normal fashion, the recent administration of antibiotic therapy and whether there have been previous episodes during which a particular diagnosis was made.

Physical examination

Priority is given to assessment of the state of hydration of the patient. When there is moderate or severe dehydration with acute weight loss, lethargy, dry mucus membranes and poor skin tone, an intravenous infusion should be established to commence fluid resuscitation before completing the physical examination.

Inspection of the stool will reveal a consistency which varies from watery to semi-formed. Blood in the stool demands investigation. With chronic diarrhoea caused by intestinal malabsorption, the stools are large and pale and may be difficult to flush in the toilet.

With medical causes of diarrhoea, physical examination of the abdomen is usually unremarkable. There is no distension or tenderness; bowel sounds are increased in gastroenteritis.

With surgical causes, there will be abnormal physical signs on abdominal examination. Localized tenderness suggests an inflammatory process (e.g. acute appendicitis, neonatal necrotizing enterocolitis). Abdominal distension occurs with subacute intestinal obstruction (e.g. Hirschsprung's disease). In intussusception, there may be a tender palpable mass.

Perianal excoriation occurs with acute diarrhoea of any cause. Rectal examination is often unrewarding but should be performed when clinical features raise suspicion of a surgical diagnosis. With acute appendicitis, there may be an inflammatory mass in the pelvis. With Hirschsprung's disease, there may be explosive passage of flatus and stool following withdrawal of the finger.

Investigation

For the child with acute diarrhoea, some tests will help confirm a provisional clinical diagnosis.

X-ray

Radiological studies will usually be obtained when there is the possibility of a surgical diagnosis. Plain abdominal X-ray may show abnormalities such as pneumatosis, abnormal gas pattern, soft tissue mass, faecal accumulation and/or dilated bowel with fluid levels, to suggest diagnoses such as necrotizing enterocolitis, malrotation with or without volvulus, intussusception or Hirschsprung's disease. Contrast studies may follow: barium meal with follow through examination for malrotation; barium or gas enema for intussusception; barium enema for Hirschsprung's disease.

Stool microbiology and culture

A stool specimen must be sent to the laboratory when the clinical features suggest a medical cause and may be wise even when a surgical diagnosis is probable. Stool culture is particularly important if there is an apparent epidemic of diarrhoea, blood in the stool or recent overseas travel.

Extensive investigation may be necessary for children with chronic diarrhoea, especially when there is associated failure to thrive. Listed are some of the tests which may need to be considered:

- Full blood count
- Sweat electrolyte estimation — for cystic fibrosis
- Examination of stool for reducing substances
- Stool chromotography
- Chest X-ray
- Urinary catecholamine investigation
- Colonoscopy with or without biopsy
- Small bowel biopsy — for giardiasis, coeliac disease

Acute diarrhoea

The causes of diarrhoea are not the same in infancy and childhood.

In the neonatal period

Necrotizing enterocolitis. Diarrhoea (very frequently with macroscopic blood) is often the first signal of the onset of necrotizing enterocolitis but this symptom alone does not justify the diagnosis. Abdominal distension, bile-stained vomiting and general signs of sepsis soon supervene and render abdominal X-ray mandatory.

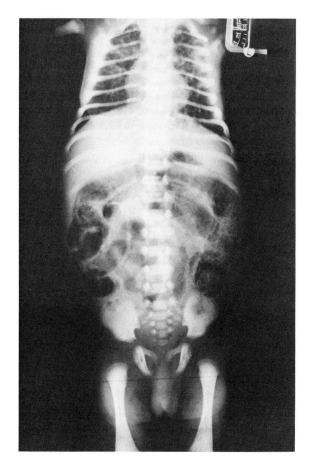

Fig. 6.2 X-ray of a patient with necrotizing enterocolitis (pneumatosis intestinalis).

The chief radiological feature of this disease is pneumatosis intestinalis (Fig. 6.2)

Neonatal necrotizing enterocolitis is a poorly understood entity which occurs in neonates who usually have been subjected to significant stress, e.g. prematurity, hyaline membrane disease, umbilical vessel catheterization, exchange transfusion, hypoglycaemia or symptomatic congenital heart disease. (See Ch. 8.)

Neonatal Hirschsprung's disease. The majority of cases of Hirschsprung's disease (see Ch. 8) become symptomatic in the newborn period and present with features of intestinal obstruction (bile-stained vomiting, abdominal distension and delayed passage of meconium). However, diarrhoea is sometimes a predominant feature, either as a spontaneous symptom or occurring in explosive fashion following withdrawal of the finger at digital examination of the rectum. The clinician may be lulled into a false sense of security when abdominal distension subsides after a loose bowel action in this situation.

Continuing diarrhoea is usually due to bacterial enterocolitis which may produce a rapid deterioration in the infant due to overwhelming sepsis, dehydration and electrolyte imbalance. Vigorous immediate treatment is necessary with fluid and electrolyte therapy, antibiotics for both aerobic and anaerobic organisms and rectal washouts pending urgent surgical decompression. Suction rectal biopsy preoperatively will clinch the diagnosis of Hirschsprung's disease.

Abnormalities of intestinal rotation and fixation. The usual manifestation of errors of the orderly return of the midgut into the abdominal cavity is subacute intestinal obstruction, usually situated in the proximal small bowel. There is bile-stained vomiting without abdominal distension. The lumen of the bowel is patent so that meconium is passed. With feeding, bowel actions continue; diarrhoea is uncommon, but can occur. Plain abdominal X-ray will show gastric and duodenal distension with a paucity of gas distally; contrast studies will establish the diagnosis. Prompt treatment is mandatory because there is a constant danger of intestinal ischaemia complicating an associated volvulus.

Gastroenteritis. Infective gastroenteritis is the common cause of diarrhoea. The most common infective agent is a rotavirus but bacterial gastroenteritis due to toxigenic *Escherichia coli*, *Shigella*, *Salmonella*, and less commonly, *Campylobacter* and *Yersinia* does occur. The diarrhoea due to *Salmonella* gastroenteritis frequently contains blood. Vomiting is a common symptom with occasional bouts of apparent colic; but abdominal pain, with abdominal tenderness and rigidity, is important in differentiating gastroenteritis from surgical causes of diarrhoea. Bowel sounds are usually increased in infective diarrhoea.

The treatment of gastroenteritis involves protein and fat restriction and correction of the dehydration which results from frequent passage of fluid stools, either by oral or intravenous fluids. Antibiotics are rarely indicated.

Carbohydrate intolerance. When carbohydrate molecules are not absorbed in the small intestine, their continued presence in the lumen of the bowel exerts an osmotic effect drawing fluid from the bowel wall and diarrhoea results.

This phenomenon sometimes occurs from birth as the result of a congenital enzyme deficiency of brush border enzymes. More commonly, the problem occurs in transient fashion following an insult to the bowel such as non-specific gastroenteritis or operation. The incidence of postoperative carbohydrate intolerance is particularly high in newborns and may complicate simple procedures such as colostomy for Hirschsprung's disease or imperforate anus, or major procedures such as laparotomy with intestinal resection and anastomosis. The motions are watery and a confident diagnosis can be made if, on testing, there is 0.5% or greater of reducing substance in the stool. Chromatography permits accurate identification of the offending carbohydrate (most commonly lactose). A change to a predigested formula or to one of low lactose content may overcome the problem. Some cases require a period of complete bowel rest with intravenous feeding until the intestinal flora and enzyme functions have returned to normal.

Congenital adrenal hyperplasia. This condition is due to an enzyme defect which interferes with the production of cortisol and aldosterone from progesterone. An excess of androgen is also produced. These infants can present in an emergency in the neonatal period, with diarrhoea and an acute salt-losing problem.

Infants and children

Acute appendicitis. Acute appendicitis occurs at all ages, but is not common in the pre-school child. There is almost always a disturbance of bowel habit with relative constipation occurring more commonly than diarrhoea.

When the inflamed appendix is in the retrocaecal position, diarrhoea often occurs early in the disease process as the result of increased colonic motility. The absence of abdominal tenderness resulting from the interposition of caecum between appendix and abdominal wall may cause the clinician to make the incorrect diagnosis of gastroenteritis initially. The psoas sign (pain and tenderness on hyperextension of the hip joint) is positive in retrocaecal appendicitis but negative in gastroenteritis.

Diarrhoea can also occur due to pelvic abscess complicating acute appendicitis. A pelvic abscess may develop when there has been delay in diagnosis, especially when the appendix is situated in the pelvic position. Pelvic abscess can also occur as a complication of appendicectomy, especially in those cases with free pus and significant local peritonitis at operation. This classically consists of fluid, mucousy stools. Digital examination of the rectum reveals a boggy mass within the pelvis.

Intussusception. Intussusception is the phenomenon of telescoping of a segment of bowel and usually occurs without a specific cause in the age group 3 months to 3 years (see Ch. 7).

There is an acute clinical illness with abdominal pain and this progresses to the features of intestinal obstruction. An early symptom in many cases is the passage of loose blood-stained stools due to exudation of fluid and minor haemorrhage from the intussuscepted segment into distal bowel. Awareness of this permits early diagnosis by ultrasound examination or contrast enema. Prompt treatment with barium or gas enema may avoid the need for operation. When surgical treatment is required, manipulative reduction is frequently successful; some cases require resection and anastomosis.

Hirschsprung's disease. In this condition chronic severe constipation can cause a spurious diarrhoea, or a superimposed enterocolitis may cause an acute diarrhoea with toxaemia (see above).

Intestinal malrotation. Small amounts of blood and mucus may be passed per anus in this condition with occasional vomiting (see Ch. 8).

Short gut syndrome. The resection of a large segment of intestine with anastomosis frequently leads to temporary disturbances of intestinal bacterial flora and intestinal enzyme function with resultant diarrhoea. Another factor is the reduced transit time which results from reduced total gut length. Massive bowel resection (especially including the ileocaecal valve) for conditions such as strangulated midgut volvulus may not leave sufficient residual bowel to allow

survival independent of intravenous alimentation. With resection of lesser magnitude, e.g. total colectomy with ileoanal anastomosis for long segment Hirschsprung's disease, the problem of frequent fluid bowel actions can be controlled with antiperistaltic medication such as loperamide.

Gastroenteritis. In infants and children, gastroenteritis is more common and less severe than in the neonate. The general management follows the lines of that in the neonate; it should always be remembered that an underlying 'surgical' cause of diarrhoea is possible.

Antibiotic therapy. Broad-spectrum antibiotic therapy has, as one of its complications, superimposed infection of the bowel by resistant organisms such as *Staphylococcus aureus* or *Clostridium difficile*. Infants or children who have been receiving such therapy and who develop diarrhoea should be suspected of such superimposed infection. Usually there is rapid improvement following cessation of the antibiotic.

Chronic diarrhoea

Intestinal malabsorption

Two common non-surgical causes of malabsorption are coeliac disease and cystic fibrosis. The child with coeliac disease passes large, pale, offensive stools and improves on a gluten-free diet. The child with cystic fibrosis has failure to thrive and chronic diarrhoea. A careful history may reveal episodes of bronchitis, pneumonia, unexplained dehydration or (important for the surgeon) intermittent rectal prolapse. The diagnosis is confirmed by the demonstration of abnormally high levels of sodium and chloride ions in the sweat. The diarrhoea in cystic fibrosis is due to deficient pancreatic exocrine secretion and is readily corrected by addition of pancreatic extract (Viokase) to the diet.

Ulcerative colitis

Ulcerative colitis is a rare but important cause of chronic diarrhoea in childhood and must always be considered in the differential diagnosis. The disease process commences in the rectum and

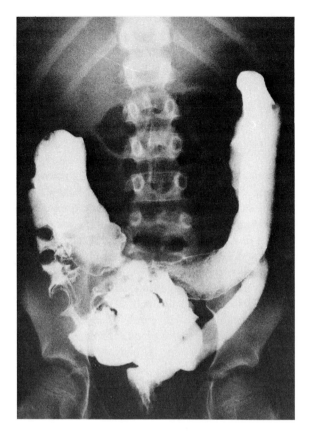

Fig. 6.3 Barium enema in a patient with advanced ulcerative colitis.

may run a benign course with the symptoms readily controlled by simple medication (Salazopyrin) over many years. Severe cases progress to involve the whole colon with ulceration and fibrosis and a characteristic barium enema appearance (Fig. 6.3). Surgical treatment (total colectomy with ileostomy or endorectal mucosal stripping and ileoanal anastomosis with the creation of a J-pouch) is sometimes necessary during teenage years.

Crohn's disease

Crohn's disease is also rare in childhood. Diarrhoea with mucus and even blood can occur as with ulcerative colitis but is not usually a predominant feature. Diarrhoea does become significant in advanced cases of Crohn's disease where the granulomatous process has resulted in internal fistula formation and intestinal hurry.

Ganglioneuroma

Tumours which arise from sympathetic nerve cells have the potential to cause chronic diarrhoea by production of catecholamines which act upon the bowel to increase peristalsis. The tumour which is particularly likely to present in this way with diarrhoea is a ganglioneuroma or ganglioneuroblastoma within the thorax. Accordingly, the routine investigation of children with chronic diarrhoea should always include chest X-ray and estimation of catecholamine excretion.

Spurious diarrhoea

Some children who present with symptoms which have been interpreted by their parents as diarrhoea (almost constant passage of small amounts of faeces) prove on history and physical examination to have chronic constipation with encopresis (see above).

NORMAL URINATION

Urine produced by the kidneys passes along the ureters into the bladder where it is stored pending micturition. As with defaecation, micturition is fundamentally a spinal reflex mediated via internal and external urinary sphincters and influenced by higher brain centres. When a critical bladder volume is reached, the internal urethral sphincter relaxes and contraction of the detrusor musculature of the bladder commences. Relaxation of the external urethral sphincter permits urine to pass along the urethra to the exterior.

The external sphincter is under voluntary control so that micturition can, if necessary, be delayed. Toilet training is completed somewhere between the age of 20 months and 3 years with bladder control usually being achieved after bowel control.

DISTURBANCES OF THE PASSAGE OF URINE

The passage of urine at times other than during a deliberate and regular act of micturition is common in childhood and is referred to as wetting.

Table 6.3   Causes of wetting

1. **Functional causes**
   Enuresis
   Giggling incontinence

2. **Organic causes**
   Urinary tract lesions
   (a) Common — phimosis
                — urinary tract infection
   (b) Rare   — posterior urethral valves
                — ectopic ureter
                — complete epispadias
                — exstrophy of the bladder
                — sphincter damage from perineal
                  trauma
   Spinal lesions
   (a) myelomeningocele
   (b) Sacral agenesis
   (c) Congenital diastematomyelia, sacral lipoma
       (tethered spinal cord)
   (d) Spinal trauma
   (e) Spinal tumours

3. **Miscellaneous causes**
   Convulsions
   Gross constipation

The most common cause is an involuntary act of micturition during sleep by children without an underlying organic problem. This may also occur during the day and is called enuresis. Most other causes of wetting (Table 6.3) are uncommon.

Retention of urine is uncommon in children but does have many possible causes. Chronic retention of urine (often with overflow wetting) occurs more frequently than acute retention.

Careful analysis of the clinical features is essential when a child presents with urinary symptoms.

History

It is important to note the sex and age of the child, past history and the duration, frequency and severity of symptoms. The acute onset of wetting in an otherwise normal child may be due to urinary tract infection, especially if the patient is unwell with dysuria. The cause for wetting will be obvious in patients who are known to have exstrophy of the bladder, epispadias, spina bifida or previous trauma to the spine or perineum. Girls with an ectopic ureter present with wetting, boys do not. Constant wetting from birth is likely to be caused by a neurological disorder.

When there is enormous variation in frequency and severity of wetting, a functional cause is likely. Wetting which occurs only at night is unlikely to have an organic cause; the history may reveal relevant contributing emotional stress factors in these patients.

Physical examination

Abnormalities such as repaired myelomeningocele, exstrophy of the bladder and epispadias will be evident from general examination. In an otherwise normal patient, inspection of the lumbosacral region may reveal a tuft of hair or sinus, raising the possibility of neurological disorder, whilst palpation there may raise suspicion of sacral agenesis. Bladder distension due to urinary retention will be evident from abdominal palpation. If gentle lower abdominal compression reveals the bladder to be expressible, a neurological disorder is likely. Physical examination in the male may reveal phimosis and in the female a wet vulva (suggesting ectopic ureter).

Investigation

Some patients will require very few or no tests, others with clinical features suggestive of an organic diagnosis will require comprehensive investigation. The following studies may be needed:

- Examination of urine
  (a) Urinalysis for sugar, protein
  (b) Microscopy and culture
- Imaging
  (a) X-ray spine — looking for abnormality of the sacrum
  (b) Abdominal ultrasound or intravenous pyelogram — to assess upper urinary tract
  (c) Micturating cystourethrogram — to assess lower urinary tract
  (d) CT scan; myelogram — if neurological diagnosis is suspected
- Cystoscopy — to asess urethra, bladder and ureteric orifices

CAUSES OF WETTING

Organic causes

Organic causes for wetting are not common, but must always be seriously considered before making a firm diagnosis of enuresis. Organic lesions which are present in very early life can usually be identified before the child reaches the age at which bladder control is normally anticipated.

Urinary tract lesions

Phimosis. Severe stenosis of the prepuce can cause wetting after micturition by virtue of the dribbling of the urine which ballooned the preputial space during voiding. This is one of the indications for circumcision. Phimosis developing in boys with a previously normal prepuce is usually caused by balanitis xerotica obliterans.

Urinary tract infection. Urinary tract infection produces wetness (largely from increased frequency of micturition and urgency) when there is inflammation of the bladder (cystitis) or urethra. For this reason, a microurine examination should be considered for children who present with wetting in order to prove or exclude urinary tract infection (see Ch. 19).

Posterior urethral valves. This condition only occurs in boys. An abnormality of development in the region of the verumontanum leads to the presence of obstructive valvular folds in the area. Most cases present in early infancy and the diagnosis is notoriously difficult to make. Non-specific symptoms such as vomiting, failure to thrive and abdominal distension may occur due to urinary tract infection or renal failure. Constant dribbling may be the presenting feature and is usually due to overflow from a chronically distended bladder. Alternatively, wetting after micturition in an older child may be due to urine drainage away from the dilated posterior urethra above the valves.

The preferred treatment is endoscopic ablation of the valves followed by an appropriate period of urinary catheter drainage.

Ectopic ureter. A relatively common congenital abnormality is for one or both kidneys to be drained by two ureters instead of one. The ureter from the upper pole of the affected kidney frequently terminates distally in an ectopic position. Wetting results when the ectopic orifice is situated distal to the internal sphincter mechanism. This situation occurs exclusively in girls. The child is constantly wet day and night despite being able to void normally at regular times during the day. On examination in the supine position, the vulva is seen to be red.

Treatment usually involves excision of the ectopic ureter and the pyelonephritic and poorly functioning renal tissue which it drains.

Epispadias. Complete epispadias (occurring without exstrophy of the bladder) is very rare and is seen more commonly in boys than girls. The basic embryological error is similar to that responsible for exstrophy. Incomplete forms of epispadias in which only a short distal segment of the anterior urethra is open dorsally usually develop normal bladder control. When the whole of the anterior urethra is involved in the abnormality (complete epispadias) urinary incontinence is the rule. The bladder is intact and of normal capacity but the bladder neck is poorly formed.

Surgical treatment when wetting is associated with epispadias is likely to require a bladder neck plasty procedure (which will include bilateral ureteric reimplantation) in addition to penile reconstruction.

Exstrophy of the bladder. Exstrophy of the bladder (Fig. 6.4) results from failure of midline fusion of mesodermal structures in the lower anterior abdominal wall. The mucosa of the bladder and urethra are open to the surface and urine constantly dribbles from the ureteric orifices which are identifiable close to the lateral borders of the exposed bladder.

Surgical treatment aims to close the bladder and produce normal urinary continence; this aim is achieved only very rarely.

Spinal lesions

Myelomeningocele. Almost all patients with myelomeningocele have a variable paralysis of the bladder musculature and urinary sphincters and therefore are constantly or intermittently wet.

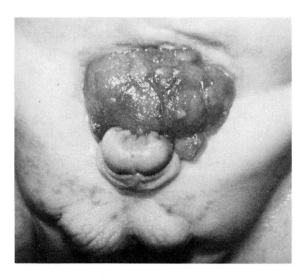

Fig. 6.4 Exstrophy of the bladder.

Their bladders may be expressible, whereas normal bladders are not.

Treatment of urinary incontinence associated with myelomeningocele poses great problems. Normal toilet training is impossible. Intermittent expression of urine from bladder is possible for some patients. A penile collecting device may be feasible for boys. Some patients can be managed with intermittent self-catheterization and be dry during the intervals. Selected patients may achieve satisfactory results from the implantation of an artificial sphincter device. These patients are no longer offered permanent urinary diversion as a method of providing artificial incontinence with a stoma.

Sacral agenesis. Disordered formation of the sacral vertebrae disrupts the parasympathetic nerve supply to the bladder and results in urinary incontinence similar to that which occurs with myelomeningocele. Most cases of sacral agenesis occur as an anomaly associated with high level anorectal agenesis. Wetting in these children may be due to sacral agenesis or, alternatively, to nerve damage during pelvic dissection at rectoplasty. Occasionally, sacral agenesis occurs as an isolated abnormality; it is for this reason that it is important to undertake careful physical examination of the sacrum and obtain appropriate X-rays in the incontinent patient who does not have an obvious diagnosis.

Other spinal lesions. The acute onset of wetting in a previously normal child may be due to a spinal lesion such as diastematomyelia or sacral lipoma with tethering of the spinal cord, spinal tumours or spinal injury. Neurological abnormalities will usually be evident on full physical examination but occasionally they may be difficult to detect. In such cases, further investigations such as myelography or CT scanning will be necessary.

Miscellaneous causes

Some children who have gross functional constipation are also troubled by wetting. Whether the wetting is due to the same factors responsible for the constipation or due to pressure effects upon the lower urinary tract from the loaded rectum is conjectural.

Functional causes

Enuresis

Enuresis is the common form of urinary incontinence in children where there is no organic disorder. All affected children wet the bed at night; some in addition, are wet by day. The frequency and severity of wetting varies enormously, with the child having some dry nights or days with other periods of almost continuous wetness. Some children have a short period out of nappies before the onset of enuresis. There is a definite incidence of spontaneous cure with age and most enuretics are dry by puberty. With some children, enuresis may simply be a delay in development in a normal physiological function; in others there may be associated psychological factors. A family history of enuresis is common.

When there is wetting with no other symptoms and no abnormalities on physical examination, the provisional diagnosis is enuresis and no investigations are required apart from examination of the urine for protein and sugar. Selected patients (e.g. those with day-time wetting or a significant period out of nappies before the onset of wetting) should have a microurine examination to exclude urinary tract infection. More comprehensive investigation is required only when there is clinical suspicion of organic disorder.

Many methods of treatment of enuresis have been described. None is thoroughly reliable and in pre-school years nothing more than simple explanation of the nature of the disorder and reassurance that spontaneous cure can be anticipated is required. A bladder distension training programme with regular delayed micturition is worth trying for children who are troubled by day-time enuresis. Restriction of fluid intake in the evening and deliberate micturition immediately before bed does not favourably influence nocturnal enuresis. Imipramine is sometimes effective but its action is not understood; side-effects are common. Hypnotherapy sometimes has transient beneficial effects.

Conditioning treatment with a pad and bell apparatus should be considered for children whose enuresis remains a problem after their sixth birthday. The child sleeps on a pad which, when wet with urine, completes a circuit and causes an alarm to ring. This awakens the child who has to get out of bed to stop the alarm and then pass urine. However, sometimes the child sleeps so deeply that other members of the family are wakened but the child is not. Any effect will be noticed within 6 weeks. If there is no improvement, it is worthwhile leaving an interval, perhaps 1 year, before trying such an appliance again.

Giggling incontinence

This is a rare phenomenon which occurs in some unfortunate children (especially girls) who have normal bladder control but who, when laughing, are plagued by dribbling or by sudden involuntary and complete emptying of the bladder. The condition is familial and there is no neurological abnormality.

RETENTION OF URINE

Acute retention of urine

Complete inability to pass urine associated with discomfort, pain and tense distension of the bladder occurs fairly frequently as a transitory phenomenon following urethral instrumentation (cystoscopy, urethral dilatation), or operations upon the external urinary apparatus such as circumcision and hypospadias repair.

Another cause of acute retention is urethral obstruction due to blood clots when there is bleeding into the urinary tract. This may occur after renal trauma, stab suprapubic catheterization of the bladder and with highly malignant tumours.

Acute retention of urine can supervene in patients with chronic retention.

Chronic retention of urine

In chronic retention of urine, the bladder is distended but painless. The patient may appear to micturate normally but the stream is usually thin and micturition is incomplete. Overflow wetting is common.

In such patients, the history may simply be one of wetting and, on examination, the distended bladder may be mistaken for a full bladder. In any case of wetting in which a palpable bladder is found on examination, the abdomen should be re-examined after micturition. If the bladder is still palpable then full investigation of the urinary tract is mandatory.

Important causes of chronic retention of urine are:

- Posterior urethral valves — see previously
- Neurogenic bladder — see myelomeningocele
- Posterior urethral stricture. The most common cause for this is rupture of the urethra with fractured pelvis from trauma
- Bladder outflow obstruction due to tumour. The most common neoplasm is rhabdomyosarcoma arising from the base of the bladder or prostate. This tumour is usually palpable on rectal examination

Management depends on the cause.

FURTHER READING

Brearly S, Armstrong G R, Nairn R, et al 1987 Pseudomembranous colitis: a lethal complication of Hirschsprung's disease unrelated to antibiotic usage. Journal of Pediatric Surgery 22: 257–259

Järvelin M R 1989 Developmental history and neurological findings in enuretic children. Developmental Medicine and Child Neurology 31: 728–736

Kleinhaus S, Boley S J, Sheran M, Sieber W K 1979 Hischsprung's disease. A survey of the members of the Surgical Section of the American Academy of Pediatrics. Journal of Pediatric Surgery 14: 588–597

Mishalany H 1989 Seven years experience with idiopathic unremitting chronic constipation. Journal of Pediatric Surgery 240: 360–362

7. Gastrointestinal bleeding

F. A. Nwako

Gastrointestinal bleeding in childhood may be due to disease localized to the gastrointestinal system or to general disease producing symptoms in the gastrointestinal system. It may present as haematemesis, melaena, bright blood per rectum or as anaemia.

Frank haematemesis or melaena is less common in childhood than in adult life, but occasionally presents as an emergency. Most commonly, gastrointestinal bleeding occurs in association with enteric infections and is a component of diarrhoea, but there are many possible causes. A careful history and physical examination will usually indicate the cause.

DIAGNOSIS

If a patient has massive intestinal bleeding the diagnosis is obvious and the first essential is resuscitation. But if the patient presents with a history suggestive of bleeding there are four basic questions to be answered.

Is the material being vomited or passed per rectum really blood?
What is the rate of blood loss?
What is the site of the bleeding?
If it is blood, is it due to local disease or general disease and what is the actual cause?

IS IT BLOOD?

Blood in vomitus or bowel content may be immediately recognizable but if chemical action has altered its appearance or if the amount is small in comparison to the volume of the containing material, it may be difficult to recognize.

The dietary history may reveal the ingestion of chocolates, dyes, tomatoes, beets, raspberries and such drugs as iron or the various salicylates, all substances likely to produce very dark red or black stools resembling melaena. If an ingested material is vomited and thought to be blood, extensive and expensive tests of the wrong sort may be ordered.

Associated features, such as progressive anaemia and reticulocytosis will confirm the presence of blood loss.

Chemical tests

Chemical tests may give some help but depend to some extent on the diet. Haemoglobin and the haem moiety possess peroxidase-like activity. They catalyse the conversion of peroxides to free oxygen which then can react with a number of dyes to produce a visible colour. These methods are not specific for haemoglobin because other dietary substances, including animal haemoglobin, certain vegetables and intestinal bacteria also contain pseudo-peroxidase activity. This is not a great problem in infants on a milk diet. In older infants or children, it is overcome by restricting the diet before testing and by choosing a less sensitive reagent for oxidation.

The most sensitive chromophor is benzidine which is no longer available for clinical use because it possesses carcinogenic properties. Ortho-tolidine is the active component of Haematest tablets and has a good level of sensitivity also. The least sensitive, and therefore most suitable chemical, is guaiac. This is the active component of the Haemoccult test.

There are also immunological tests for human haemoglobin but these are not as sensitive as guaiac-based tests for upper gastrointestinal bleeding.

RATE

This is the most crucial consideration in management. The volume of blood lost is approximately assessed from the history and, where the 'material' is available, by actual observation and measurement. Patients will always overestimate the volume, while clinicians quite often will underestimate it. Whether the loss is overt or covert, the presence of a cold, moist skin, appreciable pallor, anxiety, irritability, dyspnoea, collapsed peripheral veins with tachycardia, oliguria, hypotension and falling serial haematocrit levels suggest peripheral circulatory failure requiring urgent treatment.

SITE

Direct inspection of the blood is a useful pointer to the site of bleeding. Bright red blood arises in the anorectal region, but if there is massive upper gastrointestinal bleeding, it may induce hyperperistalsis so that unaltered or slightly altered blood is passed per rectum. Blood from the right colon is dark red while bloody mucus is suggestive of advanced intussusception. Blood from the small intestine varies from maroon to a truly dark tarry colour. The recovery of a clear or bile-stained fluid through a nasogastric tube in proven gastrointestinal bleeding suggests a lesion distal to the ligament of Treitz. In contrast, the recovery of blood in any form is indicative of upper gastrointestinal bleeding.

WHAT IS ITS CAUSE?

There is a wide variety of possible sites and causes of bleeding and the precise location and nature of the lesion must be established if possible. However, correlation of the history and physical examination will usually indicate both site and cause. A history of a well infant with

screaming on passing a hard motion and spots of blood on it, with nothing else on history or general physical examination is a local fissure-in-ano. An unwell pale child who has passed blood per rectum, and is found to have an enlarged spleen and petechiae has a general disease.

A family history of bleeding disorder or a history of easy bruising or prolonged bleeding from superficial cuts and abrasions suggests general disease, while a juvenile polyp may be felt on rectal examination.

Further examination may reveal stigmata of the causative lesion. These include jaundice, spider naevi (in the upper part of the trunk and face), palmar erythema ('red hands') and ascites in liver disease; melanin spots in the oral mucosa in Peutz-Jegher's syndrome; hereditary telangiectatic lesions on the lips, tongue and ears; or cervical lymphadenopathy in lymphoma and other reticuloses of the upper gastrointestinal tract. The usefulness of a nasogastric tube in gastrointestinal bleeding has been discussed.

DIAGNOSTIC TESTS

These are used to determine the extent, cause and site of the bleeding.

Blood tests

The haemoglobin level will give an indication of the extent of the loss except in the immediate phase and serial haemoglobin and haematocrit levels are useful in monitoring continued bleeding. Leukocytosis may occur in acute haemorrhage though a remarkable rise is suggestive of lymphoma or leukaemia in a child. A reduction in the neutrophils and platelets may be associated with the secondary hypersplenism of hepatic disease.

Barium studies

Barium contrast studies have a low identification level in active lesions. It is rapidly losing ground to endoscopy and angiography in specialized centres. However, a barium study of the upper or lower gastrointestinal tract is a useful screening procedure and may be diagnostic, e.g. duodenal ulcer, or both diagnostic and therapeutic, e.g. intussusception (Figs 7.1 and 7.2).

Endoscopy

Examination with standard instruments such as the oesophagoscope and sigmoidoscope are useful in diagnosing lesions within their reach, but have been superseded by fibreoptic endoscopy using a flexible fibreoptic gastroscrope or colonoscope and these are often useful in the acute phase to identify the site of the bleeding.

Nuclear isotope scan

This is particularly useful for the identification of peptic mucosa in a bleeding Meckel's diverticulum (Fig. 7.3). It can also be used to detect the site of active bleeding within the intestine.

Liver function tests

These assess the extent of hepatocellular dysfunction and only give indirect evidence of the possible cause and site of the bleeding.

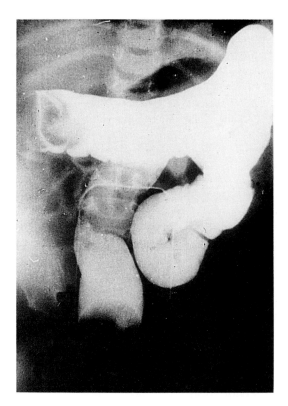

Fig. 7.1 Barium enema showing the filling defect of the intussusceptum in the right transverse colon and the 'coiled spring' sign of barium seeping around it.

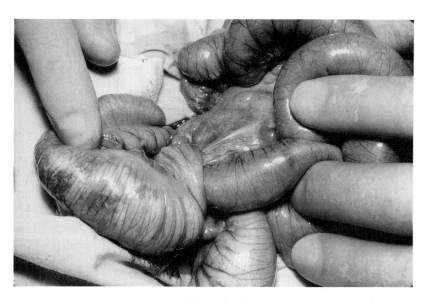

Fig. 7.2 Ileocolic intussusception. The bulk of the intussusception is clearly seen.

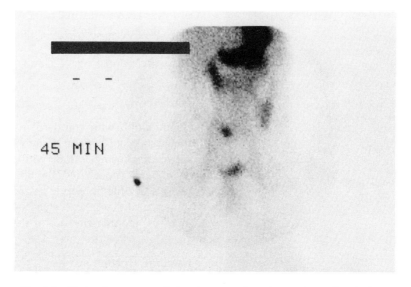

Fig. 7.3 Technetium scan outlining the stomach and a Meckel's diverticulum. Excreted technetium is shown in the bladder.

Splenoportography and angiography

Percutaneous splenoportography, as an elective procedure, will diagnose oesophagogastric varices while emergency splenic pulp manometry will identify portal hypertension in most cases. Isotopic and splenoportographic studies are useful in portal hypertension without evidence of a collateral circulation.

Angiography will identify about 90% of actively bleeding arterial lesions but it is less useful in venous lesions. However, it has been used to arrest gastrointestinal bleeding by the infusion of vasoconstrictive agents. This procedure has numerous complications and is now rarely used.

Laparotomy

Exploratory laparotomy may be both diagnostic and therapeutic. It can reveal many intra-abdominal lesions such as cirrhosis, erosions, ulcers and neoplasms and at the same time it may allow appropriate treatment for some lesions. However, it should only be used as a last resort since nothing may be found and the patient will have had an unnecessary laparotomy.

UPPER GASTROINTESTINAL BLEEDING

The causes of upper gastrointestinal bleeding include:

- Reflux peptic oesophagitis
- Oesophageal varices
- Acute gastric lesions
- Peptic ulcer
- Trauma, e.g. nasogastric tube
- Swallowed blood
- Gastritis, e.g. with pyloric stenosis

Reflux peptic oesophagitis

Gastro-oesophageal reflux is common in infants but is rare in older children. Reflux peptic oesophagitis with bleeding may occur in association with this and there may sometimes be an associated hiatus hernia.

Oesophagitis without hernia or with a sliding hiatus hernia frequently presents as occult bleeding. 'Coffee ground' vomitus is often associated with the uncommon paraoesophageal hernia in the older child due to the retention of acid contents and vascular congestion within the incarcerated gastric pouch. Epigastric tenderness may also occur. Diagnosis is confirmed by barium swallow and endoscopy. Dysphagia or discomfort on swallowing suggests a foreign body, a hiatus hernia with oesophagitis or, rarely, a neoplasm.

Treatment of reflux depends on the age. The infant should be nursed prone with the head of the cot raised up and the feeds thickened. In childhood, antacids and Gaviscon are the mainstay of treatment with dietary management as a helpful adjunct, though Gaviscon causes problems with constipation. Occasionally surgery will be necessary to help to control reflux or, rarely, to reduce a paraoesophageal hernia or a sliding hernia. Fundoplication, in which the fundus of the stomach is plicated around the abdominal oesophagus, with or without tightening of the oesophageal hiatus, is commonly used.

Oesophageal varices

Portal hypertension is the underlying cause for oesophageal varices and it results from obstruction of the blood flow from the portal venous system into the inferior vena cava. Bleeding varices constitute about 90% of massive haematemeses in children. Extrahepatic obstructive lesions are far more common than intrahepatic and are due to thrombophlebitis of the portal vein.

The causes of portal vein thrombophlebitis are:

- Omphalitis (often suspected but unproved)
- Umbilical catheterization
- Intra-abdominal trauma
- Congenital abnormalities of the portal venous system
- Peritonitis
- Pancreatitis
- Parasitic infestation (schistosomiasis causes periportal fibrosis)
- Undiscovered causes

Such obstruction allows the development of collaterals of which the clinically significant are the oesophagogastric varices. Trauma, even minor, to these varices results in torrential and spectacular haematemesis and often melaena. The less common intrahepatic lesion results from biliary atresia (hypoplasia) or other causes of cirrhosis such as hepatitis of toxic, infective or dietary deficiency origin, or of cystic fibrosis. Both infective and nutritional hepatitis occur commonly in the developing countries of the world.

Diagnosis is by barium swallow and endoscopy. Treatment can be by sclerotherapy, compression therapy, vasopressin (pitressin) therapy, embolization or surgery (see Ch. 9).

Acute gastric lesions

Acute mucosal lesions should rightly include all superficial lesions of the stomach and duodenum that are not true ulcers, such as 'stress' ulcers, erosive gastritis and duodenitis.

'Stress' ulcers, eponymously related, include Curling's ulcers in burns and Cushing's ulcers in neurological trauma and inflammations. They are usually of rapid onset, single and punched out with minimal inflammatory changes. Similarly, erosive lesions and bleeding are associated with the ingestion of steroids and salicylates (e.g. aspirin).

Peptic ulcer

True peptic ulceration is characterized by a well-defined periodicity of the symptoms of epigastric pain with the fasting–pain–eating–relief cycle. Often, however, the features are atypical, particularly in the 5 to 8 years' age group when there are emotional difficulties at home and at school. Haemorrhage is only one of many complications of peptic ulcers.

A rare variant of the true ulcer is the Zollinger-Ellison syndrome characterized by gastric hyperacidity and hypersecretion of non-beta islet cell tumours of the pancreas. The resulting ulcers are intractable, recurrent and atypically sited (e.g. the stomach, second and third parts of the duodenum). Diarrhoea occurs and there is elevated serum gastrin.

Treatment

True peptic ulceration in children is initially treated conservatively; so also are the acute mucosal erosions. The role of the organism, *Helicobacter pylori*, in the causation of peptic ulcer is still a matter of dispute. Many believe that it is the main cause of gastritis in antrum-type mucosa and that it causes a similar inflammatory response in metaplasia of the duodenal mucosa, leading to peptic ulcer. Treatment with amoxicillin and metronidazole, and continuing treatment with bismuth preparations are said to be curative in a significant number of patients. These may be combined with treatment with H_2-receptor blocking agents, such as cimetidine and ranitidine. The place of omeprazole in the treatment of peptic ulcer disease in children has not been established.

A complication such as haemorrhage is initially treated conservatively. However, in massive bleeding as revealed by a large volume of obvious blood vomited or passed per rectum, or signs of shock or the proven loss of about 20% of the total circulatory blood volume within a 24 hour period, the possibility of surgery will need to be considered. The aim is to detect and ligate the bleeding lesion. Resection is occasionally necessary if ulcers are multiple but circumscribed, though blind resection is to be deplored. Vagotomy with a drainage procedure is often the recommended procedure.

Other causes

Other bleeding lesions of importance in the stomach and duodenum include traumatic lesions, swallowed blood and gastritis from such things as pyloric stenosis. Other possible causes include neoplasms (the reticuloses, leiomyomas and sarcomas); polyps (single or multiple and familial) and in particular Peutz-Jegher's syndrome; vascular lesions (the various hamartomas including the Rendu-Osler-Weber syndrome); and various bleeding disorders. Prolapsing gastric mucosa and duodenal diverticula may rarely undergo ulceration and produce significant haemorrhage.

Abdominal trauma (especially blunt), multiple liver abscesses and bleeding into hepatomas and hepatoblastomas may produce haematobilia. In the above lesions with a lacerated or destroyed liver harbouring a central or subcapsular haematoma, blood enters the bile duct resulting in colicky right upper quadrant abdominal pain and haematemesis. Haematobilia may also occur in cholecystitis, cholelithiasis and passage of calculi, disorders not frequently encountered in children.

LOWER GASTROINTESTINAL TRACT BLEEDING

Some possible causes of lower gastrointestinal bleeding are:

- Gastroenteritis/enterocolitis
- Anal fissure
- Rectal prolapse
- Intussusception
- Polyp
- Meckel's diverticulum
- Duplication
- Chronic inflammatory disease
- Volvulus

The commonest cause is infective gastroenteritis. Of other causes, in the jejunum and ileum, intussusception and Meckel's diverticulum are common while in the colon and rectum the commonest other causes are fissure-in-ano, prolapse, trauma, intussusception, polyps, milk sensitivity, parasitic infections and various types of colitis.

Parasitic infectious diseases of surgical importance include helminthiasis such as hookworm or ascaris infestation, shigellosis, amoebic dysentery, schistosomiasis, actinomycosis and histoplasmosis, all of which may produce protocolitis. Rarer causes are lymphomas or other reticuloses, mesenteric thrombosis following septicaemia and haematological disorders.

Many of the above are well covered in medical texts.

Fissure-in-ano

This is the commonest cause of blood on a motion. In early infancy it may be caused by shallow splits in the anal mucosa caused by the passage of a large motion, without an identifiable fissure, while in later infancy and childhood it is caused by a large hard motion tearing an anal valve and causing a split in the anal mucosa. Pain on passing a motion is a distinguishing feature and the blood is on the outside of the motion though it may not always be possible to make this distinction. Pain on defaecation inhibits defaecation, causing further constipation so that a vicious cycle may develop.

Treatment consists of emptying the rectum and keeping the motions soft and regular with faecal softeners and aperients. In the initial stages, short-term applications of a local anaesthetic may be helpful if the parents can judge when a stool is about to be passed.

Chronic fissures will often have an associated skin tag and may need dilatation and occasionally excision. Multiple indolent fissures suggest an underlying general disease such as Crohn's disease or tuberculosis.

Rectal prolapse

The abnormal protrusion of the rectum through the anus may be partial, involving only the mucosa, or complete involving the full thickness rectal wall (procidentia). It is an obvious, common and troublesome condition during the first 2 years of life. Basically, there is lack of rectal support normally provided by the peritoneal reflexion, the superior and middle haemorrhoidal vessels and the sigmoid mesocolon. Subsequently, the excessively mobile rectum slides easily through a stretched and lax levator sling. In addition, organic causes seen in some patients include the redundant mucosa following anoplasty for anorectal anomalies, paralysis of anal sphincters in myelomeningocele or sacral agenesis, malnutrition states, cystic fibrosis, or exstrophy of the bladder with diastasis of the symphysis pubis and the divarication of the puborectalis muscle arising from it.

Injury to the prolapsed mucosa is usually responsible for the rectal bleeding; however, sigmoidorectal prolapse in which telescoping of the lower sigmoid mucosa occurs into the rectum is another cause of self-limiting haemorrhage.

Most patients recover spontaneously, especially if a predisposing lesion can be relieved. However, in patients who have a chronic prolapse without predisposing conditions treatment is essentially individualized. Various treatments have been used and these include sclerosant injections into the submucosa; the placement of a wire or nylon suture around the anus in the subcutaneous layer and its snug approximation around the operator's finger temporarily inserted into the anal canal (the Thiersch operation); electrofulguration of the rectum; or the induction of retrorectal fibrosis with hypertonic saline, Sterispon or Gelfoam with subsequent adherence of the rectum to the sacrum.

Patients with intractable procidentia may ultimately require sigmoid colon resection with various types of rectal fixation (rectopexy).

Intussusception

Intussusception is a condition in which a proximal part of the bowel telescopes into an adjacent distal part of the bowel (Fig. 7.2). It is common in childhood and is usually ileocolic and idiopathic in children before the age of 2 years.

The classical clinical features are:

- Colicky abdominal pain
- Vomiting
- Abdominal mass

It is associated with the classical red current jelly stool in advanced cases. The diagnosis should be made before this on the story of acute recurrent colicky pain, characterized by screaming bouts, often with drawing up of the legs, followed by pallor and exhaustion. Vomiting is common, though it is not frequent or profuse, unless complete intestinal obstruction occurs. A mobile abdominal mass will be palpable in about 80% of cases, usually in the right side of the abdomen but it may be felt anywhere along the line of the colon. An irritable infant with abdominal discomfort may resist abdominal examination and it may not be possible to feel the mass. Delay in diagnosis leads to intestinal obstruction, strangulation and a significant mortality.

Investigation

A story suggestive of intussusception is an indication for an immediate diagnostic enema with air or contrast material such as barium or gastrograffin (Fig. 7.1). This will show in a typical case, a colonic filling defect with a 'coiled-spring' sign of the contrast material infiltrating between the colonic wall and the intussusceptum. It is often possible to reduce the intussusception by hydrostatic pressure using air controlled by a pressure gauge, or a barium or gastrograffin reservoir about 1 m above the patient connected to the enema catheter in the rectum. If this is unsuccessful, operative reduction is used.

Enema reduction is contraindicated if the length of the history is more than 24 hours and if there are any signs of peritoneal irritation, shock or intestinal obstruction.

Juvenile polyp

This is a small hamartomatous lesion which, unlike true polyps, is not premalignant. It is a smooth pedunculated lesion, is single and in 70–80% of cases is situated in the rectum. Intermittent bleeding per anus, or prolapse with a bowel action, are the two common methods of presentation. These polyps are ordinarily within reach of the sigmoidoscope or may be seen on a contrast enema. Those within reach of the anus are removed by excision. Those more proximal are removed by colonoscopy or laparotomy.

Meckel's diverticulum

Meckel's diverticulitis with ectopic gastric mucosa causing ulceration of adjacent ileal mucosa, though uncommon, is perhaps the most frequent cause of substantial small-gut bleeding. This classically causes acute massive melaena with a fall in haemoglobin, in an otherwise healthy asymptomatic toddler.

A definitive diagnosis is made by a technetium nuclear scan (Fig. 7.3), which outlines the abnormal gastric mucosa in the diverticulum. On occasions, if the nuclear scan is negative and there is recurrence or evidence of continued bleeding, a laparotomy is justified. Treatment is by excision.

A duplication anomaly, either as a segment of bowel or as a cyst, may also contain ectopic gastric mucosa and cause a similar syndrome. It is also diagnosed by a nuclear scan (see Ch. 8).

Chronic inflammatory disease

Ulcerative colitis

This is a form of inflammatory bowel disease primarily affecting the mucosa of the colon and rectum. It is uncommon in childhood but it can occur at any age. The presentation is that of a progressive diarrhoea with blood and mucus in the motions, with later onset of symptoms of general disease such as malaise and weight loss. Diagnosis is by barium enema, colonoscopy and biopsy. Treatment in the acute phase with steroids and salazopyrin is ordinarily effective but because of exacerbations of the disease and the long-term risk of carcinomatous change, all of these patients will eventually have some form of proctocolectomy.

Crohn's disease

Regional enteritis (transmural granulomatous enterocolitis) is associated with slight bleeding in 25% and severe melaena in 7% of patients. There is great variability in its presentation from bleeding, recurrent abdominal pain or general malaise with non-specific symptoms, to anal disease. Anal fissures or fistulae occur in 78% of children with this disease.

Volvulus

See Chapter 8.

Other causes

Neoplasms and hamartomas may be associated with gastrointestinal bleeding. Neoplasms of the small gut, though rare, are accompanied by bleeding in 50% of cases. The lesions include polyps — single or multiple (familial polyposis), polyps of the Peutz-Jegher's syndrome and leiomyoma, leiomyosarcoma, lymphomas and occasionally carcinoid tumour. Hamartomas, including haemangiomas and hereditary telangiectasia, are uncommon causes of bleeding.

SYSTEMIC DISEASES CAUSING GASTROINTESTINAL BLEEDING

Platelet disorders

Disorders of platelet function other than those induced by aspirin are uncommon but may cause haemorrhage from mucous membranes, including gastrointestinal haemorrhage. Thrombocytopenia, of any type, is the common cause. Most often, haematemesis or melaena follow epistaxis with the swallowing of blood but pure gastrointestinal bleeding can occur.

Coagulation defects

With the exception of haemorrhagic disease of the newborn, gastrointestinal bleeding is much less common in disorders of coagulation such as haemophilia or Von Willebrand's disease than in platelet disorders.

Haemorrhagic disease of the newborn, which is due to reduced levels of prothrombin complex towards the end of the first week of life, used to be the commonest cause of haematemesis and melaena at this time, but has been very much reduced by the routine use of vitamin K analogues to prevent this disorder. It may be distinguished from apparent gastrointestinal bleeding due to swallowing of maternal blood by the Apt test — maternal blood solutions will be decolourized by 10% sodium hydroxide solution, while fetal haemoglobin is alkali resistent.

With a reduction in haemorrhagic disease of the newborn, the commonest cause of gastrointestinal bleeding in the newborn had become necrotizing enterocolitis (see Ch. 8).

Vascular disorders

Henoch-Schönlein purpura is the commonest vascular cause of gastrointestinal bleeding in childhood. In this condition, the diffuse vasculitis causes a characteristic skin rash, multiple joint pains with periarticular bleeding and haemorrhage into and from the mucosa of the small bowel. The gastrointestinal bleeding is usually recognized because of the occurrence of bouts of abdominal pain, occasionally with small bowel intussusception. Renal complications with glomerulonephritis are common, particularly in the older child.

Other vascular disorders causing gastrointestinal bleeding in childhood are uncommon, but include familial telangiectasia.

TREATMENT OF GASTROINTESTINAL BLEEDING

Life-threatening bleeding from the gastrointestinal tract is more common in infants partly due to the causative lesions at this time of life and also partly due to the small volume of circulating blood. In such infants, and in the occasional child with severe bleeding, the primary aim is to save life as in any emergency situation. The patient should be admitted to an intensive care unit or be accorded 'special care' in a general ward.

Initial measures are to provide circulatory and general supportive care pari passu with the diagnostic work-up. This support includes nasogastric suction (diagnostic and therapeutic purposes — see earlier); rapid intravenous infusions while waiting for compatible blood; blood transfusions; central venous pressure monitoring and accurate charting of the vital signs (temperature, pulse, respiration) and hourly urinary output (see Ch. 2).

An intensive search is then mounted for the bleeding lesion. In a minor or chronic haemorrhage the search is routine; in massive bleeding, diagnostic procedures are more urgent.

Once the bleeding lesion is identified, the treatment will depend on its site and type.

FURTHER READING

Graham T 1980 Gastrointestinal bleeding. The clinical presentations of acute upper gastrointestinal bleeding. British Journal of Hospital Medicine 22: 333–337
Spencer R 1964 Gastrointestinal haemorrhage in infancy and childhood: 476 cases. Surgery 55: 718–734
Venables C W 1980 Gastrointestinal bleeding. Advances in the management of gastrointestinal bleeding. British Journal of Hospital Medicine 23: 338–346

8. Intestinal obstruction

R. A. MacMahon

The problem that faces the clinician is to decide whether this infant or child has intestinal obstruction, and if so, of what type. Further management follows from these decisions.

FEATURES OF INTESTINAL OBSTRUCTION

Vomiting

In infancy, vomiting may be a symptom of many diseases, and is not necessarily a symptom of a problem in the gastrointestinal tract. It is a major symptom of intestinal obstruction and is usually the presenting feature of the infant or child with this condition. The characteristic of the vomiting which above all others suggests an intestinal obstruction is that it is bilious, i.e. green-stained. This indicates obstruction below the ampulla of Vater, while obstruction above this level causes vomiting of milk alone. Bilious vomiting may also be caused by sepsis, central nervous lesions or necrotizing enterocolitis and is almost always suggestive of a serious underlying problem.

Abdominal distension and constipation

These are prominent features of low small bowel, or large bowel obstruction. They are not features of high lesions because the oesophagus, stomach and duodenum are deflated easily by regurgitation or vomiting and the secretions of the long length of bowel below the obstruction can be passed per anus.

Abdominal pain

This is a difficult symptom to diagnose in the neonate but becomes a prominent feature in later infancy and childhood.

Two types of abdominal pain are seen in intestinal obstruction, one caused by distension and increased peristalsis of the intestine, the other caused by peritoneal irritation.

Distension and increased peristalsis of a loop of intestine causes splanchnic pain which is poorly localized and referred segmentally to the abdominal wall; foregut to epigastrium; midgut centrally around the umbilicus; and hindgut to the hypogastrium. This pain is classically intermittent and colicky and may be described as such by the older child. In infancy it is diagnosed from a history of regular intermittent screaming bouts, associated with drawing up of the legs, and pallor and listlessness following such a bout.

The onset of peritoneal irritation is a later sign, and may be localized, e.g. when the contents of an obstructed hernia become ischaemic; or generalized, when a viscus has perforated into the peritoneal cavity. It is associated with marked tenderness over the site of irritation so that tenderness may be localized or generalized.

Modifying factors

The degree and type of vomiting, abdominal distension and constipation will depend on the site or type of obstruction and on whether it is partial or complete. Complete obstructions, such as those due to atresia of a segment of the bowel, give symptoms soon after birth, but other lesions may not give symptoms until infancy, childhood or adult life. Intermittent partial obstruction may present as failure to thrive.

83

PHYSICAL EXAMINATION

A complete physical examination is essential, not only to assist in diagnosing the cause of the symptoms but to diagnose or exclude other congenital abnormalities, since it is common for abnormalities of several systems to occur in the same infant. A complete adequate physical examination can only be performed in infancy when the infant is naked and, if possible, relaxed and quiet. The conditions for examination should be optimal including a warm environment, good light and appropriate instruments. In particular, every orifice and the inguinal region must be examined.

INVESTIGATIONS

Fluids and electrolytes

Estimation of the fluid, electrolyte and acid–base status of infants or children with suspected intestinal obstruction is usually necessary, and zeal for establishing a diagnosis should not be allowed to delay investigation and management of fluid and electrolyte imbalance. Infants in whom the obstruction has been diagnosed in the first day of life and in whom vomiting has not been a feature, e.g. those with oesophageal atresia, may not need such investigations.

Radiology

In the investigation of a suspected gastrointestinal lesion, a plain X-ray of the abdomen, both supine and erect, is usually sufficient to include or exclude mechanical obstruction. The radiological signs of obstruction are dilated loops of intestine, sometimes with fluid levels. Depending upon the site of obstruction there will be a few or many dilated loops. The number and size of the dilated loops depend on how far down the intestine it is obstructed and whether the obstruction is complete, partial or intermittent.

Further investigations will depend on the presumptive diagnosis at this stage. Contrast material introduced either into the upper or lower gastrointestinal tract will frequently give the diagnosis.

AETIOLOGY

Intestinal obstruction most commonly occurs in the neonatal period and is usually the result of a defect in the embryological development of the gastrointestinal tract. These obstructions may be complete or partial and, like other hollow tube obstructions, may be caused by a lesion which is intraluminal, intramural or extramural. The type of defect determines the resultant disordered physiology which in turn determines the symptomatology.

EMBRYOLOGY

The foregut and hindgut

In the developing embryo, the gastrointestinal tract is formed by the lengthening and infolding of a flat plate of cells to form a tube, which then undergoes modification and division (Figs 8.1 and 8.2).

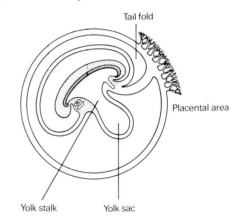

Fig. 8.1 Early embryo developing from a laminar disc.

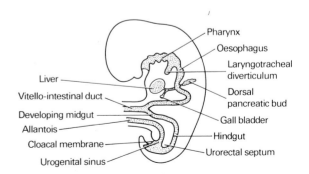

Fig. 8.2 Organs developing from the primitive gut.

A trilaminar embryonic disc has formed by the third week of development and by the fourth week the embryo folds in both longitudinal and transverse planes. During this folding, part of the yolk sac is taken up into the embryo as the foregut, part as the hindgut and, as the lateral and ventral body walls form, part of the yolk sac forms the primitive midgut. The terminal part of the hindgut dilates to form the cloaca which ends blindly at the cloacal membrane.

The primitive foregut and the hindgut cloaca both divide into two tubes. The foregut divides by a laryngotracheal groove appearing in the caudal end of the primitive pharynx, and this groove deepens into a diverticulum which later becomes separated from the foregut by the tracheo-oesophageal septum into the ventral trachea and dorsal oesophagus.

The hindgut cloaca develops into a dorsal rectum and ventral urogenital sinus by the formation of a urorectal septum which moves caudally towards the cloacal membrane; this membrane later ruptures to form the urethral and anal openings. In the female the fused Mullerian ducts that will form the uterus and vagina migrate down the urorectal septum and come to separate the urinary and intestinal systems.

It is obvious that if a teratogenic influence interferes with this development, there may result atresia, stenosis and fistulae between systems.

The midgut

Much of the early growth of the midgut takes place outside the abdomen in the extraembryonic coelom; during the 10th week of intrauterine life the midgut returns to the abdomen, undergoes an anticlockwise rotation of 270° and then fixation to the posterior abdominal wall. Many varieties of malfixation and malrotation can occur at this time, and these anomalies may cause clinical symptoms at any age, though they often occur in the first few months of life.

Embryological causes of obstruction

Anomalies of rotation and fixation are often associated with abnormal peritoneal bands. For instance, an epigastric caecum may be fixed to the posterior abdominal wall on the right side by bands which lie across the duodenum; these bands may cause obstruction of the duodenum by compression from outside, and in addition may be associated with a duodenal diaphragm, causing intraluminal obstruction.

Interference with the blood supply to a segment of bowel during rotation and fixation, or later in intrauterine life, may lead to atresia of a segment or segments of intestine.

The lumina of both the oesophagus and the duodenum become obliterated by proliferation of endodermal cells in their early development, followed by recanalization. Failure of this recanalization may contribute to obstruction.

The yolk sac, which was attached to the midgut by the vitello-intestinal duct, normally completely disappears, but the common embryological remnant of this system is a Meckel's diverticulum. Other remnants include a persistent vitello-intestinal duct attached to the umbilicus or a fibrous band connecting a Meckel's diverticulum to the umbilicus. These are all possible causes of intestinal obstruction either in the neonatal period or later in life.

Because of the complex nature of the embryological development of the gastrointestinal tract, many other rare anomalies can occur. The major types of obstruction are listed in Table 8.1. The common problems are obstructed inguinal hernia, pyloric stenosis and intussusception. The relative frequency of abnormalities are discussed in Chapter 22.

OESOPHAGEAL ATRESIA

Features of oesophageal atresia include:

- Vomiting — early, saliva and milk
- Abdominal distension — not usually a feature but may be marked if a large tracheo-oesophageal fistula is present
- Constipation — not a feature
- Polyhydramnios of pregnancy is present in 25–30% of cases

The infant with oesophageal atresia will be 'mucousy' after birth with excess frothy saliva at

Table 8.1   Major types of intestinal obstruction

1. Oesophageal atresia

2. Pyloric stenosis

3. Duodenal obstruction
   (a) Atresia
   (b) Stenosis
   (c) Diaphragm
   (d) Malrotation with bands or volvulus
   (e) Annular pancreas

4. Obstruction of the jejunum and ileum
   (a) Obstructed inguinal hernia
   (b) Intussusception (see Ch. 7)
   (c) Atresia
   (d) Stenosis
   (e) Meconium ileus
   (f) Long-segment Hirschsprung's disease
   (g) Peritoneal bands or herniae
   (h) Duplication cysts

5. Large bowel obstruction
   (a) Hirschsprung's disease
   (b) Anorectal anomalies

6. Necrotizing enterocolitis

7. Adhesion obstruction following surgery,
   e.g. post-appendicectomy

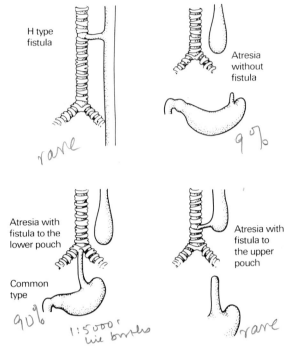

Fig. 8.3   Types of oesophageal atresia.

the lips. Attempted feeding will produce choking or cyanotic attacks which may mimic a congenital heart lesion. Attempted feedings with fine bore tubes, with small amounts of feed, may appear to be tolerated since fine bore tubes curl up in the upper pouch of the oesophagus which can hold several millilitres of fluid. If the infant is premature, the respiratory distress syndrome may complicate the clinical picture.

The common type of oesophageal atresia has a blind upper pouch (Fig. 8.3) with a fistulous connection between the lower oesophagus and the trachea, usually at the carina. As a result, fluid may enter the lungs, either by aspiration of saliva or milk from the blind upper pouch, or by regurgitation of the acid gastric juice from the stomach via the fistula; aspiration pneumonia will result.

If the tracheo-oesophageal fistula is large, especially if the baby cries and strains, air will be blown into the stomach and intestine causing gaseous abdominal distension, the so-called pseudo-Hirschsprung's presentation. In oesophageal atresia without a fistula, there is no intra-abdominal gas and the abdomen is scaphoid.

Types of oesophageal atresia

Since oesophageal atresia with or without tracheo-oesophageal fistula results from a disturbance of the division of the single foregut tube into tracheal and oesophageal tubes, the possible types can be worked out. The common form (90%) is that described above, with an upper pouch ending blindly and a tracheo-oesophageal fistula to the lower pouch. The second commonest is atresia without fistula, almost 10%. The remaining few per cent are made up of atresia with a fistula from the upper pouch, atresia with a double fistula, or H-type fistula without atresia (see Fig. 8.3).

Associated malformations

These are common and may be only minor, such as vertebral or rib anomalies, but 30–40% will have major defects such as congenital heart disease or imperforate anus.

Investigations

The basic investigation when this diagnosis is

suspected is the passage of a blunt-ended, large (10 French gauge) firm catheter through the mouth and down the oesophagus. This will be arrested at the bottom of the atretic pouch at 10 cm from the gum margin. A plain X-ray of chest and abdomen is necessary to distinguish between atresia with or without a fistula by the presence or absence of intestinal gas and to assist in the diagnosis of the commonly associated lesions of aspiration pneumonia, congenital cardiac disease and other gut atresias. Ultrasound examination of the cranial contents, heart and renal tract will define lesions in those organs.

Treatment

During transport, or while the associated lesions are being treated, the infant should be nursed prone to reduce the risk of aspiration of acid gastric contents into the lungs. A tube is inserted into the pouch and frequent suction applied to remove mucus and saliva.

General principles of the care of the sick neonate, such as control of temperature, apply to these infants, many of whom are premature.

The surgical correction depends on the type but for the common variety, a thoracotomy and end-to-end anastomosis is performed.

CONGENITAL HYPERTROPHIC PYLORIC STENOSIS

Features of congenital hypertrophic pyloric stenosis include:

- Vomiting — prominent, projectile
- Visible peristalsis — left to right, upper abdomen
- Palpable pyloric tumour
- Loss of weight
- Dehydration
- Alkalosis
- Distension — upper abdominal, intermittent
- Constipation — later, progressive

In this condition there is hypertrophy of the muscle wall of the pylorus. The infant with pyloric stenosis (Fig. 8.4) is usually an otherwise healthy infant aged 4–6 weeks who commences to vomit milk feeds. Initially this may seem to be no more than the normal possetting of infancy but the vomiting continues and increases in amount and strength. The prominent feature of the vomiting is its force — projectile vomiting, though this may occur in other conditions. There is no bile in the vomitus but if there is delay in diagnosis it will contain some brown material from altered blood, due to an associated gastritis.

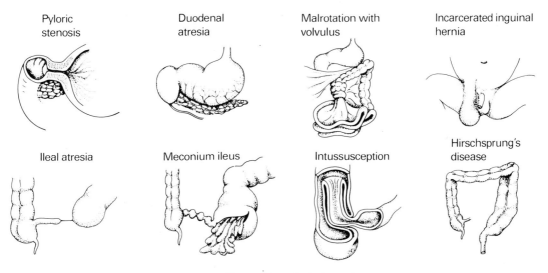

Pyloric stenosis   Duodenal atresia   Malrotation with volvulus   Incarcerated inguinal hernia

Ileal atresia   Meconium ileus   Intussusception   Hirschsprung's disease

Fig. 8.4 Types of intestinal obstruction.

In the early stages the infant feeds hungrily and will take another feed immediately after vomiting but with continued vomiting there is dehydration with marked loss of hydrochloric acid and electrolytes, producing a metabolic alkalosis (see Table 2.5). The infant then loses weight and becomes sleepy and lethargic.

The onset of symptoms is rare before the second week of life or after the second month. There is no generalized abdominal distension but the distended stomach may produce upper abdominal fullness. Constipation is not an early feature, but is usually seen later in the course of the illness. Strong gastric contractions may be seen in the upper abdomen, passing as slow intermittent peristaltic waves from left to right.

Signs of dehydration may be present, associated with a failure to gain weight or a loss of weight.

The clinical diagnostic feature is a palpable nodule at the pylorus. This may be difficult to feel, and the circumstances of palpation are important. The infant needs to be relaxed, which is best achieved by examining during a feed, while the pylorus is palpated from the left side of the infant with the left hand and the tumour is felt deep to the right rectus muscle. The position of the tumour may vary from the right edge of the rectus to the mid-line.

Jaundice due to glucuronyl transferase deficiency occurs in about 10% of these infants. This resolves spontaneously following surgery.

Aetiology

The cause is not known. It is common, occurring in approximately three infants per 1000 live births. It is more common in males, 4:1, but siblings and offspring of an affected female have a much greater risk of also having this problem than those of affected male infants.

Investigations

Electrolyte and acid–base status should be investigated. Alkalosis is usual but not invariable. No other investigations are usually necessary but if there is a suggestive clinical story and the tumour cannot be felt, a barium meal examination will show marked hold-up at the pylorus, with an elongated and sometimes narrowed pyloric canal — the 'string' sign — typical of this condition. Ultrasound can be used instead of X-ray examination in such cases. The stomach needs to be outlined with fluid, if necessary by inserting a nasogastric tube, and the size of the pylorus is measured. A pylorus greater than 1.5 cm in diameter, or a muscle width of 4 mm, is highly suggestive, and a pyloric muscle length equal to or greater than 1.9 cm is diagnostic.

Treatment

Fluid, electrolyte and acid–base status are returned to normality or near normality before operation is undertaken; otherwise a respiratory alkalosis following the mechanical respiration during anaesthesia is superimposed on the metabolic alkalosis of the condition. This may cause major problems in re-establishing spontaneous respiration. Surgical treatment consists of laparotomy and longitudinal incision of the serosa and muscle wall of the pylorus, without opening into the lumen. This procedure (Ramstedt's operation) is curative and there are no long-term problems.

DUODENAL OBSTRUCTION

The features of duodenal obstruction include:

- Vomiting — early, profuse
- Dehydration and electrolyte imbalance — early and prominent
- Distension — upper abdominal, not obvious
- Constipation — present but not a prominent feature

Table 8.1 lists the various types of duodenal obstruction. The usual clinical problem is a newborn infant aged 1–2 days who begins to vomit green-coloured fluid, but the symptoms and signs depend on whether the obstruction is partial or complete, on whether there is an associated volvulus with strangulated bowel and on whether delayed diagnosis has allowed dehydration and electrolyte imbalance to become marked.

Vomiting in complete obstruction is early, profuse and bile-stained, while in partial obstruction it is intermittent and variable and may only occasionally show some green staining or green flecks.

Generalized abdominal distension is not a feature unless peritonitis supervenes with malrotation and volvulus. However, there may be some upper abdominal fullness.

Constipation is not an early feature.

The symptoms and signs of dehydration and electrolyte imbalance appear early in complete obstruction but are variable in intermittent or partial obstruction.

Intrinsic duodenal obstruction (atresia, stenosis, diaphragm or annular pancreas) differs from extrinsic obstruction in that it is common to have a history of hydramnios in the mother, 50% of the infants are premature, a third of the patients have Down syndrome and two-thirds have at least one other abnormality.

Atresia, stenosis and diaphragms of the duodenum (see Fig. 8.4) usually occur in the region of the ampulla of Vater, the site of entry of the common bile and pancreatic ducts. In such cases, instead of there being a single common bile–pancreatic duct opening into the duodenum, there may be several, with orifices above and below or on the obstruction. This accounts for the variable presence of bile in the vomitus.

Malrotation occurs if the midgut loop, on its return from the extraembryonic coelom, does not undergo complete rotation and fixation (see above). An epigastric caecum may cause duodenal obstruction by bands or if there is complete absence of fixation, the midgut loop is suspended within the abdominal cavity by the superior mesenteric vessels and may rotate on this axis.

Volvulus of the midgut obstructs the duodenum and may give an initial clinical and X-ray appearance of duodenal obstruction, but interference with the blood supply to the midgut loop soon dominates the picture. Bloody diarrhoea, blood or mucus in the stools or 'burgundy' coloured stools occur and this symptom, together with vomiting, may produce a picture difficult to distinguish from necrotizing enterocolitis in the neonate, or acute dysentery or intussusception in the older infant or child. Progression of the vas-

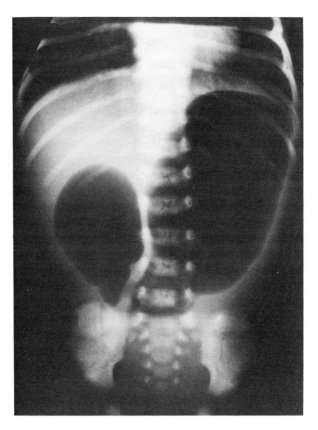

Fig. 8.5 The 'double-bubble' seen on plain abdominal X-ray in duodenal obstruction.

cular obstruction leads to gangrene, perforation, peritonitis, septicaemia and shock.

Investigations

Estimation of electrolyte and acid–base status will be necessary in any infant in whom there is any delay in diagnosis.

Plain X-ray of the abdomen will usually be diagnostic in complete obstruction; there is the characteristic 'double-bubble' (Fig. 8.5) appearance of air in the distended stomach and proximal duodenum. In partial or intermittent obstruction, this 'double-bubble' appearance may not be obvious and a barium meal examination is necessary to show a duodenal stenosis or diaphragm. A barium enema will show malposition of the caecum, indicating malrotation.

Chromosomal studies are indicated in patients with possible Down syndrome.

Treatment

In any infant or child who is vomiting, there is a danger of aspiration. The insertion of a nasogastric tube with immediate and continued aspiration of the stomach contents is the first step in treatment. Intravenous therapy is required for dehydration, electrolyte and acid–base imbalance. Obstruction of the duodenum from external compression, such as a peritoneal band, can be corrected easily at laparotomy. Mural and intra-luminal lesions such as atresia, stenosis, membrane or annular pancreas, are usually at the site of entry of the bile ducts and can only be treated by duodenoduodenostomy or duodeno-jejunostomy, to bypass the obstruction.

The treatment of a volvulus is a surgical emergency. Initial rapid resuscitation should be followed by immediate surgery to untwist the volvulus and, if possible, to prevent gangrene of the midgut loop.

OBSTRUCTION OF JEJUNUM AND ILEUM

These may be partial or complete and features include:

- Vomiting — early, profuse and bilious
- Abdominal distension — marked and generalized
- Dehydration and electrolyte imbalance — early features
- Constipation — a feature but usually overshadowed by the vomiting and abdominal distension
- Colicky central abdominal pain — a feature in older infants and children

Physical examination does not usually give any particular diagnostic information, apart from the signs of dehydration and abdominal distension, except in obstructed inguinal hernia, meconium ileus and duplication cysts (see later). Intestinal obstruction is a late complication of intussusception, but the abdominal distension makes it very difficult to feel an intussusception mass.

Atresia, stenosis or diaphragm

These occur much less frequently in the jejunum and ileum than in the duodenum, but give

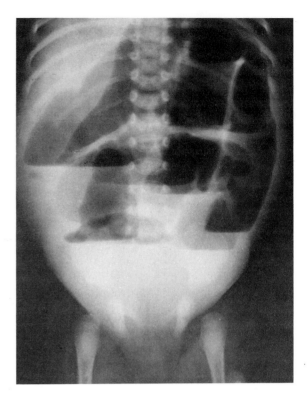

Fig. 8.6 Plain X-ray showing multiple distended loops of bowel with fluid levels in ileal atresia.

a similar presentation with early vomiting and, in addition, generalized abdominal distension (see Fig. 8.6).

Incarcerated inguinal hernia

This is a common cause of partial or intermittent obstruction, particularly in the first 6 months of life and it is mandatory to examine the hernial orifices for an irreducible lump whenever examining a patient of any age with intestinal obstruction (Fig. 8.4).

Meconium ileus

This obstruction of the lumen of the ileum is due to thick inspissated meconium. It occurs in 10% of patients with fibrocystic disease and is caused by the viscid mucus and lack of pancreatic enzymes characteristic of that disease.

The terminal ileum and colon are small and collapsed (microcolon) (Fig. 8.4) and filled with pale pebbles of inspissated mucus. Such infants have a markedly distended abdomen at birth. The distended loops of small bowel filled with thick meconium are often both visible and palpable. Of infants with complete obstruction, 50% will have an associated atresia. The associated respiratory problems are the main cause of morbidity and mortality. *) diaphragmatic splinting

Meconium peritonitis

As its name implies, this is due to the escape of meconium from a perforation in the bowel, either during intrauterine life or in the perinatal period. If this has occurred in intrauterine life, these infants, like those with complete obstruction from meconium ileus, are born with a markedly distended abdomen. The peritonitis is not bacterial but chemical. The perforation is usually associated with some pathological lesion of the intestine, such as meconium ileus, atresia of jejunum or ileum, Hirschsprung's disease or intrauterine volvulus.

Meconium peritonitis should not be confused with meconium ileus.

Duplication cysts

These may occur anywhere in the alimentary tract and always occur on the mesenteric border. If such a cyst is large and tense it may cause intestinal obstruction or volvulus, while the presence of ectopic gastric mucosa may produce bleeding or perforation. The cystic mass is sometimes palpable.

Investigations

These are similar to those for suspected duodenal obstruction. Fluid, electrolyte and acid–base disturbances occur early and are marked, and need immediate treatment.

Plain X-rays of the abdomen will show multiple dilated loops of bowel (Fig. 8.6). In the case of a high jejunal obstruction there will be only a few dilated loops visible but in low ileal obstruction there will be many. The X-rays may also show plaques of calcification in meconium peritonitis, or the 'ground-glass' appearance of meconium ileus. A barium enema will show the 'microcolon' appearance (Fig. 8.7) of the unused

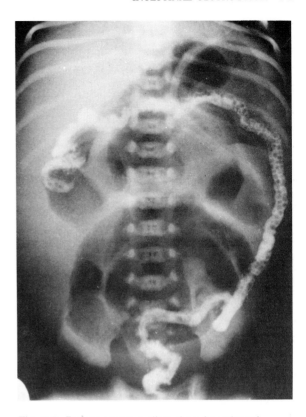

Fig. 8.7 Barium enema outlines the microcolon of meconium ileus or low small bowel atresia.

colon of low ileal atresia or meconium ileus, or malposition of the caecum in cases of intermittent volvulus.

In uncomplicated meconium ileus, a diagnostic gastrograffin enema may be curative by removing the meconium plugs from colon and terminal ileum and by making the thick tenacious contents of the dilated ileum more fluid, allowing it to be passed per anus.

Suspected associated lesions, such as fibrocystic or Hirschsprung's disease, will need investigation.

Treatment

A nasogastric tube is inserted and the stomach contents emptied to prevent vomiting and possible aspiration. Intermittent suction is continued until the problem is relieved.

Intravenous therapy is needed to correct any dehydration, electrolyte or acid–base imbalance and for continued therapy and possible intravenous feeding.

If there is a possibility of strangulated bowel, suggested by shock, bloody diarrhoea and abdominal tenderness, emergency surgical treatment is necessary after immediate resuscitation. In other cases the treatment depends on the cause.

Extrinsic obstruction by bands or herniae are easily relieved at laparotomy. Atresia is treated by end-to-end anastomosis though this may be complicated by gross distension of the proximal segment. Meconium ileus, if uncomplicated, may be treated by evacuation of the intraluminal contents by gastrograffin enema, or by laparotomy and evacuation of contents or by temporary ileostomy.

LARGE BOWEL OBSTRUCTION

The features of large bowel obstruction include:

- Abdominal distension — early, marked
- Constipation — prominent
- Vomiting — late, intermittent
- Spurious diarrhoea — occasional

Because these are low obstructions, vomiting is a relatively late symptom and abdominal distension is marked. Failure to pass meconium or delay in its passage is a prominent feature.

Large bowel obstructions usually occur in the neonatal period and fall into two main groups. Hirschsprung's disease and anorectal anomalies.

Hirschsprung's disease

This is one of the commonest causes of intestinal obstruction in infancy. The usual presentation is an acute or subacute obstruction in the neonatal period. Alternatively, there may be episodes of constipation in the neonatal period progressing to marked constipation with abdominal distension in later infancy and childhood, sometimes associated with failure to thrive. If enterocolitis supervenes, unremitting diarrhoea and septicaemia will be the main features.

Rectal examination may show a narrow anal canal and rectum, but is more often unremarkable. Sometimes this examination produces a

rapid passage of meconium and flatus with relief of symptoms and the condition may then be labelled a meconium plug syndrome.

The meconium plug syndrome is common in very small premature infants, possibly due to delayed maturity of ganglion cells, but can also occur in meconium ileus and in some otherwise normal infants. Hirschsprung's disease should be excluded in full-term infants who have any features of the meconium plug syndrome.

Associated lesions are not as common with Hirschsprung's disease as with some other gastrointestinal abnormalities such as oesophageal atresia. It is associated with a number of syndromes which also involve hearing problems, renal problems, cleft palate, brachydactyly or polydactyly and heart defects. Down syndrome is the most frequently encountered associated abnormality.

Pathology

Hirschsprung's disease is caused by an abnormality of the innervation of the terminal bowel, with absence of ganglion cells in the submucous and myenteric plexuses, extending proximally from the line of the anal valves for a variable distance. It is due to the interruption of the caudal migration of the neuroblasts from the cranial end of the alimentary tract and the length of the aganglionic segment depends on the stage at which this interruption took place.

The rectum only is involved in 25% of cases, the rectum and sigmoid in 50% and in 5% the whole colon is affected. The aganglionic segment extends into the small bowel in 1–2% of cases.

Familial incidence

Hirschsprung's disease has a definite familial incidence. Several siblings in a family may be affected and several mother–child cases have been reported. Short segment cases — to the rectosigmoid — are much more common in males than females in a ratio of 5:1, whereas long segment cases, i.e. in which the aganglionic segment extends proximal to the rectosigmoid, have an equal sex distribution. The risk for siblings with a short segment distribution is 1 in 30 overall, with a higher risk for brothers than for sisters. In the long segment cases, there is a risk of 1 in 10 for sisters and 1 in 6 for brothers.

Investigations

If the presentation is that of acute intestinal obstruction, then fluid and electrolyte investigation is of prime importance.

Plain X-ray of the abdomen shows gaseous distension of the whole gastrointestinal tract (Fig. 8.8), though it is sometimes possible to see that the lower colon is mainly affected. Colonic fluid levels may also be visible. Barium enema typically shows the 'ice-cream cone' appearance (Fig. 8.9) of the dilated, hypertrophied normal proximal colon narrowing to the abnormal segment in the region of the rectosigmoid junction. In long segment disease and in patients in whom there has been

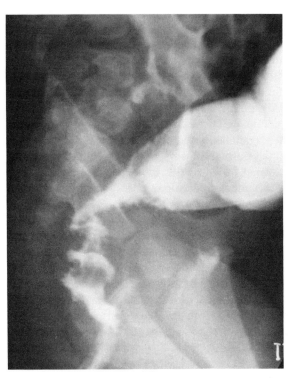

Fig. 8.9 The 'cone' seen on barium enema in Hirschsprung's disease.

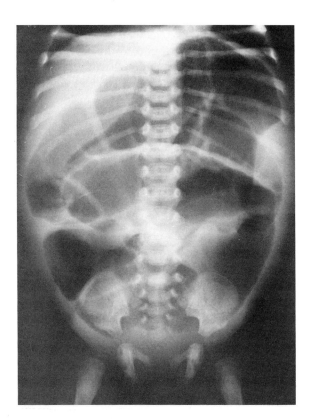

Fig. 8.8 Diffuse gaseous distention of plain X-ray of the abdomen in Hirschsprung's disease.

vigorous washing-out of the terminal bowel, this cone may not be apparent. The X-ray appearances, both plain and contrast, can be variable in Hirschsprung's disease and may be misleading. The cone may not be visible and is only of significance if definite and in the region of low colon and rectum.

Definitive diagnosis is made by a rectal biopsy, usually suction biopsy, in which a small piece of mucosa and submucosa is removed from the rectum by a suction biopsy instrument introduced via the anus. This is done without anaesthesia. Histological examination demonstrates the absence of ganglion cells in the submucosal plexus, characteristic of this disease. Large abnormal nerve trunks may also be present and are a positive diagnostic feature. Acetylcholinesterase staining of the tissues of the mucosa is abnormal and is also a positive feature of the disease.

Manometry (Ch. 6) can also be diagnostic but is not widely used due to difficulties in interpretation.

Treatment

As always, if there is acute intestinal obstruction, insertion of a nasogastric tube, aspiration of the stomach and insertion of an intravenous line for fluid and electrolyte therapy, are the first therapeutic steps.

The definitive treatment consists of excising the aganglionic segment and mobilizing the proximal normal bowel so that an anastomosis of normal bowel to the anus can be made. If there is a short aganglionic segment, it is often possible to evacuate the terminal bowel with enemas to allow an early formal operation without the need for a preliminary colostomy. However, if there are doubts about the length of the aganglionic segment, or in the presence of enterocolitis, or in the presence of gross dilatation of the proximal bowel in the older patient, a defunctioning colostomy is the first step, with later resection and anastomosis.

Anorectal anomalies

The basic problem in these anomalies is an abnormality of the site and/or type of anal opening and this should be diagnosed at birth in the standard physical examination of the newborn infant. The unrecognized case and the one in which there is a delay in treatment will develop the symptoms and signs of large bowel obstruction.

The anal opening may be completely absent, or there may be a stenosed opening in the normal site or more commonly in an anterior ectopic site (Fig. 8.10). If an anal opening cannot be found on standard clinical examination, there may be a fistula from the end of the bowel to the vagina in the female, or to the urethra or more rarely the bladder in the male. If there is an ectopic opening visible it will be an anocutaneous fistula in the male, or an anocutaneous or anovestibular fistula in the female.

These anomalies result from arrest or aberration of the normal development of the cloaca into a dorsal rectal tube and a ventral urinary system. These developmental effects result in atresia, fistula or stenosis and are complicated by the intervention of the Mullerian system in the female. It is obvious that there are many possible

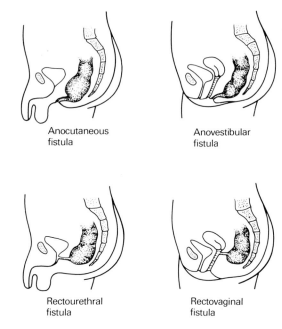

Anocutaneous fistula

Anovestibular fistula

Rectourethral fistula

Rectovaginal fistula

Fig. 8.10   The basic types of anorectal anomalies.

types of defects that may occur and extensive classifications can be found of the various types.

Clinically, anorectal anomalies fall into two main groups — high anomalies and low anomalies — depending on the relationship of the distal limit of the bowel to the levator ani muscle. This is the muscle of major rectal continence. If the bowel ends at or above the puborectalis, the upper segment of the levator ani, it is called a supralevator or rectal anomaly and if it ends below the puborectalis, it is called a translevator or anal anomaly. The bowel in either group may end as an atresia (rare in the anal group) or may continue as a fistulous opening as mentioned above. This fistulous opening is above the puborectalis in the rectal group and below it in the anal group (Fig. 8.10).

The clinical distinction between the two groups depends on whether a fistulous opening can be identified from below. These can, on occasions, be difficult to identify because the opening may be small and hidden in the vestibule or there may be a covered fistulous track marked by a line of small whitish nodules. If the fistula is found, the infant belongs to the anal anomaly group and if it is not found, the infant almost certainly belongs to the rectal anomaly group. The distinction is of fundamental importance in that the anal and rectal groups are very different in both treatment and prognosis.

Associated malformations

Almost two-thirds of these infants will have one or more associated malformations, with the rectal anomalies having twice the incidence of the anal anomalies. The most commonly associated malformations are genitourinary and vertebral and less common are alimentary, cardiac and central nervous malformations. Major sacral abnormalities can be associated with neural abnormalities affecting the nerve supply to both bladder and bowel. There is also an increased incidence of prematurity. Serious associated abnormalities are a major factor in mortality and morbidity.

Treatment and prognosis

Low anal lesions can be treated in the neonatal period by dilatation and/or simple incision to enlarge the opening. The high rectal lesions require a colostomy in the neonatal period and a definitive pull-through of the terminal bowel. There is still some controversy on the most appropriate age of operation for this group but most have the operation early in the first year of life via a sacroperineal approach. The aim is to place the pulled-through bowel within the remnant of the sphincter complex.

Normal continence will be obtained in most of the low group, while 50% of the high group would be expected to be mostly continent, 25% to have fair continence with energetic measures to control bowel function and 25% would be incontinent, though this group can be controlled usually with daily bowel washouts. High imperforate anus patients are rarely normally continent but are usually content with their degree of function, with appropriate management.

NECROTIZING ENTEROCOLITIS

This is a disease of unknown aetiology affecting mainly very small premature infants, particularly those who are very ill in the perinatal period with such conditions as hyaline membrane disease or jaundice requiring exchange transfusions. It is often associated with the use of in-dwelling intravascular catheters.

Symptoms and signs

These suggest a combination of sepsis and partial bowel obstruction. Volvulus is a common differential diagnosis.

Lethargy and refusal to feed is usually the first indication of the disorder. Abdominal distension is generalized and in severe cases may be associated with some redness and oedema of the abdominal wall. Vomiting is common and often bile-stained, but is intermittent and not profuse. Blood is passed per rectum in 25–50% of cases.

The diagnosis is suspected when an infant at risk develops these symptoms and it is confirmed by plain X-ray abdominal examination which shows bubbles of intramural bowel gas (see Fig. 6.2). Full blood examination and blood and bowel cultures are necessary to define the extent of the illness.

Acidosis is a prominent feature, with associated sepsis, anaemia and some dehydration.

Treatment

Initial measures are to stop oral intake, feed intravenously, give broad-spectrum antibiotics and treat dehydration and acidosis. If the infant's condition deteriorates with the above or if there is evidence of perforation with widespread peritonitis, operation will be necessary. Late strictures in the colon, after recovery from the acute illness, also occur.

FURTHER READING

Breaux C W, Hood J S, Georgeson K E 1989 The significance of alkalosis and hypochloremia in hypertrophic pyloric stenosis. Journal of Pediatric Surgery 24: 1250–1252
Gutman F M, Braun P, Bensoussan A L, Desjardins F G, Collin P-P 1975 The pathogenesis of intestinal atresia. Surgery, Gynecology and Obstetrics 141: 203–206

9. Jaundice, hepatosplenomegaly and diseases of the pancreas

P. Upadhyaya

JAUNDICE

Jaundice in the newborn is quite common. Its nature may vary from the simple self-correcting physiological jaundice to complex problems of obstructive infantile cholangiopathy — the neonatal hepatitis–biliary atresia complex.

Causes

These may be divided for convenience into medical and surgical causes (see Table 9.1).

Some degree of physiological jaundice is seen in 50% of full-term and 80% of premature babies. The jaundice is of the unconjugated type of hyperbilirubinaemia, appears on the second or third day of life and disappears within 2 weeks.

A common cause of conjugated hyperbilirubinaemia in young infants is severe infection. However these infants are acutely ill. In contrast to this, jaundice which appears in otherwise healthy infants in the second or third week of life and which is clearly cholestatic (conjugated type) poses a serious diagnostic and therapeutic problem. A good clinical examination and relevant screening tests readily rule out the medical causes listed in Table 9.1.

After excluding sepsis, the two most common causes of conjugated hyperbilirubinaemia in neonates are neonatal hepatitis and biliary atresia. These two entities have similar clinical, biochemical and histological features and very often it is difficult to distinguish one from the other.

Traditionally, extrahepatic biliary atresia has been described as correctable or incorrectable (Fig. 9.1). Recent advances in surgical technique offer a high cure rate even for 'incorrectable' biliary atresia, provided it is treated before 8 weeks of life. It is, therefore, of utmost importance to diagnose this condition early, i.e. before this critical period of 8 weeks.

Table 9.1 Causes of jaundice in infancy

Medical
1. Haemolytic
   (a) Physiological
   (b) Rh incompatibility
   (c) ABO incompatibility

2. Severe infections

3. Viral infections
   (a) Cytomegalic disease
   (b) Toxoplasmosis
   (c) Rubella
   (d) Herpes simplex virus

4. Neonatal hepatitis

5. Congenital syphilis

6. Galactosaemia

7. Alpha-1 antitrypsin deficiency

8. Rare diseases, e.g. Gilbert's, Gaucher's and Neimann-Pick

Surgical
1. Biliary atresia

2. Biliary hypoplasia

3. Inspissated bile syndrome

4. Choledochal cyst

Biliary atresia

Biliary atresia is defined as a condition in which extrahepatic bile ducts are non-patent and instead consist of atretic fibrous cords incapable of transporting bile. Its incidence is 1 in 10 000 live births.

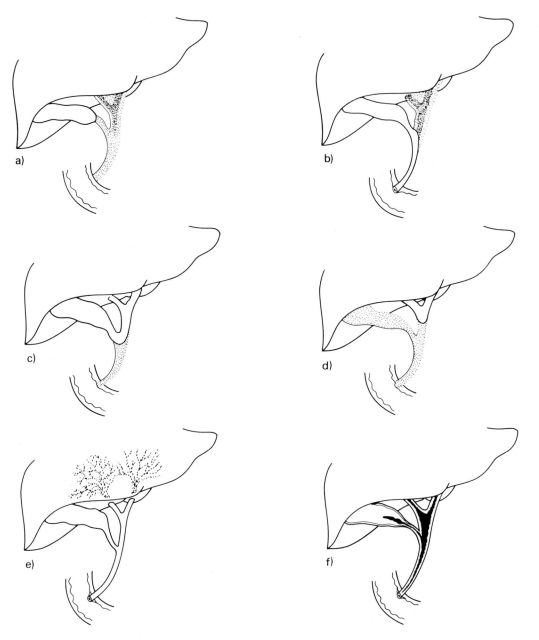

Fig. 9.1 Types of biliary atresia. A and B: Incorrectable atresia: A: involving all extrahepatic ducts. B: The right and left and common hepatic ducts. C and D: Correctable atresia: the proximal bile ducts are patent. E: Intrahepatic atresia. F: Inspissated bile syndrome.

In the past it was believed that biliary atresia was a true congenital malformation — a failure of development of patency in the extrahepatic bile ducts. Recent studies, however, have conclusively shown that non-patency of ducts is due to destruction and subsequent fibrosis of preformed bile ducts caused by intrauterine or perinatal viral infection, the probable causative agent being reovirus type 3. The inflammatory process actually affects not only the extrahepatic bile ducts, but also the liver parenchyma in a manner similar to that of neonatal hepatitis.

Before 3 months of age, the fibrous tissue mass at the porta hepatis contains many patent bile ductules varying in diameter from 20 to 800 μm. These channels are utilized for internal drainage of bile in Kasai's operation of hepato-portoenterostomy. If operation is delayed the channels become progressively atretic, diminishing the chances of a surgical cure.

Currently, it is believed that neonatal hepatitis, biliary atresia and choledochal cyst are the result of varying grades of intrauterine viral inflammation of the liver and its intrahepatic and extrahepatic bile ducts, producing a similar clinical picture of obstructive cholangiopathy.

Clinical features

- Jaundice — appears 2 to 3 weeks after birth or there is persistence of what was considered to be physiological jaundice
  — conjugated hyperbilirubinaemia: bilirubin, 137–376 μmol/L (8–12 mg/dL)
- Liver — soft, slightly enlarged
  — gradually becoming firmer and more enlarged due to rapidly developing fibrosis
- Stools — pale, clay coloured, absence of bile pigments
- Spleen — becomes palpable at 3 to 4 months

In early cases, the general condition is good and the infant is feeding well and gaining weight. In late cases, ascites appears by 9–10 months. If not treated, death occurs due to liver failure, usually before the second birthday.

Anatomical types of biliary atresia (Fig. 9.1)

- Extrahepatic — incorrectable
  — correctable
- Intrahepatic

Correctable biliary atresia is seen in less than 20% of cases. In these cases the common hepatic duct (and sometimes the gall bladder and part of the common bile duct also) are patent. In the 'incorrectable' type the proximal part of extrahepatic ducts or the entire extrahepatic ductal system is atretic. Intrahepatic biliary atresia is diagnosed by liver biopsy which shows absence of intrahepatic bile ducts.

Diagnosis

Valuable time should not be wasted in doing a battery of tests, which are of doubtful value. The following investigations have been found very useful. These should be completed before the infant is 8 weeks old.

- Liver function tests
- Ultrasonography
- Radioisotope excretion studies (using technetium-99m IDA (iminodiacetate) agents)
- Percutaneous liver biopsy
- Operative cholangiogram

Radioisotope (^{99m}Tc-IDA) scanning is most valuable in differentiating neonatal hepatitis from biliary atresia. Technetium-tagged organic derivatives of iminodiacetic acid are taken up by hepatocytes and excreted into the biliary tracts. Excretion of the radionuclide in the intestine rules out the possibility of biliary atresia. However, absence of excretion is seen in biliary atresia as well as some cases of neonatal hepatitis. Specificity of the test improves by giving phenobarbital for a week before the isotope excretion study.

If a radioisotope excretion study has failed to confirm patency of the extrahepatic ducts, an operative cholangiogram is done by injecting radioopaque contrast medium into the gall bladder.

Management

A correctable type of atresia is treated by choledochojejunostomy using a Roux-en-Y anastomosis (Fig. 9.2A). In incorrectable biliary atresia, the fibrosed extrahepatic ducts from the porta hepatis to the upper border of the duodenum (Fig. 9.2B) are excised and Kasai's portoenterostomy is done. Bile coming out of the

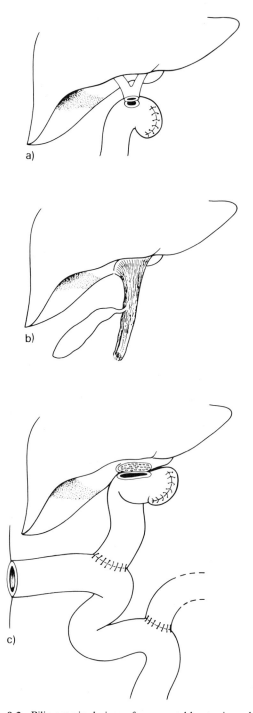

Fig. 9.2 Bilio-enteric drainage for correctable atresia and incorrectable atresia. A: Common hepatic duct anastomosed to a Roux-en-Y loop of jejunum. B: Complete atresia of extrahepatic bile ducts, which are replaced by fibrous tissue. C: Roux-en-Y loop anastomosed to the porta hepatis (after excision of the fibrosed ducts and anastomosis to the skin (Kasai's operation).

patent bile ductules, opened by the dissection at porta hepatis, is internally drained into the jejunal loop (Fig. 9.2C).

Prognosis

If portoenterostomy is attempted before 8 weeks of life, drainage of bile into the intestine can be achieved in 80% of cases. However, long-term jaundice-free survival is seen in only 40 to 50% of infants.

If the operation is delayed beyond 3 months the success rate is significantly lowered and biliary cirrhosis may develop in spite of free drainage of bile. Complications include repeated attacks of ascending cholangitis, fever, progressive biliary fibrosis and portal hypertension. A higher incidence of hepatic malignancy has been reported.

Liver transplantation

This has been successfully carried out in a large number of children who developed liver failure months and years after Kasai's portoenterostomy. However, donor infant livers are uncommon and an adult liver may need to be reduced in size to fit the infant abdomen. Alternatively, a lobe of the liver of a live donor may be transplanted. Success rates are reasonable.

Biliary hypoplasia

In this condition the extrahepatic biliary ducts, although radiographically patent, are severely narrowed, producing obstructive jaundice. It is possibly a variant of the same generalized hepatobiliary disease as neonatal hepatitis and biliary atresia.

Inspissated bile syndrome

Rarely, severe haemolysis due to Rh or ABO incompatibility, leads to blockage of the extrahepatic bile ducts with inspissated biliary sludge. Treatment consists of saline irrigation of bile ducts via the gall bladder.

Choledochal cyst

Choledochal cysts are localized cystic dilatations of the bile duct, usually its supraduodenal portion (Fig. 9.3). Bile stagnation in the cysts frequently leads to stone formation. Nearly 75% of cases are infants or children; four out of five are females. A large number have been reported from Japan and other Asian countries.

Usually there is a fusiform dilatation of the whole of the common bile duct except for its distal end which is stenosed. The intrahepatic ducts are distended. Liver parenchyma varies from normal to cirrhotic. The capacity of the cysts varies from a few millilitres to 2000 mL. The wall of the cyst may be as thick as 1 cm, or so thin that bile shines through it. It is usually composed of fibrous tissue with inflammatory cells and there is no definite epithelial lining.

Aetiology

The exact cause is not known. Two theories commonly put forth are:

1. Congenital segmental weakness of the wall
2. Inflammatory degeneration of the wall of the bile duct by pancreatic reflux

Clinical features

The classical clinical triad is:

1. Abdominal pain, right upper quadrant
2. Mass in the right upper abdomen
3. Obstructive jaundice

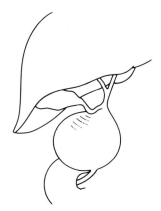

Fig. 9.3 Choledochyl cyst.

Symptoms are due to stasis of bile in the cyst leading to intermittent biliary obstruction. Superimposed bacterial infection causes ascending cholangitis manifesting as jaundice with chills and rigors. The classical clinical triad is present in only 30% of cases, the remaining children having only one or two of these features.

Diagnosis

The diagnosis can be easily established by:

- Ultrasonography or CT scan
- Radioisotope scanning using ^{99m}Tc-IDA
- Cholangiography — preoperative, percutaneous or endoscopic (retrograde) in order to further define the intrahepatic and extrahepatic cysts

Treatment

Best results are obtained when the entire cyst is removed and a Roux-en-Y choledochojejunostomy performed (Fig. 9.2A). If the cyst is thick walled and grossly adherent to surrounding structures a long Roux-en-Y anastomosis is performed between the side wall of the cyst and the jejunum. However, the long-term results are not satisfactory, as 50% develop anastomotic stricture, recurrent cholangitis or risk a malignancy.

GALL BLADDER DISEASE IN CHILDREN

Gall bladder disease is uncommon in childhood, but both acute cholecystitis and cholelithiasis/cholecystitis occur, particularly in older children. Acute cholecystitis is usually misdiagnosed as acute appendicitis, while cholelithiasis presents as recurrent bouts of abdominal pain with vague gastrointestinal symptoms and right upper quadrant tenderness in an acute bout. An overweight child and a family history of gallstones suggest the diagnosis, which is confirmed by cholecystogram and ultrasound examination for stones. Treatment is by interval cholecystectomy.

Haemolytic disease such as hereditary spherocytosis, sickle cell anaemia and thalassaemia may precipitate stone formation so that ultrasound examination of the gall bladder for stones should be performed if splenectomy is being considered. The surgeon should also examine the gall bladder at splenectomy. The gallstones are pigment stones within a normal gall bladder and jaundice is rare. Children with ileal dysfunction and a long history of parenteral nutrition may also develop gallstones presumably due to bile stasis.

HEPATOSPLENOMEGALY

Enlargement of the spleen or liver or both constitute nearly 50% of abdominal masses in children and may be due to a variety of conditions in which surgery has a role.

SPLENOMEGALY

The spleen may be just palpable on inspiration in normal infants and young children on routine examination. It is often palpable if the infant or young child has an acute intercurrent infection.

The splenomegaly of disease is usually due to its reticuloendothelial function. The common presenting symptoms are jaundice, abdominal pain, bruising or bleeding.

Function of the spleen

The spleen is an important part of the reticulo-endothelial system. Its red pulp, consisting of splenic cords and sinusoids, is concerned with sequestration and phagocytosis of senescent blood cells, particulate matter and bacteria. The white pulp, made up of lymphocytes, plasma cells and macrophages arranged around the central arterioles, takes part in antibody formation. In hypersplenism the red pulp functions of the spleen become abnormally exaggerated leading to anaemia, leucopenia and thrombocytopenia. Splenectomy helps, rather indirectly, by prolonging the life of abnormal red blood cells in spherocytosis, and of platelets in thrombocytopenia.

Severe post-splenectomy infections in children have highlighted the spleen's role in the immune defence mechanism. The spleen produces opsonins and IgM. Bacteria agglutinated and immobilized by the antibodies are trapped and phagocytosed in the spleen. In the absence of the spleen the antibody response to severe blood borne infection, particularly to *pneumococci* and *Haemophilus influenzae*, may be markedly impaired. The resultant overwhelming infection has a 50% mortality. Splenectomy should, therefore, be undertaken only when essential and preferably not before 5 years of age.

Diagnosis

Enlargement of the spleen may occur in a variety of diseases, only a few of which will involve the surgeon. Mostly, splenectomy is only a palliative method to treat haematological and/or mechanical complications of splenomegaly. Extensive laboratory investigations, including haematological work-up, may be necessary to arrive at a diagnosis and decision to remove the organ. Indications for splenectomy are listed below.

- Hereditary spherocytosis
- Idiopathic thrombocytopenic purpura
- Thalassaemia
- Hypersplenism
- Portal hypertension
- Primary diseases of the spleen, e.g. cysts, tumours, splenic trauma not amenable to conservative management

Congenital haemolytic anaemia (hereditary spherocytosis or acholuric jaundice)

The basic defect lies in the cell membrane of the erythrocytes, which becomes spherical in shape and has an increased osmotic fragility. The abnormal red cells are trapped and haemolysed in the red pulp of the spleen. The disease is inherited as an autosomal dominant trait and is suggested by a strong family history. In some cases it may occur as a spontaneous mutation.

Clinical features

- Anaemia
- Splenomegaly
- Episodic haemolytic crises — jaundice
  — abdominal pain
  — fever

The symptoms usually start in later childhood, but may sometimes occur in infancy. The severity of anaemia varies greatly. In mild cases there is a chronic anaemia and the spleen is enlarged slightly. These children have a good prognosis and normal life expectancy. In severe cases periodic episodes of haemolytic crisis may occur, producing abdominal pain, fever, vomiting, severe anaemia, acholuric jaundice and marked splenic enlargement. There is an increased incidence of biliary calculi in children above 10 years of age.

Treatment

Splenectomy gives excellent results; in the absence of the spleen the abnormal red blood cells are able to complete their lifespan. Splenectomy should be done as an elective procedure, when the acute crisis has been tided over by careful blood transfusions. The operation should not be done in children under 5 years of age. Prior to operation, an ultrasound examination of the gall bladder should be performed to detect gallstones. At operation the gall bladder is palpated for stones and the abdomen searched for accessory spleens, which should be removed if present.

Other haemolytic anaemias

In other haemolytic anaemias such as thalassaemia, acquired haemolytic anaemia and paroxysmal nocturnal haemoglobinuria, splenectomy is not as useful as in hereditary spherocytosis. However, if the enlarged spleen is trapping the red blood cells and worsening the anaemia, as shown by shortened lifespan of radioisotope-tagged transfused normal cells, it should be removed. Splenectomy may benefit to the extent of reducing the frequency of blood transfusions.

Idiopathic thrombocytopenic purpura

This is a rare condition, an autoimmune disorder, characterized by a decrease in the number of circulating platelets, more frequently seen in female children.

In 80% of cases the disease manifests as an acute purpuric attack preceded by a mild systemic infection. Usually the course is self-limiting and complete recovery occurs in 1–2 months. In the remaining cases it may take a chronic course prolonged over several years. The spleen is usually not enlarged.

Platelets, although produced in adequate number, are abnormally sequestered in the spleen due to their sensitization by a circulating anti-platelet IgG antibody. Thrombocytopenia (less than 50 000/μL) and increased capillary permeability produce spontaneous haemorrhage in the skin (petechiae and extensive bruising) and mucous membranes.

Acute forms may rarely be complicated by:

- Extensive internal haemorrhage needing blood transfusion
- Submucosal bleeding in the gastrointestinal tract mimicking intussusception and sometimes actually leading to it
- Haematuria due to intrarenal haemorrhage
- Intracranial bleeding — the most dreaded complication — leading to serious brain damage and even death

Treatment

If the attack is mild no active treatment is needed as spontaneous recovery usually occurs. If there is severe loss of blood the acute attack may be tided over by giving platelet transfusions or transfusion of fresh blood. Administration of corticosteroids over a short period may increase the platelet count and avert the crisis.

Splenectomy is indicated in a small number of selected cases which have:

1. Failure to respond to conservative measures
2. Intracranial haemorrhage
3. Life-threatening haemorrhage
4. A chronic state persisting for over a year

Splenectomy, when indicated, gives lasting remission of clinical symptoms, although platelet count returns to normal in only 60–70% of cases.

Hypersplenism

This is a non-specific term incorporating a variety of conditions in which the spleen becomes over-active in trapping and destroying one or more of the formed elements of the blood. The bone marrow shows increased production of the blood elements destroyed by the spleen.

Causes of hypersplenism

Hypersplenism may be primary or secondary.

Primary hypersplenism occurs when the spleen itself is normal, but has become overactive due to trapping of abnormal blood elements as in hereditary spherocytosis and idiopathic thrombocytopenic purpura.

Secondary hypersplenism occurs when the splenic enlargement is secondary to a coexisting disease such as portal hypertension, Hodgkin's disease, Gaucher's disease, histoplasmosis, reticuloendotheliosis or malaria. Splenectomy often helps in correcting anaemia or pancytopenia. The mortality of splenectomy for secondary hypersplenism is more than four times higher than splenectomy with a normal spleen.

Overwhelming post-splenectomy infection

The commonly held view that the spleen can be removed without any ill effects is incorrect. Recently it has been shown that overwhelming fulminant sepsis may occur in over 4% of cases weeks, months or years after splenectomy. It proves fatal in nearly 50% of cases. The risk is highest in infants and small children under 5 years of age, or when the spleen has been removed for a serious underlying disease such as Coombs' disease, Gaucher's disease, thalassaemia or Hodgkin's disease.

It is, therefore, necessary to remember that splenectomy should be done in children only when it is unavoidable. Every effort should be made to conserve the spleen following its rupture due to blunt trauma.

After splenectomy, prolonged prophylactic penicillin therapy (2–3 years) should be given in high-risk cases. Active immunization may be achieved against pneumococcal infection by using polyvalent pneumococcal vaccine.

PORTAL HYPERTENSION

Portal hypertension is due to an obstruction to the flow in the portal venous system. This results in varicosities in the weak-walled vessels of the lower oesophagus.

Clinical symptoms

- Haematemesis
- Melaena
- Chronic anaemia
- Splenomegaly and hepatomegaly

The older infant or child who presents with a major haematemesis should be considered to have portal hypertension until proved otherwise. The attack of severe haematemesis or melaena is usually preceded by mild fever and upper respiratory tract infection or by ingestion of drugs like aspirin. There is splenomegaly with or without liver enlargement.

Pathology

Portal hypertension may be due to extrahepatic or intrahepatic causes.

Extrahepatic

In children, portal hypertension is usually due to an extrahepatic block. The portal vein becomes thrombosed following umbilical sepsis or umbilical vein catheterization in early infancy. The thrombosed portal vein is surrounded by a complex meshwork of collaterals, erroneously called a cavernoma. The liver is essentially normal.

Intrahepatic

Only in 5 to 10% of cases is portal hypertension due to biliary cirrhosis or portal cirrhosis or to other causes such as congenital hepatic fibrosis and the Budd-Chiari syndrome.

Investigations

The order of the investigations will vary depending on whether there is an acute or chronic presentation.

1. Complete haematological examination: Hb%, packed cell volume, leucocyte and platelet counts to detect hypersplenism, if any
2. Prothrombin time
3. Barium swallow to outline oesophageal varices. It must be remembered that varices may be collapsed for some time after a severe bout of bleeding
4. Endoscopy — a fibreoptic oesophagogastroscope may show the site of bleeding as well as the grade of oesophageal or gastric varices
5. Liver function tests
6. Grouping and matching of blood
7. Ultrasonography
8. Percutaneous splenoportography — which also gives a renal pyelogram

Management

Haemorrhage from oesophageal varices is an emergency and is managed conservatively by:

- Blood transfusion
- Sedation
- Nasogastric intubation for aspiration and gastric lavage with iced saline
- Nursing in a propped up position
- Penicillin parenterally for any upper respiratory tract infection
- Frequent, regular monitoring of the central venous pressure, pulse rate, blood pressure, urinary output, haemoglobin and packed corpuscular volume levels
- Vitamin K and calcium injections

In almost all the children, bleeding will stop with these measures. However, if the bleeding continues intravenous injection of Pitressin may be tried.

Oesophageal tamponade using a Blakemore-Sengstaken tube is not advocated in children. The tube is difficult to pass and poorly retained in small babies; moreover, there is a definite risk of regurgitation of accumulated saliva into the tracheobronchial tree.

Endoscopic sclerotherapy

Recently, endoscopic injection of sclerosing agents into the varices has been effectively used. In a significant number of cases the varices can be successfully sclerosed avoiding the need for portosystemic shunt.

Portosystemic shunt surgery

A splenorenal shunt is the most commonly used shunt but if the splenic vein is not large enough, a mesocaval shunt is used. Shunt surgery should, as far as possible, be delayed till the child is 8–10 years of age by which time the veins to be used attain an adequate size. Till that time conservative measures including sclerotherapy should be tried. In some cases adequate collaterals may develop with the passage of time and a shunt may not be required. Shunt patency can be easily assessed by urinary fructose examination, after fructose loading, before and after shunt.

HEPATOMEGALY

A variety of conditions may produce liver enlargement. Most of these are 'medical' causes. Surgery is indicated in the following groups of conditions:

1. Liver abscess — amoebic or pyogenic
2. Liver cysts — parasitic or neoplastic
3. Liver tumours
   (a) Benign: haemangioma, haemangio-endothelioma, hamartoma
   (b) Malignant:
   Primary — hepatoblastoma, adenocarcinoma
   Secondary — neuroblastoma, Hodgkin's disease, lymphoma, leukaemia, Wilm's tumour

Liver abscess

Abscess of the liver is relatively uncommon in children. In the developing countries, a liver abscess is more often amoebic than pyogenic.

Amoebic abscess

The child with an amoebic abscess has malaise, a diminished appetite, fever, intercostal tenderness, right upper abdominal pain and mild jaundice. The abscess may produce a smooth and tender enlargement of the liver. It may occasionally rupture into the right pleura or the abdominal cavity. Infection is caused by drinking contaminated water or by ingestion of uncooked green vegetables. In less than half the cases there is a history of amoebic dysentery preceding the liver abscess. Entamoeba histolytica travels from the gut to the liver via the portal vein radicles. The posterior superior part of the right lobe of the liver is most commonly involved. The abscess cavity is devoid of a fibrous wall and, therefore, it easily collapses after aspiration.

Diagnosis. Presence of mobile amoebae in stools and a positive amoebic serology confirm the diagnosis. Ultrasonography accurately localizes the abscess and helps in following the effects of treatment. Needle aspiration will produce the so-called anchovy sauce pus, the microscopic examination of which may show trophozoites.

Treatment. Metronidazole orally or intravenously in the dosage of 7.5 mg to 10 mg/kg of body weight, 3 times a day for 8–10 days is the preferred mode of treatment. The pus is evacuated by needle aspiration, which may need to be repeated. Antibiotics are administered if secondary infection is present.

Pyogenic liver abscess

Pyogenic liver abscess is rare but occasionally seen in immunocompromised children. High fever with chills and rigors and a raised leucocyte count are often seen. There is continuous pain and acute tenderness in the right subcostal region. Jaundice, if present, is mild and the liver function tests are only slightly deranged. There may be an associated pleural effusion. Ultrasonography, CT and radioisotope scanning of the liver not only clinch the diagnosis, but also delineate the size and location of the abscess. At times there are several abscesses.

The bacteria responsible may enter via the lymphatics as in cholangitis, via the portal tract as in omphalitis, appendicitis or acute enteritis and via the bloodstream as in cases of subacute bacterial endocarditis. *Staph. aureus, Esch. coli, Salmonella typhi, Proteus* and *Pseudomonas* are the usual causative organisms. The possibility of anaerobes such as *Bacteroides*, either alone or in combination with pyogenic bacteria, must be kept in mind. Opportunistic fungal infections should also be considered.

Treatment. Surgical drainage is essential. Unlike amoebic abscesses, aspiration alone is inadequate and may, indeed, prove hazardous. Pyogenic liver abscesses carry a 50% mortality. Causes of death include rupture and peritonitis, septicaemia and interference with liver function, often due to inadequate drainage.

Liver cysts

Congenital cysts of the liver

These may be:

- Solitary simple cysts — hamartomatous mesenchymal cyst
- Multiple cysts — polycystic disease of the liver

Simple solitary cysts are filled with clear serous fluid and hardly ever communicate with intrahepatic biliary channels. They present as painless liver swellings. It is often possible to remove the cyst by cystectomy or wedge excision.

Polycystic disease is an inherited autosomal defect which may coexist with polycystic disease of the kidneys.

Hydatid cyst

Hydatid cysts of the liver are caused by the helminth *Echinococcus*. An older child may present with 'liver enlargement' which may be smooth or irregular. There may be some abdominal pain or discomfort. Rarer presentations are as biliary colic and jaundice due to passage of cysts into the common bile duct or as acute abdomen due to sudden bursting of the cysts into the peritoneal cavity with concomitant shock.

Diagnosis. The methods of diagnosis include:

1. The Casoni intradermal test and indirect haemagglutination tests for hydatid disease are diagnostic, but false negatives are common
2. Plain X-ray of the abdomen may show calcification in the cyst wall
3. Ultrasonography
4. Radionuclide scanning of the liver

Treatment. The cysts consist of an outer fibrous wall (exocyst) belonging to the host and an inner parasitic cyst (endocyst). The inner membrane of the endocyst bears the scolices and the daughter cysts. At laparotomy the fluid is aspirated from the cysts, after taking due precautions to avoid seepage of the fluid containing daughter cysts into the peritoneal cavity. It is replaced by an equal amount of hypertonic saline or 95% alcohol to kill the residual scolices inside the cyst prior to removal. After 5 minutes a small incision is made in the cyst wall and when the cyst collapses a little it is enucleated intact. If this is not possible the contents are evacuated by suction and with spoon. Calcified and infected cysts need excision of the entire cyst. Before closing, the abdomen is searched for extrahepatic cysts which may be in the omentum, spleen and at times in the common bile duct. Long-term treatment with mebendazole has been found useful for the treatment of hydatid cysts.

Liver tumours

Benign tumours are rare. They may be epithelial, mesodermal or teratomatous in origin. Epithelial tumours are adenomas arising from liver cells or bile ducts. Mesodermal tumours are mesenchymal hamartomas or vascular tumours such as haemangiomas and haemangioendotheliomas: they are not premalignant conditions.

Vascular tumours (cavernous haemangioma or haemangioendothelioma) are seen in early childhood. They present as hepatomegaly often with congestive heart failure.

A tumour-like lesion, 'focal nodular hyperplasia', has been described which must be distinguished from malignant tumours by an open biopsy.

Malignant tumours of the liver

These may be primary tumours or metastic deposits, usually from neuroblastoma or Wilm's tumour. Primary malignant tumours are rare and are mostly of two types, hepatoblastoma and rarely hepatocarcinoma (see Ch. 4).

PANCREAS

Pancreatic disorders are rather uncommon in children. Among the developmental anomalies, the commonest is annular pancreas, presenting as duodenal obstruction in the newborn. Other anomalies are very rare.

Pancreatitis

This is a very uncommon condition in childhood. It presents in one of the following forms:

- Acute pancreatitis or haemorrhagic pancreatitis
- Chronic relapsing or recurrent pancreatitis
- Traumatic pancreatitis, often forming a pseudocyst

Acute pancreatitis

This is more common than the chronic form. The condition often remains undiagnosed till a laparotomy is performed. Its milder form, seen as a complication of mumps, can be confused with appendicitis or peritonitis. The symptoms subside after a few days without any active treatment.

Acute fulminant or haemorrhagic pancreatitis presents as acute abdominal pain, jaundice, tachycardia, peripheral circulatory failure and coma. There is oedema, haemorrhage and at times septic infarction of the pancreas. The patient may have a preceding history of some acute febrile illness or vomiting, dehydration, diabetic acidosis, corticosteroid therapy, major surgery or thermal burns.

Other predisposing factors include hyperlipidaemia, cystic fibrosis and polyarteritis nodosa. However, in nearly two-thirds of cases no aetiological factors can be identified. Unlike this disease in adults, there is no obstruction due to stenosis or stones at the sphincter of Oddi. When associated with septicaemia, coliform organisms have been isolated from the infarcted pancreas.

Diagnosis. Serum and urinary amylase may be elevated to 3–5 times normal. Peritoneal tap reveals dark fluid with a considerably raised amylase level.

Treatment. The methods of treatment include:

1. Relief of pain by analgesics such as pethidine or pentazocine.
   Morphine produces spasm of the sphincter of Oddi and is contraindicated
2. Nothing by mouth and nasogastric suction, to reduce pancreatic secretion
3. Anticholinergic drugs
4. Intravenous fluids and electrolytes to replace losses in the peritoneal cavity, around the pancreas and in the paralysed gastrointestinal tract. Calcium supplements are given to replace calcium lost to saponification of necrotic tissue
5. Adequate parenteral nutrition
6. Treatment of shock. Monitor pulse, haematocrit, urinary output and central venous pressure
7. Antibiotics to combat infection

If the diagnosis is not clear, laparotomy is performed and the lesser sac is drained. Associated predisposing factors are investigated.

Chronic pancreatitis

This is due to a variety of causes producing obstruction to the flow of pancreatic juice. The presentation is in the form of recurrent attacks of abdominal pain radiating to the lumbar spine and weight loss. There may, at times, be associated steatorrhoea and diabetes. A chronically inflamed pancreas has a hard, fibrosed, nodular feel. There may be segmental dilatation of the pancreatic duct with evidence of stasis due to stricture or stenosis of the duct, a stone in the ampulla or a choledochal cyst.

Investigation. Radiological examination of the gastrointestinal and biliary tracts are mandatory. An upper gastrointestinal series may show some widening of the duodenal loop due to an oedematous pancreas. Direct cannulation of the pancreatic duct using a flexible fibreoptic gastroduodenoscope shows areas of stricture alternating with segmental ectasia. Surgery aims at instituting a free ductal drainage by removing or bypassing the obstruction.

Pseudocysts of the pancreas

Although congenital and neoplastic cysts are known, they are rare; most cysts of the pancreas are pseudocysts. Pseudocysts are produced by the collection of pancreatic juice in the lesser sac following blunt abdominal trauma or acute pancreatitis. Classically, a bicycle handle-bar injury crushes the pancreas against the lumbar vertebrae resulting in seepage of the juice from the severed duct. This history of blunt injury may be several weeks and at times a few months before the appearance of symptoms such as epigastric pain, loss of appetite, vomiting and upper abdominal distension.

Barium meal examination shows a retrogastric collection, displacing the stomach upwards, transverse colon downwards and widening the duodenal loop. Ultrasonography and CT scan of the abdomen provide an adequate localization of the cyst.

Treatment

Internal drainage of the cyst into the posterior wall of the stomach (cystogastrostomy) or Roux-en-Y cystojejunostomy give very good results.

Pancreatic neoplasia

There are three main groups, non-beta islet cell tumours producing the Zollinger-Ellison syndrome, islet cell adenoma (insulinoma), and carcinoma. These are extremely rare and will not be discussed further.

FURTHER READING

Altman R P, Stolar C J H 1985 Pediatric hepatobiliary disease in: Symposium on Pediatric Surgery Part I. Surgical Clinics of North America 65: 5, 1245–1268
Eichelberger M R, Hoelzer D J, Koop C E 1982 Acute pancreatitis. The difficulties of diagnosis and therapy. Journal of Pediatric Surgery 17: 244–254
Eraklis A J, Filler R M 1972 Splenectomy in Childhood. A review of 1413 cases. Journal of Pediatric Surgery 7: 382–388

Fonkalsrud E W 1980 Surgical management of portal hypertension in childhood. Archives of Surgery 115: 1042–1045

Mitra S K, Kumar V, Datta D V, et al 1978 Extrahepatic portal hypertension. A review of 70 cases. Journal of Pediatric Surgery 13: 51–54

Robertson J F R, Carachi R, Sweet E M, Raine A P M 1988 Cholelithiasis in childhood. A follow-up study. Journal of Pediatric Surgery 23: 246–249

10. Conditions causing deformities of the skeleton

W. K. Chung

Deformities of bone and joint may be dynamic or structural, static or progressive. They may be the result of skeletal deformation, soft-tissue contractures, muscular imbalance or simply postural. Management begins with the identification of the nature and causation of a deformity.

These conditions can be classified into two main groups: congenital disorders and disorders of posture and gait.

CONGENITAL DISORDERS

The common causes of congenital disorders are shown in Table 10.1.

Table 10.1 Congenital disorders

1. **Local congenital disorders**
   Congenital hip instability
   Congenital talipes equinovarus
   Infantile torticollis
2. **Generalised congenital disorders**
   Skeletal dysplasia
   Arthrogryposis multiplex congenita
   Down syndrome
   Muscular dystrophies
   Marfan syndrome
   Osteogenesis imperfecta

LOCAL GONGENITAL DISORDERS

Congenital hip instability (congenital dislocation of the hip)

The congenitally unstable hip, which manifests in varying degrees of instability, is the result of genetic and environmental factors. The incidence varies considerably amongst different racial groups, being in the order of 3 per 1000 live births in Australia, North America and northwest Europe. The incidence is much higher in Japanese, Navajo Indians and Yugoslavs. It is uncommon in the Chinese. The ratio of girls to boys is 6:1 and of unilateral to bilateral 2:1. Breech births and first borns are more vulnerable. The incidence is higher in children born with significant postural or structural foot deformities, e.g. calcaneovalgus, congenital club foot, torticollis and infantile scoliosis. Genetically, the risk to a succeeding sibling of an affected child is 6% where the parents are normal, and 36% when one parent suffers from the condition.

There is variable influence from genetic and environmental factors. Two physical attributes, joint laxity and acetabular dysplasia, are seen to be related to the production of congenital hip instability. Joint laxity is a factor in neonatal instability and may be due to transient influence of maternal 'relaxin' hormones. Acetabular dysplasia is a factor in hip dislocations diagnosed after the neonatal period.

Diagnosis

Diagnosis of the unstable hip is clinical. Every infant should be examined soon after birth and again before discharge from hospital. The infant should not be crying or irritable during the examination. It is better to return later for a re-examination if ideal conditions cannot be obtained. The examination should be performed on a firm surface, not in the baby's cot or mother's lap. Inspect for groin, thigh or gluteal asymmetry and the posture of the lower limbs. The presence of an excessively turned out leg, foot deformities or torticollis should heighten suspicion of an abnormal hip.

111

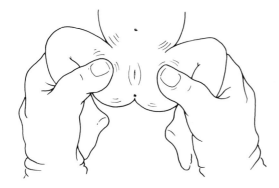

Fig. 10.1 Examination of the hip in a neonate for congenital dislocation.

The leg to be examined is flexed at the hip and knee (Fig. 10.1). The examiner's thumb overlies the lesser trochanter, the middle finger supports the greater trochanter. With the opposite hand the pelvis is steadied by holding the buttock and anterior pelvis between fingers and thumb respectively. The hip is then abducted and adducted gently. The examiner palpates for a sensation of dislocation when adducting the hip and of relocation when abducting the hip. In a dislocatable hip, a visible and palpable jerk can be felt when the hip dislocates with adduction. When this hip relocates with abduction a visible, palpable and often audible 'jerk of re-entry' is elicited (Ortolani's sign).

Lesser grades of instability (subluxation) produce less dramatic signs and require more sensitivity in the examination. A subluxatable hip will not produce a visible jerk or an audible clunk, rather it gives a sensation of insecurity of the hip in adduction. 'Clicks' not associated with palpable movement of the femoral head out of the hip socket are innocent and do not require treatment. At the other end of the spectrum is a hip that is dislocated at birth and will not relocate with the usual manual examination. This represents a teratological dislocation and will usually require operative reduction at some stage.

X-rays in the first 3 months of life are of little value. Ultrasonography is increasingly used as an aid in diagnosis. There seems little doubt that when the investigation is performed properly and by a skilled ultrasonographist, it is a reliable tool. It is a very useful investigation to confirm proper reduction of a hip when the child is in a brace or hip spica.

Neonatal screening programmes carried out in Australia and other parts of the world have not eliminated late diagnosis of congenital dislocation of the hip (CDH). It reflects the difficulty in establishing the presence of an unstable hip in the neonatal period.

Many hips are unstable (either subluxatable or dislocatable) at birth due to joint laxity. Most of these will stabilize spontaneously over the first week. In fact, about one in 100 neonates will show signs of hip instability when examined soon after birth. Without treatment most of these children will have normal hips after a week or two. Those who still have abnormal hip signs represent true congenital hip dislocations.

Except for the teratological dislocation, neonates, even with hip dislocations, usually have a full range of hip motion. Untreated true cases of CDH will develop contracture of the adductors by the age of 3 months and at that stage limitation of abduction in flexion represents an important physical sign. In fact, all infants with asymmetrical or absolute loss of abduction should be examined clinically and radiographically for hip instability. A leg length discrepancy will be present if the hip is constantly dislocated and other features such as delay in walking and waddling gait will manifest in the child over a year old.

Besides the neonatal examination, all children with a resolved hip instability or who are in the high-risk category (positive family history, foot deformities, infantile torticollis) should have a further clinical and radiographic examination at 4–6 months of age. By this age there is ossification of the upper femoral epiphysis and radiographs are far more reliable than they were in the neonatal age.

Treatment

The goal of treatment is essentially to obtain a stable and concentric reduction of the femoral head in the acetabulum. This is consistently achieved (95%) within the first 6 months by positioning and maintaining the hip in a reduced physiological position of flexion and abduction.

A variety of braces can be used though the Pavlik harness is most popular at the present time. This particular brace is attractive in that it is not a static brace and permits movements of the hip within the 'stable zone' (the range of abduction and flexion within which the hip remains stable in reduction). Regardless of the type of brace used, treatment is not without the potential risk of osteonecrosis of the femoral head. Osteonecrosis or avascular necrosis is the result of vascular embarrassment to the femoral head. Even the normal hip is vulnerable to this complication whilst in a brace.

Excessive abduction (more than 45°) has been shown to interfere with blood flow to the femoral head, and must be avoided. Flexion is safe and most hips should be braced in at least 60° of flexion and not more than 45° of abduction. Bearing in mind the risk of avascular necrosis and the high percentage of neonatal hip instability that resolves spontaneously, treatment should not be embarked on lightly. As the majority of unstable hips discovered during the neonatal period will stabilize without treatment, it is reasonable to actively treat only those that are grossly unstable or who already have some limitation of abduction. The rest may be re-examined in 3 weeks and if they are found to still have signs of instability, they may then receive brace treatment. Double nappies have no useful role in the management of CDH.

A stable reduction must be achieved with the brace within a month, otherwise a closed reduction and plaster spica immobilization is necessary. Ultrasonography is particularly useful in this context as it reduces the need for X-rays. Occasionally it is difficult to know if a reduction is concentric. In such situations, an arthrogram is indicated. An arthrogram will outline the cartilaginous femoral epiphysis and its relation to the acetabulum and labral cover. A reduction is not concentric or complete if there is soft tissue interposing between the femoral head and acetabulum. A femoral head that fails to seat deep into its acetabulum will not develop properly. A properly reduced hip will generally stabilize after 2–3 months of brace treatment depending on the age at which treatment is commenced. Children who achieve stable reductions will need to be followed up till they have started walking.

Brace treatment can be effective up to the age of 6 months after which children who present with CDH will usually have developed significant soft-tissue contractures. Such contractures prevent the safe and effective reduction of the hip. The majority up to the age of 2 years can still be managed successfully by closed methods which generally involve the use of prereduction traction followed by a closed reduction (under general anaesthetic) and immobilization in a hip spica. An adductor tenotomy is usually required to relieve tightness of the contracted adductor muscles. Persistent adductor tightness increases the risk of avascular necrosis during treatment in a plaster spica. If a concentric reduction is obtained, the hip is sufficiently stable after 3 months for the plaster spica to be removed and for an abduction brace (e.g. Denis-Browne abduction brace) to be applied in its place till adequate acetabular development is seen to have occurred. This treatment programme takes at least 6 months to complete. If reduction has been unsuccessful or imperfect, an open reduction is required. At times a femoral osteotomy is required to stabilize a reduction. If the acetabulum is dysplastic, a pelvic osteotomy, such as the innominate osteotomy, may be required.

The missed congenital dislocation

The older child (after the age of 2 years) who presents with CDH will generally require operative treatment. Those who present after the age of 4 years remain a major challenge in paediatric orthopaedics. Unilateral dislocations in this group should be actively treated as their limp from leg length discrepancy and hip instability is quite unacceptable. Serious consideration needs to be given before embarking on complex surgery to treat an older bilateral CDH. The incidence and severity of complications are high. Osteonecrosis is a common complication of late surgery. Incomplete reduction results in conversion of a dislocation to a subluxation and with it the risk of osteoarthritis in early adult life.

As the dislocations are established for some years, the femoral head and acetabulum are malformed, the femoral head rides up high on the pelvis and the soft tissues, including the long muscles around the hip, are severely shortened. To achieve the reduction of such hips, extensive release of the soft tissues is required and in spite of this, the femoral head cannot be readily brought down into the acetabulum. The femur is surgically shortened (Klisic procedure) to allow the femoral head down to the level of the acetabulum. The acetabulum is underdeveloped (acetabular dysplasia) and is shallow, lacking its normal concavity. The acetabulum has, therefore, to be reconstructed by some form of acetabuloplasty (e.g. innominate osteotomy). The end result may be a stable reduction but hardly ever a normal hip.

Congenital talipes equinovarus

Congenital talipes equinovarus (clubfoot) invariably requires active treatment to achieve an anatomically acceptable foot. The incidence amongst Caucasians is approximately 1 per 1000 live births. It is 300 times more common in monozygotic twins, 25 times more common in first degree relatives and 5 times more common in second degree relatives. The Chinese and Japanese have a lower incidence but the condition is common amongst Polynesians. It affects males twice as often as females.

The basic cause of clubfoot is not known. Diverse theories about its aetiology reflect the difficulty of separating the primary or essential malformations from secondary adaptive changes. It is clear that the deformity is established in utero and that there is malformation of the talus, variable degrees of ankle, subtalar and midtarsal joint deformities, as well as soft-tissue contracture. Although there is some controversy, it is likely that clubfoot is most often of multifactorial aetiology with possibly a major gene effect as well.

The deformity combines equinus and varus of the hindfoot with adduction and supination of the forefoot (Fig. 10.2). The presence of hindfoot deformity differentiates clubfoot from innocent metatarsus adductus. The foot is stiff. This discriminates clubfoot from postural and paralytic equinovarus feet. The calf is thin and the heel

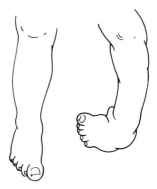

Fig. 10.2 Normal right foot compared with a left talipes equinovarus foot.

looks small and is difficult to palpate. There is obvious asymmetry with reduction in foot size, calf girth and leg length. A general examination for associated abnormalities such as hip dysplasia, torticollis and deformity of the opposite foot is essential.

X-rays are of no value in the diagnosis of the condition.

Treatment

Approximately 50% can be successfully treated without surgery. The non-operative treatment of congenital clubfoot should begin on the day of diagnosis. With the exception of neonates requiring complex intensive care, there is no excuse for deferring passive correction and splintage. This ensures that stretching and manipulation coincides with the maximaun pliability of ligaments conferred by maternal hormones. Manipulative correction of the clubfoot deformity is better described as gradual closed reduction of the malaligned joints. It should be frequent, repetitive and gentle. There is no doubt that over-enthusiastic wrenching of the foot, as practised in the past, leads to bone and cartilage deformation and joint stiffness. The foot may be splinted in plaster slabs, full plaster casts or arrangements of slings and strappings (strap and buckle method). Such splints may be gradually weaned when full correction of all components of the clubfoot deformity is achieved. It is then necessary to maintain correction with special shoes or boots fitted to external rotation bars

(Denis-Browne boots and bars) to be worn in the evenings.

Soft-tissue surgery is indicated for those patients in whom a supple, mobile correction is not obtained within the first 6 months. Persistent hindfoot equinus and varus usually indicate the need for operative treatment. There is no general consensus on either timing of surgery or selection of operative procedures. Differences in treatment protocols reflect the diversity of views regarding what constitutes a satisfactory result and the extent of surgery necessary to achieve good results. Where possible, soft-tissue surgery commences before 6 months and involves the release of such soft-tissue constraints as are necessary to effect correction of the subtalar, ankle and midtarsal joint deformities. Following operative treatment the foot is kept in maintenance plasters for 2 to 3 months after which special shoes or boots are prescribed. Operative treatment then is merely an incident in the ongoing corrective treatment programme.

Final assessment of treatment cannot be made until the foot is skeletally mature. Relapses are frequent and evolve from incomplete initial correction. For late-diagnosed or relapsed cases, treatment is directed at salvaging a plantigrade foot and semblance of normality. The parents of a newborn child with talipes equinovarus can be assured that, if successful, treatment will bestow a perfectly adequate degree of agility and athletic ability, although it is unlikely that these patients will achieve top class performance in explosive athletic events.

Infantile torticollis

Wryneck or torticollis describes a tilting of the neck and head towards one shoulder. This may be the result of irritative, mechanical or neurological lesions. Congenital anomalies, particularly those involving the occipitocervical junction, e.g. atlanto-occipital fusion or Klippel-Feil syndrome, may cause mechanical restriction of motion and present with torticollis. Viral or bacterial pharyngitis, cervical osteomyelitis, soft-tissue or skeletal injury of the neck are causes of irritative torticollis. Children with skeletal dysplasia, Down syndrome and juvenile rheumatoid arthritis

should be examined carefully for atlanto-axial instability if they present with a wryneck. Tumours of the posterior fossa, spinal cord and vertebrae are often accompanied by torticollis. Infantile torticollis represents the most common form of torticollis (see Ch. 3). An important association in this group is congenital hip instability (20%).

GENERALIZED CONGENITAL DISORDERS

These are well described in standard texts and only key features will be mentioned here.

Skeletal dysplasia

Constitutional diseases of bone and cartilage are broadly grouped under skeletal dysplasia. Achondroplasia represents the classic form of short-limb dwarf. Today over 100 conditions are recognized and separable into dysplasias, dysostoses and dystrophies. Although specific enzyme defects have been recognized in some skeletal dysplasias and better genetic characterization achieved with others, diagnosis is generally made clinically on the basis of recognizable features and abnormalities. Accurate and early diagnosis is necessary to allow prediction of ultimate height, deformities, other medical problems and for genetic counselling.

Achondroplasia

This is the most common and best known skeletal dysplasia. It is transmitted by autosomal dominant inheritance. The principal orthopaedic concerns are with deformities of the spine and limbs. Thoracolumbar kyphosis, if persistent and progressive, may lead to cord compression. Lumbar spinal stenosis becomes a clinical problem in adulthood and may require spinal decompression. Genu varum is the most common deformity to require treatment. Osteotomy of the tibia combined with shortening or epiphyseodesis of the fibula is required to correct a significant deformity.

Other dysplasias

A wide spectrum of skeletal abnormalities is seen in skeletal dysplasias. One should look for alteration in stature, proportion, deformities of the spine, ligamentous laxity, joint instability, angular deformities of the limbs, changes in bone density and premature joint degeneration. The most serious complications are the result of thoraco-lumbar kyphosis and instability of the cervical spine.

Arthrogryposis multiplex congenita

Arthrogryposis is taken from two Greek words to describe 'curved joints'. It is now recognized that any lesion affecting the final neuromuscular pathway during the formation of the limbs in utero can result in congenital contractures. The syndrome of arthrogryposis multiplex congenita therefore represents a heterogenous group of conditions causing non-progressive, congenital joint contractures with frequent dislocations. It occurs once in 3000 births. As the aetiological and genetic basis is varied, genetic counselling is difficult. Deformities of the extremities may be in flexion or extension. In the classical case, the upper limbs are internally rotated, the elbows stiff in extension, the hands and wrists flexed, there is flexion contracture of the knees and severe clubfoot deformities. Treatment to restore function is technically difficult, with significant incidence of relapse and may include early surgical releases, prolonged splintage, osteotomies and tendon transfers.

Down syndrome

This is the best known of chromosomal abnormalities. It is usually due to trisomy 21. These children have delayed physical milestones, but will achieve independent ambulation. Their orthopaedic problems relate to ligamentous laxity. The most important consideration is with their potential for atlanto-axial instability (20%). All children with Down syndrome should have periodic cervical spine X-rays. Where significant instability is demonstrated, stabilization by an atlanto-axial fusion is required. Even those children with no demonstrable instability should be kept away from body contact sports. Painless and often voluntary hip dislocations are seen with these children. Such dislocations are easily relocated but are not stabilized by usual conservative measures such as plaster spicas and braces. Operative treatment is not necessarily indicated where closed treatment fails. Occasionally surgical tightening of the lax, redundant hip capsule may be required (capsulorrhaphy). Osteotomies of the femur or pelvis are less frequent requirements.

Muscular dystrophies

This is a collection of genetically inherited, primary, skeletal muscle diseases. The most common muscular dystrophy is the Duchenne type, others being the limb girdle and facio-scapulo-humeral types.

Orthopaedic treatment is aimed at keeping the child ambulant as long as possible and then to minimize uncomfortable contractures of the extremities and deformities of the spine.

Marfan syndrome

The main orthopaedic problems are in the feet and spine. Progressive scoliosis occurs in 10–20% of cases and brace treatment is often unsuccessful. Children with Marfan syndrome have long and thin feet which make shoe-fitting difficult. These feet are severely flat and rolled out (plano-valgus). They may become stiff and painful later and may require surgical treatment in the form of a triple arthrodesis.

Osteogenesis imperfecta

This connective tissue disease is characterized by congenital osteoporosis, fragile bones (osseous fragilis), abnormal tooth development (dentino-genesis imperfecta), short stature and hearing deficit. It is genetically heterogenous and about half the cases are the result of mutation.

The child born with multiple fractures of broad, crumpled long bones and ribs is unlikely to survive (90% mortality) and if he/she does, will not walk. Those born with fractures but who have less abnormal looking long bones and ribs, generally survive but growth is quite severely affected, and they are eventually wheelchair dependent. Parents of children with birth fractures do not usually suffer the disease.

Fractures in these children heal normally and are treated by reduction and splintage. Deformities of the weight-bearing limbs may require surgical splintage. Spinal deformities are common and are difficult to manage. Kyphoscoliosis is the usual deformity. Brace treatment is not effective due to the softness of the rib cage. Spinal fusion with instrumentation may be required but is technically difficult.

DISORDERS OF POSTURE AND GAIT

Parental concern regarding a child's posture or gait constitutes one of the most common causes for consultation with a paediatric orthopaedic surgeon. Often the complaint is non-specific — 'my child walks funny' or '. . . stands crooked'. Even when the complaint is localized to a specific region of the body, a systematic examination is necessary as the apparent fault may originate from a distant deformity, e.g. a flexible scoliosis may be due to leg length inequality, or, as in the case of in-toeing, the problem is often that of rotational deformity of the hips.

The common causes are shown in Table 10.2.

SPINAL DEFORMITIES

Scoliosis

Scoliosis is an abnormal lateral curvature of the spine. Non-structural curves are flexible and they disappear on forward flexion while structural curves do not (Fig. 10.3). Flexible curves may be postural or due to leg length inequality. A sci-

Table 10.2 Disorders of posture and gait

1. **Spinal deformities**
   Scoliosis
   Juvenile kyphosis
   Spondylolisthesis

2. **Torsional deformities of the lower limb**
   Persistent femoral anteversion
   Internal tibial torsion

3. **Angular deformities of the lower limb**
   Genu varum
   Genu valgum

4. **Aberrations of foot shape and arch**
   Postural calcaneovalgus
   Metatarsus adductus/varus
   Pes planus
   Pes cavus

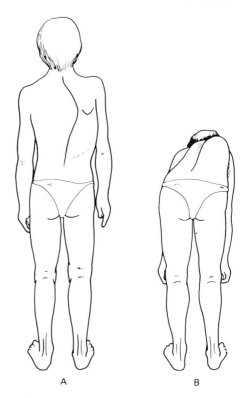

A B

Fig. 10.3 Scoliosis. **A**: Spinal curvature. **B**: Rib hump prominence on flexion.

atic scoliosis is not truly structural, but may not disappear on bending because of stiffness and pain. Such curves are the result of irritative lesions in the spine, e.g. an acute prolapse of the intervertebral disc.

There are two essential components to the structural scoliotic curves: lateral deviation and rotation. The lateral deviation results in a tilt of the shoulder or pelvis. The rotational deformity causes a rib hump when the curve is thoracic, or a paravertebral muscle hump with lumbar curves. The deformity is best assessed in an erect posteroanterior roentgenogram.

Idiopathic adolescent scoliosis is the most common variety of scoliosis, but other causes of the deformity must be excluded first. A scoliotic deformity may be the result of congenital vertebral anomaly, e.g. hemivertebrae, incomplete segmentation. Some curves are due to muscle imbalance and a spectrum of neuromuscular diseases need to be considered, e.g. poliomyelitis, cerebral palsy or syringomyelia.

A degree of scoliosis is detectable in 5% of the

adolescent population. The vast majority of curves are mild and of no consequence; 85% of significant curves occur in girls. Such curves appear during the prepubertal period, usually coinciding with the growth spurt.

The aetiology of idiopathic scoliosis is unknown. There is certainly a familial tendency and a multifactorial inheritance is suggested. Curves are to the right or left according to the convexity; they are thoracic, lumbar or thoracolumbar or double according to site. Eighty per cent of the thoracic curves are to the right and the same proportion of lumbar curves are left-sided. Thoracolumbar curves are commonly to the right.

Minor curves are common (5 to 15°) and most do not progress much. Minor curves do not require active treatment but should be observed until skeletal maturity. A curve is most likely to progress if it is more than 20°, or if the patient is young. The adolescent growth spurt starts about a year before menarche for girls and most growth ceases 2 years after menarche. Curves of moderate severity (20 to 40°) in patients who are actively growing require control in a brace.

A variety of braces are available and are chosen according to the location of the deformity. Braces are maintained till growth ceases. More severe curves cannot be controlled effectively by bracing and may require surgical stabilization. Useful correction can be achieved with a variety of modern instrumentation and the correction is maintained by means of spinal fusion. The consequences of severe, untreated scoliosis amount to more than the cosmetic blemish. Thoracic curves of more than 60° affect cardiorespiratory function adversely and severe lumbar curves lead to chronic back pain in later adult life.

Juvenile kyphosis

An abnormal increase of thoracic kyphosis with compensatory increase of lumbar lordosis is seen occasionally in the adolescent. This topic is discussed in Chapter 11.

Spondylolisthesis

This condition presents usually as a cause of backpain but is more conveniently discussed in this section.

Spondylolisthesis is an abnormal forward slip (olisthesis) of the vertebrae. It occurs predominantly at the lumbosacral level and is usually the result of a defect in the pars interarticularis. There are several types of spondylolisthesis recognized by conventional classification according to causation, though some types are not seen in paediatric patients, e.g. degenerative spondylolisthesis. Isthmic spondylolisthesis represents the main category and here the basic defect is in the pars interarticularis. It is an acquired condition in most patients, although there seems to be a genetic predisposition in the development of a pars interarticularis defect.

Children and adolescents involved in sports such as gymnastics and football are much more likely to develop a spondylolisthesis than is the public at large. Repetitive hyperextension stress to the pars interarticularis is felt to cause fatigue fractures and subsequently an olisthesis. An acute fracture of the pars, if recognized, is treated by appropriate immobilization with prospects of healing. A less common variety is dysplastic spondylolisthesis in which there is no defect of the pars, but there is instead congenital abnormalities of the upper sacrum or arch of the fifth lumbar vertebra. In this type of spondylolisthesis neurological problems can arise even with relatively minor degrees of slip.

The condition is often asymptomatic but is a relatively common cause of lumbar back pain in the adolescent. The pain is usually localized to the low lumbar area but may be referred to the posterior thigh. Compressive radiculitis is uncommon in this age group.

The patient with spondylolisthesis has a typical posture characterized by increased lumbar lordosis. A palpable and occasionally visible step is present at the level of slip. The hamstring muscles are often tight and hyperextension of the lumbar spine reproduces pain. The degree of olisthesis is best demonstrated in an erect, lateral X-ray of the lumbar spine. Oblique views show up the pars defect best.

Although spondylolisthesis may progress during childhood, progression is uncommon. The treatment depends on symptoms and degree of slip. In most instances, conservative treatment is effective. Operative treatment in the form of spinal fusion is indicated where pain is intractable or if there is progressive slip.

TORSIONAL DERFORMITIES OF THE LOWER LIMB

Gait and posture during the toddling and early childhood years tend to be subjects of many parents' concern. In-toeing or pigeon-toeing is the most common complaint. The cause of in-toeing can be simply determined by an organized clinical examination.

The most convenient and effective way to examine a child for in-toeing is to lie the child prone with the knees to 90° and ankles set at neutral. The examiner looks from above the feet. From this position it is possible to determine the shape of the feet, the rotation of the leg and to assess the range of rotation of the hips. Merely from these three observations the cause of torsional deformity can be determined.

Metatarsus adductus

Metatarsus adductus or varus, is a condition in which the forefoot is turned in (adducted) in relation to the hindfoot. The deformity is frequently seen at birth and the vast majority disappear within the first 2–3 months. It probably represents a postural persistence of the fetal foot position. Metatarsus adductus is a flexible deformity and should be differentiated from the rare, rigid deformity of congenital metatarsus varus, which is far more recalcitrant to treatment.

The deformity seen at birth requires no treatment unless the deformity is severe, when simple plantar-medial splints are used. Those that persist after 3 months should be assessed and treatment undertaken if the deformity is significant. It is generally believed that most cases of metatarsus adductus will correct spontaneously without treatment by the age of 5 years. However, those that do persist after that age will not respond well to conservative plaster treatment. Therefore, for those feet with significant deformity after the age of 3 months it is preferable to commence early

treatment. Treatment at this stage is relatively simple and consistently effective. Serial plaster cast correction over a period of 6 weeks will correct almost all deformities. The corrected feet are then kept in special outflare shoes for about a year.

Persistent femoral anteversion

Femoral anteversion is a normal feature of the human hip joint. It is essentially the forward or anterior twisting of the proximal femora relative to the transverse axis of the knee. The degree of torsion determines the distribution of internal and external rotation available in the hip joint. Where the degree of anteversion is high, there is more internal rotation and less external rotation. Where it is excessive, the kneecaps point inwards or squint, in the relaxed, standing posture and the entire lower limb turns in when the child walks. This tendency is most obvious when the child is tired and it is a cause of clumsiness.

Femoral anteversion is present in all newborn hips, but is masked by the presence of lower femoral external torsion present also at this age. With the mechanical torque of walking this proximal femoral torsion reduces gradually over the years of growth and assumes the mild degree of adult femoral anteversion towards the end of skeletal growth. If there is an excessive degree of anteversion it will tend to manifest at around the age of 4 years. The best way to diagnose and assess the degree of femoral anteversion is to examine the range of hip rotation with the child lying prone. The adult hip rotates about 45° inwards and 50° outwards. A child whose hip rotates inwards more than 70° with a corresponding loss of external rotation has mild anteversion of the hips. If internal rotation exceeds 90°, the anteversion is severe.

Children with significant femoral anteversion will tend to sit quite comfortably in a 'W' position. This posture is not the cause of hip anteversion, but it may retard natural correction of the deformity and should therefore be discouraged. The vast majority of hips with excessive anteversion will correct spontaneously over the first 10 years. Even the occasional older children with persistent hip anteversion do not suffer significant disability. In them the problem is largely cosmetic and athletic ability is barely affected.

There is thus no need to treat the condition except in those with severe, persistent anteversion after the age of 10 years. In them there is the occasional indication for derotation by femoral osteotomy.

Internal tibial torsion

The tibia may be twisted medially in some children to cause the feet to point inwards. Internal tibial torsion is the most common cause of in-toeing in the second year of life. It is often associated with metatarsus adductus. At least 15–20% of infants have clinically apparent internal tibial torsion and as only 5% of adults have the deformity, it is obvious that spontaneous correction occurs in the majority. Most adults have, in fact, a mild degree of external tibial torsion.

The condition seen in infancy corrects rapidly without treatment in most cases. Those that persist after the age of 2 years may warrant treatment with derotation bars. Such devices are applied as night splints for 6–12 months. Correction is con-

sistent when treatment is started at this age and less effective after the age of 4 years.

There is hardly ever cause for surgical treatment because persistent deformity, even in the adult, causes no measurable disability.

ANGULAR DEFORMITIES OF THE LOWER LIMB

Most children exhibit a mild degree of genu varum or bow-leggedness during the first 2 years of life and of genu valgum — knock knees — between the ages of 2 and 5 years. The physiological bow-leg deformity may be exaggerated by associated internal tibial torsion and may concern parents. These parents can be reassured that spontaneous correction will take place over a 2 year period, and in fact their child may progress to the opposite deformity. A graph showing the normal progression from bow legs to knock knees is helpful in this explanation (Fig. 10.4).

Genu varum

Physiological genu varum of up to 30° can correct spontaneously. Persistent deformity is un-

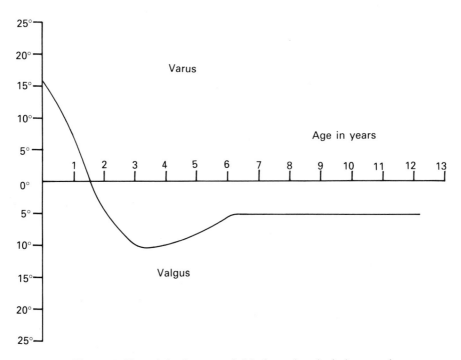

Fig. 10.4   Normal development of tibio-femoral angle during growth

common in Caucasians but is seen more commonly amongst Asian populations. A family history is usual for persistent genu varum.

The distance between the medial femoral condyles (with the child standing and the feet together) provides an objective way of assessing the deformity. A significant deformity is present if the intercondylar distance exceeds 5 cm. It is necessary to differentiate apparent bow-leggedness due to internal tibial torsion from angular deformity of the tibia. A child older than 4 years with significant or progressive genu varum may require splint treatment.

It is important to differentiate the innocent condition from a variety of pathological genu varum. Blount's disease is the most common form of pathological genu varum. This is probably a localized dysplasia of the postmedial portion of the upper tibial growth plate. The condition leads to progressive deformity and an aggressive infantile and less virulent adolescent variety is recognized. Unlike physiological and developmental genu varum, the treatment of Blount's disease is almost always surgical. Other forms of skeletal dysplasias, e.g. achondroplasia, and bone softening conditions such as rickets, cause genu varum as well.

Genu valgum

Knock-knees in children up to the age of 5 years can be safely ignored. Those that persist after the age of 7 years and are significant deformities require treatment considerations. The deformity is measured clinically by the separation of the medial malleoli (inter-malleolar distance) when the child is standing with his/her knees together. An inter-malleolar separation of 10 cm or a tibio-femoral angle greater than 15° represents a significant deformity. A full length, erect X-ray of the knees provides a more accurate assessment. The angle formed by the long axis of the tibia and femur (tibio-femoral angle) is normally below 10°.

Brace treatment is effective for lesser deformity but is cumbersome and not well tolerated at this age. Surgical treatment is usually preferred and relatively simple and effective. Growth in the medial portion of the lower femoral epiphysis can be arrested temporarily or permanently by stapling or surgical fusion. The procedures need to be timed according to the amount of remaining growth in the physeal plate.

ABERRATIONS OF FOOT SHAPE AND ARCH

Postural calcaneovalgus

Calcaneovalgus describes the foot that is dorsiflexed and everted. This is a very common deformity seen in the newborn. The deformity can be dramatic with the foot dorsiflexed against the shin, but there is always flexibility in the foot. This differentiates it from the rigid and more serious deformity of congenital vertical talus.

In the vast majority of cases, spontaneous correction occurs within the first 6 months. Treatment is not generally required though simple splinting and stretching will hasten correction in those feet that have some degree of stiffness.

Postural calcaneovalgus may be associated with a slightly high incidence of eventual pes planus. There is also a high incidence of associated congenital hip instability and a proper examination of the hip is mandatory.

Metatarsus adductus

This is discussed in a preceding section.

Pes planus

Neonatal feet appear flat due to the presence of a thick fat pad on the plantar-medial aspect and also because the medial longitudinal arch does not develop fully for the first 5 years. This apparent flatness of the foot is exaggerated by normal medial rotation of the hip and knees seen in this age range. The onset of walking will also increase the tendency for the feet to pronate and cause the feet to look even flatter. At the age of 2 years, almost 97% of normal children have some degree of flatness of the feet, but most will go on to normal arch development over the next few years. There is quite a high incidence of benign flat-feet in the general population (approximately 15–20%) and many of these have a familial predisposition.

Pes planus or hypermobile flat-feet is characterized by a loss of the medial longtitudinal arch, variable degrees of valgus of the hindfoot and pronation of the foot. The arch reconstitutes when the child stands on tip-toe, which is not the case in rigid, pathological flat-feet. The Achilles tendon may be tight and in severe and long-standing cases, the midtarsal joint mobility may be reduced.

Most cases, certainly those under the age of 5 years, do not require treatment. Treatment with orthosis can help reduce incidence of foot strain and abnormal shoe wear, but does not alter the natural history of the condition. Races that are shod and those that are unshod have similar incidence of flat-feet. Costly shoe modification is unjustified and operative treatment is rarely required and only for treatment of recalcitrant foot pain.

Pes cavus

An abnormal increase of the longitudinal arch is usually associated with some degree of varus of the forefoot and hindfoot. Cavovarus more accurately describes the deformity which may be idiopathic and developmental but more often the result of neuromuscular disease, e.g. Charcot-Marie Tooth or spinal dysraphism. A thorough neurological examination including a neurophysiological examination is necessary.

The structures on the plantar aspect of the foot, such as the plantar fascia and muscles, are contracted. The deformity it usually rigid and is often progressive and symptoms arise from abnormal weight-bearing and difficulties with shoe fitting. Operative treatment is directed at correcting the deformity and reducing pressure points for weight-bearing.

FURTHER READING

Williams P F 1982 Orthopaedic management in childhood, 1st edn. Blackwell Scientific Publications, London

11. Painful musculoskeletal conditions

W. K. Chung

Orthopaedic conditions, whether in the adult or child, present either with pain or deformity or both. In the child, skeletal growth is an additional dimension to consider in the natural history and therapy. Growth potential of the skeleton provides a mechanism for remodelling of a skeletal deformity, but where this growth potential is damaged partially or completely, shortening or asymmetry of the limb is exaggerated. This constitutes the cardinal consideration in management of paediatric orthopaedic diseases.

Sometimes obvious pain may not be the presenting symptom of a pain-causing condition. The affected limb may cease to function (pseudoparalysis) or a limp may be the source of distress. This is particularly common with younger children and infants; with them, the clinical examination will need to be more thorough and discerning. There are conditions like osteoid osteoma where few and subtle signs are evident in the early stages of the disease and pain is predominantly nocturnal.

Painful conditions of the skeleton may be idiopathic or the result of inflammatory (infections of bone and joints, rheumatic diseases), neoplastic, traumatic or idiopathic (osteochondritic) processes.

INFECTIONS OF BONES AND JOINTS

Acute osteomyelitis

Acute osteomyelitis (OM) may result from direct trauma though more usually from haematogenous spread from a distant and often unidentifiable focus. The skin, urinary and respiratory systems are possible foci of infection. Sustained intravenous cannulation in the neonate is a potential source of infection. Generally, one bone is involved and the commonest sites are the lower femur, upper tibia, the upper femur and upper humerus. The physiology and anatomy of the growing skeleton accounts for major differences between the skeletal infection of children and adults. The expanding metaphysis, the presence of a physeal plate and thickness of the immature periosteum, all contribute to the difference.

In children the infection almost invariably settles in the metaphysis due to the relative vascularity of the metaphysis, the hairpin arrangement of capillaries, and the vulnerability of growing cells to infection.

Staph. aureus accounts for the vast majority of infections (75–90%). Other causal organisms can be *Streptococcus*, *Pneumococcus*, *Esch. coli* and *H. influenza*. Infection of atypical sites, by atypical organisms or multicentricity, may suggest reduced immune capacity. OM may coexist with, and indeed mask a neoplasm, e.g. lymphoma.

A nidus of infection settles in the metaphyseal sinusoids and induces a localized hyperaemia. This phase of hyperaemia lasts 48 hours, during which time appropriate antibiotics given in adequate dosages can theoretically eradicate the illness. Soon an exudative phase follows with production of proteolytic enzymes and oedema. Tension builds within the rigid Volkmann's canals in the bone and ischaemia and pain results. Pus forms and this may break through the cortex causing a subperiosteal abscess. Redness and swelling of the overlying soft tissue is then apparent. A week may have passed since the onset of infection. Antibiotics alone will not eradicate

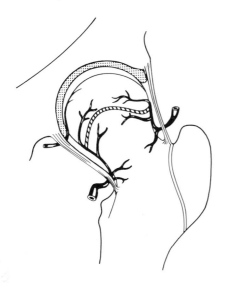

Fig. 11.1 The relationships of the epiphysis and blood supply of the upper femur to the capsule of the hip joint. All epiphyseal vessels have an intra-articular course.

the infection and surgical drainage is required. Local tissue tension and stripping of the periosteum causes ischaemia of the cortex and a sequestrum (necrotic bone) may result. Osteopenia and bone destruction seen at this stage may result in a pathological fracture. New bone forms in response to the periosteal stripping and there is thickening of the bone. If this bone formation is extensive, it constitutes an encasing involucrum which may contain holes (cloacae). The physeal plate serves as an effective barrier to extension of the infection into the epiphysis except in infants where terminal branches of nutrient arteries perforate the plate; this may allow an infection to cross the growth plate to cause an infective apophysitis and even septic arthritis. Septic arthritis may also follow OM of an intra-articular metaphysis, e.g. hip (Fig. 11.1).

Clinical features

The main clinical features are:

- Malaise
- Pyrexia
- Local pain

There is usually a few days of malaise and pyrexia followed by a rapidly increasing pain of the involved part. This pain is not relieved by rest and the child will tend not to move or use the limb (pseudoparalysis). Even in this early stage acute localized bone tenderness can be elicited. In the younger child or infant, the presentation is often more dramatic with gross systemic features due to septicaemia. When soft-tissue swelling and redness is present there is usually a subperiosteal abscess. Antibiotics will often alter this classical presentation and delay diagnosis.

In the neonate there is a non-septicaemic form of osteomyelitis with major bone destruction developing without general symptoms or signs and with minimal local symptoms and signs. Low levels of IgA have recently been reported in some affected neonates and this may persist into later childhood.

Investigations

A leukocytosis is present. The sedimentation rate is often above 55 mm/hr. Blood cultures will be positive in less than 50% of cases but should be routinely performed before starting antibiotics. Localization may be a problem and a technetium or gallium scan is the best method of localization in the early stages. There is no specific radiographic change for up to 10 days. The first sign may be that of soft-tissue swelling and this is not present for at least 48 hours, by which stage antibiotics alone are insufficient therapy. Localized rarefaction is next seen and at a later stage marginal sclerosis occurs as nature attempts to ward off the infection. Sequestrum and involucrum are late changes. Given appropriate and prompt treatment, most cases today should resolve without ever developing X-ray changes.

Differential diagnosis

Cellulitis, erysipelas, rheumatic fever, acute rheumatoid arthritis and sickle cell crisis may be difficult to differentiate from osteomyelitis. Septic arthritis, particularly in the infant, may confuse; indeed the infection may have arisen in bone and spread to the joint. Ewing's sarcoma may present with systemic and local signs similar to those of acute osteomyelitis. However, the presence of grey 'pus' at exploration and the finding of mononuclear cells with no organisms at exploration should arouse strong suspicions of Ewing's sarcoma.

Management

The diagnosis is clinical and treatment must be prompt. Where diagnosis is made within the first 36–48 hours, antibiotics in adequate doses can effect eradication of the disease. Antibiotics should be started once blood cultures have been taken. As most infections are due to *Staphylococcus*, flucloxacillin is the antibiotic of choice. Amoxycillin is given in addition in children between the ages of 4 months and 4 years to cover for *H. influenzae*. Appropriate adjustments are made after culture results are obtained. Effective antibiotics should cause reduction of pain and general clinical improvement within 24 hours. Where little or no improvement results, consider the possibilities that an abscess has formed (and surgical drainage is required) or that alternative antibiotics may be required.

Surgical treatment is required if an abscess is suspected. Where the focus is well defined and accessible, trephine needle aspiration may suffice. More often it is necessary to perform a formal open drainage. Where a subperiosteal abscess is present, a simple evacuation of this abscess is required. Cortical drilling is carried out where an intraosseous abscess is discovered which has not responded to antibiotics. The affected limb together with adjacent joints is splinted either by traction or plaster support to prevent joint contractures and pathological dislocations (where septic arthritis has occurred). Such splints are maintained till irritability of the limb settles.

Optimal duration of antibiosis is not firmly established. Factors that influence treatment duration include characteristics of the infecting organism, duration of established infection, extent of bone destruction, and host resistance. In general, paediatric patients require less sustained antibiotic treatment than adults. Where treatment had been prompt and minimal bone destruction has occurred, antibiotics are given for 6 weeks.

Complications

Septicaemia, metastatic infection, septic arthritis, an effect · on the adjacent physeal plate with resultant growth disturbance, overgrowth of bone due to metaphyseal hyperaemia and chronic osteomyelitis, all occur.

Chronic osteomyelitis

Chronic OM may occur either as a sequel to acute OM or may have an insidious onset. OM of the latter category such as tuberculosis will not be discussed in this chapter.

Where chronic OM follows acute OM it represents a failure to fully eradicate the primary illness. Often there is residual dead organic material (sequestrum) and the local tissue is dysvascular. There may be persistent cavitation of bone and in some chronic sinuses are present.

The dormant bacteria lead to recurrent flare-ups of infection characterized by local pain, swelling, redness and stiffness of the affected limb. There is usually pyrexia and even mild toxicity. The abscess may break through spontaneously to the surface and leak chronically through an established sinus track. Occasionally a sequestrum will discharge, leading to abatement of the acute infective episode. Where a sinus discharges chronically, the bacterial flora are mixed. *Streptococcus* accounts for many acute on chronic flare-ups.

Management

Management of chronic OM is generally conservative. Operative treatment is wisely restricted to specific goals as eradication of the disease by surgical treatment is unpredictable. Acute flare-ups are treated by bacteriological sampling, splintage, antibiotics and where a discharging sinus is present, with local irrigation and dressings to encourage decompression, extrusion of sequestrum and granulation. Patients with chronic OM often have had multiple courses of antibiotics and a short course of antibiotic to combat the acute situation is all that is necessary. There is little point in multiple long courses of antibiotics.

Surgical treatment is undertaken where there is a clear chance of eradicating the infection or where an abscess cavity or sequestrum is responsible for recurrent episodes of flare-ups. A simple incision, drainage and lavage is all that is required in most cases. Surgery directed at excising the chronic sinus track without successful eradication of the underlying bone disease is pointless.

Subacute osteomyelitis

The child is usually over the age of 8 years and presents with deep bone pain over the metaphyseal end of a long bone. Characteristically, the condition is silent for years and then there is episodic flare-up. There may be some local soft-tissue swelling during the symptomatic phase and an oval radiolucency is seen in the metaphysis. A variable margin of sclerosis is present. Treatment is surgical. The abscess is unroofed and the sclerotic abscess wall curetted. The abscess content is usually sterile.

Septic arthritis

Acute suppuration of joints may result from a penetrating injury (especially the knee), retained foreign body, spontaneous evacuation of an intra-articular focus of osteomyelitis or as a result of blood spread from a distant focus of OM. *Staphylococcus* is the most frequent offender. *H. influenza* accounts for 20–30% of infections between the ages of 4 months and 4 years, since up to the age of 4 months maternal antibodies confer protection. There is also a higher incidence of the organism in children with agammaglobulinaemia.

Gonococcus should be considered in the sexually active adolescent. *Candida albicans* is seen in multiple joint disease in children with immunodeficiency.

Management

When a diagnosis of septic arthritis is made, blood cultures are taken and parenteral antibiotics commenced. The child is then given a general anaesthetic and the joint needled for pus. A large bore (16 gauge) spinal needle is required. Successful entry into the joint must be confirmed by lavage technique. Bacteriological samples are taken and the joint washed out thoroughly. If cleansing of the joint is impeded by debri or viscosity of the pus, an arthrotomy should be per-

formed. Improvement is expected within several hours.

Antibiotics are given parenterally for at least a week and for as long as necessary to control the acute toxicaemia. Flucloxacillin (200 mg/kg/day) is the antibiotic of choice. Amoxycillin is given in addition to children under 4 years. Oral antibiotics are given for another 3 weeks if there is no associated OM. The joint and limb is splinted for the duration of limb/joint irritability.

Complications

The aftermath of unsuccessfully treated septic arthritis can be crippling. Painful joint stiffness, leg length discrepancy and post-septic joint degeneration are conditions that will require expert orthopaedic treatment for many years.

RHEUMATIC DISEASES

Quite numerous conditions under this banner are encountered in childhood, e.g. juvenile rheumatoid arthritis, rheumatic fever, ankylosing spondylitis, Henoch-Schönlein purpura, systemic lupus erythematosus, scleroderma and Reiter's syndrome. Whilst most of these are medical conditions, they may present as subacute, chronic or occasionally, acute arthritis. They may be confused with septic joint diseases and viral-related arthralgias. Rheumatic fever is less frequently seen today but is still encountered as an acute, migratory polyarthritis following a group A beta-haemolytic streptococcal infection. Its migratory, transient form of arthritis differs from juvenile rheumatoid arthritis (JRA).

Separation of JRA into three major groups on the basis of clinical manifestations (viz., systemic, polyarticular and pauciarticular), remains a useful classification. Newer groupings that take into account the presence of immune complexes and histocompatibility antigen more closely reflect the disease spectrum. The systemic form of JRA presents dramatically with pyrexia, rashes, hepatosplenomegaly and lymphadenopathy. It may be confused with septic arthritis. One in four develop crippling, chronic arthritis. Destructive arthritis is common in JRA with positive rheumatoid factor. This disease is similar in form to adult type rheumatoid arthritis and occurs mainly in older girls.

Treatment generally consists of splintage to prevent deformity, physical therapy to maintain mobility of joints, synovectomy where medical control is inadequate, soft-tissue releases and realignment surgery to correct recalcitrant deformity and finally reconstructive joint surgery where the arthritis is destructive.

NEOPLASTIC CONDITIONS

Bone tumours may occasionally present as a deformity, e.g. the bony prominence of a large or superficial osteochondromata, but, far more often, they present with pain which is deep seated and mainly nocturnal. A pathological fracture following relatively minor trauma may announce the presence of a bone cyst or, less commonly, a malignant tumour. There may be systemic symptoms as in the case of Ewing's sarcoma, or the local signs may mimic an osteomyelitis as is sometimes the case with lymphomas.

The commonest benign bone tumours are:

- Osteochondroma
- Simple (unicameral) bone cyst
- Aneurysmal bone cyst
- Non-ossifying fibroma
- Enchondroma
- Osteoid osteoma

The malignant bone lesions seen in childhood are:

- Osteosarcoma
- Ewing's sarcoma
- Fibrosarcoma
- Histiocytosis X

It is beyond the scope of this chapter to deal with each tumour type. It should also be remembered that bone is a common site of involvement for leukaemia and secondary deposits.

Diagnosis is on suspicion and X-rays are always required to define the lesion. Where standard projections give insufficient information of the character and extend of the lesion, CT and MRI scans are indicated. Bone scans are useful for characterization of the primary lesion and identifying other distant foci of spread.

Benign lesions are not associated with inflammatory changes of the overlying skin and soft tissue, a phenomenon which should suggest an aggressive lesion. X-ray changes at the margins of the lesion reflect bony adaptation to slow expansion, such as well-defined sclerotic margination, cortical thickening and a lack of trabecular destruction or youthful new bone formation under the periosteum. The lesion is always well-defined and its core may be radiolucent (fluid), semi-opaque, groundglass (fibrous tissue) or spotted with flecks of calcification (cartilaginous). Many benign lesions have characteristic roentgenographic appearances and when this is considered with the site of the lesion and the age of the child, a strongly suggestive diagnosis can be made even before biopsy.

Aggressive lesions show features common to their counterparts in other organ systems: destruction, local and distant spread. In bone the effect of tissue destruction is radiographically manifest as osteolysis. Rapid expansion of the lesion causes the envelope of periosteum to be elevated and this in turn results in formation of subperiosteal new bone, classically called the 'Codman's triangle'. Repeated elevation of the periosteum as seen in Ewing's sarcoma leads to an appearance of 'onion skin' as several generations of new subperiosteal bone is laid one on top of the other. Tumours like osteosarcoma produce malignant osteoid which gives the appearance of patchy sclerosis. Malignant bone tumours may spread up and down the medullary canal, beyond local bone confines into the surrounding soft tissues or to distant foci, most often the lung.

Where a lesion presents classically and is known to behave non-aggressively, perhaps to natural resolution, it can be observed without requiring a biopsy, e.g. fibrocortical defects and some simple bone cysts. A biopsy is generally required and often part of an excisional procedure.

Treatment

Benign lesions are generally treated by curettage or en bloc excision (with or without bone grafting) depending on the size and known biological behaviour. Sometimes no treatment is necessary. Malignant lesions are staged to determine prognosis and resectability. Limb preservation is often possible with modern chemotherapy, but amputation may be necessary.

IDIOPATHIC CONDITIONS

Conditions which affect either epiphysis or apophysis and cause apparent fragmentation, are broadly classified as osteochondroses or osteo-chrondritis. The essential pathological process is believed to be an avascular necrosis though the aetiology is not known. Trauma is believed to be at least a factor in a number of these conditions and genetics have a role in some. Osteo-chondroses have been described in over 50 sites but the common ones will be described.

Perthes' disease

Perthes' disease is an avascular necrosis of the head of the femur due to an, as yet, unknown cause. It is currently believed that the condition results from more than one episode of bone in-farction. What triggers the infarction is not known and theories concerning increased venous hypertension, synovitis, increased blood viscosity, and intrinsic bone defects have been raised but largely discounted. It quite clearly occurs more often in children of low birthweight, low socio-economic group, small stature and decreased bone age. A deficiency of somatomedin (a growth hormone metabolite) observed in some children with the condition is of particular interest.

A part or all of the femoral head may be af-fected by the ischaemia. The infarctions occur in the bony epiphysis and retard development of the ossific mass. The joint space thus appears wid-ened as the ossific nucleus is diminished (Fig. 11.2). This is the earliest radiographic change. Bone scan abnormalities appear before X-ray changes and in the early stages an area of de-creased radionuclide uptake reflects the segmental avascularity of the femoral head. The size of this 'cold' area may not correlate with the extent of femoral head involvement. This limits the prognostic value of a bone scan. MRI may prove a more useful investigation in providing

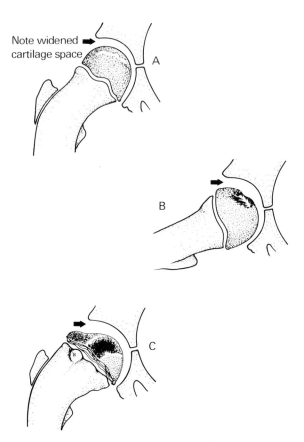

Fig. 11.2 Changes in the hip seen in Perthes' disease.
A: Early anteroposterior view. **B**: Early lateral view.
C: Advanced disease with some repair.

imaging of the articular configuration of the head as well as the distribution of dead and live marrow.

As the disease evolves, the affected portion of the bony epiphysis crumples giving the radio-graphic appearance of fragmentation and collapse. The femoral head may then flatten from mechanical loading of the weakened epiphysis (Fig. 11.2). As biological repair occurs, there is localized hyperaemia which stimulates perichon-drial growth causing an increase in size of the cartilaginous epiphysis. An extrusion of the en-larged head beyond the confines of the aceta-bulum leads to an appearance of subluxation of the femoral head. The femoral head is then more vulnerable to mechanical deformation.

Where the disease is minimal the femoral head will heal without deformity. As the femoral head remains vulnerable to deformation until sufficient mechanical strength is restored through repair, the rate of healing influences the outcome as much as the extent of head involvement. Thus, the young child (under 4 years of age) will generally do well even without active treatment as biological repair is rapid. On the other hand, the older child, particularly those over the age of 8 years, will tend to do poorly even with treatment. Although Perthes' disease has often been held to have minimal effect on the longevity of the hip, a recent study indicates that a high proportion of cases developed degenerative hip disease in later years and many required total hip replacements. This is particularly true for those who sustained the disease after the age of 8 years. In spite of obvious femoral head deformities, most will not have significant hip pain for at least the first 30 years of their lives. Symptomatic arthritis generally manifests in the fifth decade.

Clinical presentation

Boys are more commonly affected and usually between the age of 4 and 10 years. Sufferers present with a very gradually increasing limp. The discomfort is usually felt in the knee, thigh or groin. The child is generally well and abnormal findings are confined to the affected hip which is irritable and stiff. Abduction and adduction in flexion and internal rotation are movements most consistently restricted. With painful inhibition of the abductor muscles, there may be a positive Trendelenburg sign. Full blood count and ESR are normal.

Management

Treatment of Perthes' disease remains controversial if not confused. This results from lack of controlled and comparable studies. However, it is generally agreed that few children under the age of 4 years require active treatment, as the eventual outcome is almost always good. It is also a common belief that little can be done to help the child with a disease commencing after the age of 8 years, as the prognosis is poor regardless of treatment modality. This latter belief may prove to be erroneous as newer regimens of treatment are tried.

A high proportion of patients do not need treatment other than measures to reduce hip pain, e.g. local rest and non-steroidal anti-inflammatory agents. These are patients who are young or have minimal head disease. There are those who present late with established deformities of the femoral head and with signs of re-ossification. These hips cannot benefit from treatment.

Treatment of Perthes' disease is based on the principle of containment, i.e. it is directed at preserving roundness of the femoral head during the period when it is vulnerable to deformation. To achieve this the femoral head has to be kept under protective cover of the acetabulum. Containment can be by means of an abduction brace in which the head is kept under cover of the acetabulum by restricting motion within a selected range, or by surgically redirecting the femoral head (femoral osteotomy) or acetabulum (innominate osteotomy) to provide the cover. There is little to choose between operative and non-operative treatment in terms of eventual results and there are advantages and disadvantages with both methods of treatment. Regardless of the chosen method of treatment, mobility of the hip joint has to be maintained throughout the duration of treatment. Recurrent bouts of painful stiffness and recalcitrant loss of motion indicate a poor end result.

The duration of treatment by bracing varies with the age of onset of the disease and to some extent the degree of femoral head involvement. With brace treatment splintage is maintained for at least 2 years but possibly up to 3 years in the older child. Children with significant disease are kept from impact sports till such time as the head is fully reconstituted.

Scheuermann's disease

Scheuermann's disease is excessive thoracic kyphosis of unknown aetiology and frequently presents as a problem of poor posture. Pain is not a consistent symptom. Pain is uncommon in thoracic deformities and frequent in thoracolumbar kyphosis. The location of the kyphosis is as important as the severity of deformity. Scheuermann's disease in the lumbar and thoracolumbar spine is associated with low back pain in 78% of patients.

There is considerable variation in the degree of thoracic kyphosis in normal individuals (20–40°). In Scheuermann's disease there should be more than 50° of kyphosis and wedging (in excess of 5°) of at least three adjacent vertebrae. There is a defect of the anterior portion of the cartilage growth plate of the vertebral body and resultant growth retardation of the anterior part of the vertebrae. Disc material herniates into the vertebral body and this change is seen on lateral radiographs as defects in the upper or lower parts of the body (Schmorl's nodes).

Significant kyphosis when present in the skeletally immature is best treated in a Milwaukee brace. Treatment is effective and correction often rapid. Brace treatment should be maintained for at least 18 months. A less cumbersome underarm orthosis may be prescribed for a thoracolumbar kyphosis. Surgical correction and fusion is rarely indicated and only for severe (more than 60°) curves that are persistently painful.

Osgood-Schlatter disease

This is one of the most common cause of anterior knee pain in the growing child. It is typically seen in the 10–15 year old boy, during a period of active tibial apophyseal growth. It is commonly described as an osteochondritis of the tibial tubercle though it is more likely to be due to fatigue failure of the growing apophysis. The child presents with complaints of pain over the tibial tubercle during or after physical activities and there may be swelling of the area due to increased prominence of the tubercle. The condition is characterized by focal tenderness over the tubercle. The condition will settle in the vast majority without interventional treatment when the apophyseal growth slows or ceases. Reassurance and advice are generally all that is required. Complete abstinence from sports is unnecessary and undesirable. The child is advised to titrate his/her level of activities to the symptom level and occasionally adjustment of sport type is required for short periods. Hamstring stretching is also beneficial for those with tightness of these muscles. A small number of patients will remain persistently

symptomatic and in them a separated piece of apophysis is recognized to be the source of continued irritation. Removal of this unstable fragment will cure the pain.

Sever's disease

This is a self-limiting condition of pain localized to the calcaneal apophysis. Classified as an osteochondrosis, it has been misinterpreted as an avascular necrosis of the calcaneal apophysis. The increased density and apparent fragmentation of the apophysis is now recognized to represent the normal pattern of ossification. The apophysis appears variably between 5 and 10 years and is first seen as a fleck of calcification. Several centres of ossification are often present which eventually fuse to form the mature os calcis.

The condition is again more frequent in boys who are athletically active. There is a strong association with repetitive impact type sports, e.g. basketball. Occasionally a stress fracture through the apophysis can be recognized and should be treated by an appropriate period of rest as for other acute skeletal injury. Generally the condition is treated expectantly with advice to restrict heavy impact sports during periods of significant symptoms. The condition consistently settles over a period of several months and active treatment is hardly ever required.

Köhler's disease

Classified as an osteochondrosis of the navicular bone, Köhler's disease is probably the result of mechanically induced avascular necrosis of the immature naviculus. The navicular bone is the last tarsal bone to ossify. Its ossification centre appears just before 2 years in girls and about 6 to 12 months later in boys in whom the condition predominates. The late appearance of this ossification centre makes the naviculus more vulnerable to compressive forces of weight-bearing and may explain the susceptibility of this bone to avascular change.

The condition appears in boys of about 5 years and younger girls of 4 years. Its presentation is characterized by painful weight-bearing and findings of inflammation around the naviculus. It can be mistaken for osteomyelitis. The naviculus appears dense and flattened in roentgenograms. The principle of treatment here is similar to that for management of other skeletal avascular necrosis and consists of rest and protection from mechanical stress of the affected part. A below-knee walking plaster moulded to support the medial longitudinal arch is applied for 2 months. This shortens the recovery considerably and on the average most cases recover after 3 months with plaster treatment, whilst those treated without protection may take up to 15 months to settle. Given appropriate treatment the naviculus reconstitutes over a period of 2 years. Where a persistent and significant deformity is present, a permanent loss of the foot arch results and secondary midtarsal arthritis may occur later in life.

Slipped upper femoral epiphysis

This is a condition that occurs during puberty in which the upper femoral epiphysis slips backwards on its metaphysis. The separation takes place in the growth plate, at the level of the zone of hypertrophied cartilage cells. This separation may occur suddenly (acute slip) or insidiously (chronic slip). The majority, however, present with acute on chronic slips. The backward displacement of the epiphysis causes the femur to externally rotate and at a later stage migrate upwards. This accounts for the characteristic clinical findings of loss of internal rotation, resting external rotation of the leg and slight shortening.

The cause of the disorder is not known but because it occurs during puberty, at a time of rapid growth, sexual maturity and hormonal changes, much attention has been focused on hormonal aspects of the disease. It has been suggested that an imbalance of sex hormones (which stabilize the growth plate) and growth hormone (which decreases shear strength of the growth plate) may be a cause of weakness in the growth plate. The condition is most often encountered in children with adiposogenital physique and not infrequently in tall, thin children with a history of sudden rapid growth.

There is an increased familial incidence and black people are more frequently affected than whites. Males are affected twice as often as females. Both hips are involved in one-third of cases, usually found on diagnosis. Delayed slips in the opposite hip occur within a year.

Clinical presentation

Children who present with acute slips do not have previous complaints and the onset of pain and limp follows an episode of trauma. Pain is usually sufficient to prevent weight-bearing. More commonly there is a history of vague aches and pains either in the groin or medial aspect of the knee for some weeks or months prior to a sudden increase in pain brought on by a fall or similar injury. In this mode of acute on chronic presentation, and also with the more gradual chronic form, the diagnosis is often delayed by complaints of knee pain.

The degree of abnormal physical findings depends on the severity of epiphyseal slip and mode of presentation. Chronic slips may not be associated with significant joint irritability and if the degree of slip is minimal, diagnosis is difficult on clinical examination and even X-ray changes may be difficult to detect. In minor slips the only abnormal physical sign is often a loss of terminal internal rotation of the hip in extension. As the degree of slip increases, an increasing loss of internal rotation or even a fixed external rotation deformity and slight adduction and shortening becomes evident.

Investigations

X-rays are mandatory if the diagnosis is suspected (Fig. 11.3). An anteroposterior view of the hip in some degree of internal rotation and a frog-leg lateral view should be taken. In minimal slip, a slight widening of the joint space may be seen in the anteroposterior view and the diagnosis is made on the lateral X-ray. A tilt of the epiphyseal plate relative to the long axis of the femoral neck (epiphyseal-plate angle) allows even minor slips to be detected. With greater degrees of slip the diagnosis is also obvious in the anteroposterior view. A line drawn along the superior border of the neck normally cuts part of the epiphysis in

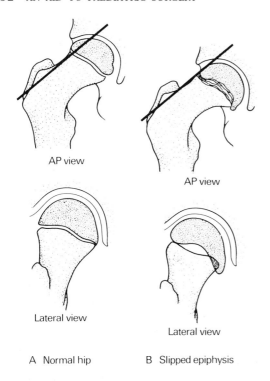

AP view

AP view

Lateral view

Lateral view

A   Normal hip

B   Slipped epiphysis

Fig. 11.3 Anterior and lateral views of the changes in slipped epiphysis. **A**: Normal hip. **B**: Slipped epiphysis.

the anteroposterior view; but in this condition the epiphysis slips below the superior neck line (Trethowan's sign).

It is suggested that a pre-slip stage can sometimes be identified with the use of bone scan. A slight broadening of the physis may be present in plain X-rays during this prodromal stage.

Management

The treatment of slipped upper femoral epiphysis has changed substantially in the past 30 years. In principle, treatment is directed at stabilizing the unstable epiphysis and inducing a closure of the physis. Previous controversies have concerned the need to reduce the deformity. Attempts at reduction of the epiphyseal slip have been associated with high risk of avascular necrosis. Recognition of such risk and the knowledge that remodelling of the proximal femur takes place to minimize even quite severe deformities, prescribes the present philosophy of 'pinning in situ'.

Children who present with acute slips of more than 50% may benefit from a period of traction to safely reduce the degree of deformity. Minor and chronic slips should not be reduced. Fixation of the epiphysis is effected by screws or threaded pins. Great care must be exercised to ensure proper placement of such pins so as to avoid penetration of the articular surface. There is strong evidence that pin penetration increases the risk of chondrolysis.

Despite the high incidence of bilateral hip disease, there is little support for prophylactic pinning of the opposite hip. Provided close supervision is possible over the next 2 years, the child with unilateral hip involvement should have the opposite hip simply observed. The risks associated with pinning of a normal hip are difficult to justify.

Complications

Avascular necrosis (osteonecrosis) is the most frequent early complication occurring in about 15% of cases. It occurs most frequently with severe acute slips where it is due to sudden traumatic disruption of the posterior retinacular blood vessels. Avascular necrosis may result also from attempts at reduction of epiphyseal slips, particularly with open reductions and osteotomies. The outcome of avascular necrosis is worse than that of untreated slipped epiphysis.

Chondrolysis, as the term implies, is a destructive disorder of the articular cartilage which leads to a stiff and painful joint. It is a complication that occurs most often in black populations and is uncommon where treatment has not been given for the slipped epiphysis. It is very likely that pin penetration increases the risk of chondrolysis. The exact mechanism of chondrolysis is not known but there are suggestions of it being an autoimmune phenomenon. The disease, once initiated, is relentless and results in a loss of articular cartilage, its replacement by fibrocartilage and eventually degenerative joint disease.

Osteoarthritis will complicate even minor hip deformities that result from slipped upper femoral epiphysis. This is a late sequela.

TRAUMATIC CONDITIONS

Dislocations and fractures

The child's bone differs substantially from the mature skeleton in its mechanical and reparative properties and in the presence of the growth plate and epiphysis (Fig. 11.1). The child's bone is plastic, which accounts for the occurrence of plastic deformation in which the diaphyseal bone bends without actually breaking. The metaphysis is more substantial in children and is the focus of the majority of fractures. Here the fractures may be: a simple buckle (torus fracture), in which the metaphyseal bone is compressed and the overlying cortex folds; greenstick, in which the cortex on the convex side of the fracture ruptures but that on the concave side remains intact (Fig. 11.4); or complete.

The child's bone has much thicker periosteal wrapping than the adult's and this confers on it an enormous potential for healing and remodelling. The periosteum forms a scaffold of new bone following a fracture and this provides early stabilization and healing of the break. Through the influences of mechanical factors, more new bone is laid and retained on the concave side of a residual deformity and this provides a mechanism for reshaping of the bone. The periosteum, being thick and strong in a child, also provides resilience to separation of fracture ends and influences the fracture characteristics. The growth plate (physis) and epiphysis are subject to compressive, distractive or shear injury and account for a third of skeletal injuries in childhood. Where the injury involves the physis and crosses into the epiphysis, growth disturbance can result if such fractures are not replaced anatomically. Compressive forces of sufficient severity can result in disturbance of growth even though a fracture may not be apparent in an X-ray. A useful classification of growth plate injuries is provided by Salter & Harris (Fig. 11.5).

Type 1: The physis is separated horizontally with the cleavage plane between the calcified and uncalcified cartilage. This injury is not common and seen mainly in infants.

Type 2: The plane of cleavage is also along the growth plate but the fracture line deviates into the metaphysis to take a fragment of bone along with the epiphysis. This is the most common injury. The distal radius is its most common example.

Type 3: The fracture occurs horizontally through part of the physis and then vertically through the epiphysis into the joint.

Type 4: The fracture extends through the epiphysis, across the physis and into the metaphysis. The lateral humeral condyle fracture is a typical example.

Type 5: The physis is crushed and there is partial or complete damage.

Bone bridges form across the damaged growth plate in type 3 and 4 fractures if the fractures are malunited. This results in disturbance of the normal growth processes. As only part of the physis is involved, the resultant growth disturbance is

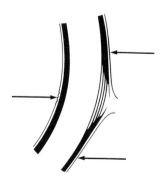

Fig. 11.4 Greenstick fracture showing the deforming force and the resultant fracture of the opposite side of the bone.

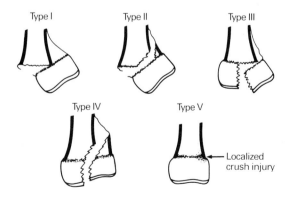

Fig. 11.5 Types of epiphyseal injury.

often asymmetrical. This results in angular deformity besides shortening of the affected bone. Therefore, accurate anatomical reduction is necessary with types 3 and 4 fractures. Where this cannot be achieved by closed manipulation, open reduction is indicated.

A major difference occurs in the child's bone in response to injury. It heals much faster (at least twice the rate) and by virtue of the growth potential, it remodels much of the deformity that may be present after healing. Remodelling by deposition of new bone on the concave side of a deformity is also present to some extent in the adult skeleton, but is enhanced in the child by differential growth stimulus. Therefore, fractures close to the growth plate remodel better than those at a distance. The skeleton is capable of remodelling angular deformities as well as correcting displacement, but will not correct rotational deformities. Deformities in the plane of motion of the adjacent joint will correct better.

Dislocations are rare in childhood because the ligaments that support a joint tend to be more resilient than the immature bone and cartilage. Avulsion fractures of apophyses and physeal separations will take place more readily than a dislocation. Indeed, most dislocations, when they occur, are associated with fractures, even if they may not be readily apparent. Dislocations that do occur take place in the elbow, hip and superior radio-ulnar joints.

Given the enormous propensity of the juvenile bone to heal rapidly and to remodel even significant deformities, few injuries require operative treatment. Most fractures can be treated effectively by closed reduction and temporary immobilization either in a splint, plaster or some form of traction device. Indeed, fractures even in major bones in the infant often do not require active treatment. The latitude offered by nature should not encourage complacency, as the same mechanism of growth which corrects residual deformity, will be a source of progressive deformity if the growth apparatus is damaged. Recognizing injuries that can lead to this eventuality is an important and early requirement in the management of paediatric fractures. Fractures in children heal quickly, even if the bone ends are significantly separated. Fractures therefore become stable within 10 to 14 days.

Attempts to remanipulate fractures after 2 weeks in order to correct deformity will require the use of great force with risk of damage to the growth plate. It is often wiser with late presenting fractures to accept the deformity and to consider a corrective osteotomy as necessary at a later date, after effective healing and a passage of time for remodelling. The use of internal fixation devices, particularly metal plates, can result in an abnormal stimulation of the growth mechanism with resultant overgrowth of the bone. Fractures involving the shafts of long bones, especially the femur, are associated in some cases with compensatory overgrowth of the bone. The mechanism of this phenomenon is not known.

Fracture management

The principles of fracture management in childhood are similar to those in the adult, with the added qualification that, because of more rapid and reliable remodelling, the effects of growth and the greater capacity for soft-tissue functional recovery, childhood fractures rarely need an open operation.

The four **R**'s of fracture management are: **R**ecognition, **R**eduction, **R**etention and **R**ehabilitation.

Recognition. A careful history will usually yield information on the mechanism of injury, though not infrequently a history of trauma is absent or uncertain and the child presents with complaints of pain or loss of use of the affected limb. Correlating history to the pattern of injuries is vital in the exclusion of child abuse.

Usually a fracture can be diagnosed on the following findings:

- Pain
- Local swelling and tenderness
- Loss of limb function
- Deformity
- Abnormal mobility
- Crepitus

Incomplete fractures (e.g. torus, greenstick) with minimal deformities may not be easily recognized but are usually suggested by the child's refusal to move or use the limb. X-rays will in most cases permit easy identification of the fracture, but must include at least two projections taken at planes perpendicular to each other (anteroposterior and lateral). Because children are still skeletally immature, some of their skeletal organs are cartilaginous and fractures through them may not be readily identified. This is particularly so with younger children and with injuries of the wrist and elbow. Comparative X-rays of the unaffected, opposite limb are very helpful and should be taken if any doubt exists.

As a general rule with the younger child, one should presume a fracture to be present (until proven otherwise) if a joint is painful and swollen following trauma. This is particularly so if blood is present in the joint (haemarthrosis). In such a circumstance an arthrogram is indicated if a fracture cannot be seen on plain X-rays of good quality.

A fracture may be: closed or open (compound). Compound fractures vary enormously in severity of tissue damage and contamination. The temptation to judge the magnitude of damage on an X-ray appearance of the fracture must be resisted. The bony elements constitute but a part of the injury which includes invariably damage to the surrounding soft tissues. Proper evaluation of muscle, tendon, nerves, vessels and skin must be carried out. A pin-hole wound may mask serious contamination, as the contaminated bone end may have retracted into the depth of the wound. Such wounds must be explored, debrided and cleansed as with all cases of compound fractures. Wound swabs should be taken for bacteriological studies and prophylactic antibiotics, e.g. penicillin and cloxacillin, commenced and maintained for at least 2 weeks. Only wounds that receive prompt treatment (within 6 hours) and are completely cleaned and without risk of further soft-tissue necrosis or haematoma formation, should be closed primarily. Doubtful wounds can generally be closed after 5–7 days.

Reduction. Children under the age of 10 years will tolerate quite significant angular deformity (of up to 10°) through a mechanism of remodelling, yet there are certain fracture types, e.g. types 3 and 4, which require anatomical reduction regardless of the age of the child. Therefore, many children's fractures do not require reduction and a knowledge of the principles outlined earlier helps with decision-making.

Reduction of a fracture can be achieved by one of the following methods:

- Traction
- Manipulation
- Open reduction

Traction is employed to reduce and retain reduction of some fractures. Traction treatment can be simply the use of gravity (e.g. hanging cast for treatment of humeral shaft fractures) or the use of weights applied to the end of an injured limb. When weights are used they are attached to the limb either by means of adhesive tapes (skin traction) (Fig. 11.6) or through a pin driven through the bone (skeletal traction).

Manipulation is the usual method of achieving reduction of most fractures and dislocations. An anaesthetic is usually required, though in some instances oral sedation is sufficient, e.g. greenstick fractures in infancy, recurrent shoulder dislocations. In upper limb fractures regional or intravenous blocks can be considered, but in most cases general anaesthetic is preferred. Manipulative reduction begins with identifying the deformity in three planes and understanding the mechanism of injury. Traction is applied along the line of existing deformity, then the distal fracture fragment is manipulated to line up with the proximal fragment by a reversal of the deformity. Malrotation must be corrected. Some residual angulation or overlap can be tolerated.

Open reduction is indicated if:

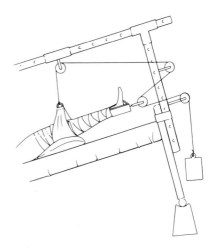

Fig. 11.6 Hamilton-Russell traction for a fractured femur.

1. Closed reduction is impossible, e.g. soft-tissue interposition
2. Closed reduction is not adequate — most commonly with intra-articular fractures where accuracy is mandatory
3. Compound fractures

Retention. Once reduction of a fracture is achieved it needs to be held in the reduced position till sufficient union has taken place. Retention can be achieved by one of several methods:

1. External fixation
   (a) Traction
   (b) Plaster cast
   (c) Percutaneous skeletal pins with external frame fixation
2. Internal fixation
   (a) Intramedullary pins or rods
   (b) Onlay metallic plates
   (c) Interfragmentary screws or wires

In a child, internal fixation must be used judiciously and there is no place for excessive use of metal implants. Healing in children takes place rapidly and only very temporary fixation is required. Furthermore, non-union in uncomplicated fractures is not encountered. It is a highly commendable practice to employ minimal internal fixation and to supplement such fixation with a plaster cast, rather than to use metallic plates and screws in a child's fracture.

Rehabilitation. Juvenile fractures heal much faster than adult fractures. Typically, an upper limb fracture will unite sufficiently in 3 weeks to allow removal of plaster cast. Union should be sufficiently solid by 6 weeks to allow a graduated return to normal activities. Lower limb fractures generally take twice as long to heal.

In the absence of neurovascular injury or severe soft-tissue damage, the child will recover normal mobility and use of the limb in a matter of weeks without the benefit of organized physical therapy. In fact, aggressive and inappropriate physical therapy, especially massage and passive manipulation, can result in myositis ossificans. Myositis ossificans is the heterotopic ossification occurring after trauma to a joint, bone or muscle. The elbow is particularly vulnerable to this complication and loss of motion is the consequence.

Upper limb fractures and dislocations

Clavicle fracture

In children,. the clavicle is the most frequently broken bone and fractures of the shaft are commonest. These fractures do not need active treatment and a sling is given for comfort. Malunion is invariable with deformed fractures and may be unsightly for the first year.

Elbow dislocation

Elbow dislocations are almost always associated with fractures in children. The commonest associated injury is a fracture of the medial epicondyle. In the young child minimally ossified fracture fragments are difficult to identify, as are fragments entrapped within the joint.

Supracondylar fracture

This common elbow injury results usually from a fall on the hand with the elbow bent. The humerus breaks just above the humeral condyles, at a level where the bone is broad but thin. Complete fractures therefore tend to displace and have little natural stability. The fracture also occurs adjacent to important nerves and vessels, and injuries to these structures directly (by bone ends) or indirectly (Volkmann's ischaemia) must always be looked for. Undisplaced fractures are treated by flexion of the elbow and a collar and cuff support. Even in this group, swelling can be severe and close observation is necessary, particularly to confirm that distal pulses are still present after elbow flexion.

The vast majority of fractures displace backwards, twisting inwards and shifting medially at the same time. There is usually severe bruising, swelling and deformity. A careful examination of the circulation and neurological function in the hand is mandatory. Ischaemia from increased flexor compartment pressure (Volkmann's ischaemia, closed compartmental syndrome) is a surgical emergency and it serves well to remember the sequential onset of signs and symptoms. These are: *Disproportionate Pain.*

Disproportionate **Pain** (in the ischaemic compartment)	
Paralysis	**Pallor**
Paraesthesiae	**Pulselessness**

Treatment of ischaemia begins with:

- Relief of all encircling bandage and wrappings
- Reduction of deformity
- Relief of compartmental pressure by fasciotomy (if preceding measures fail)

The fracture should be reduced under general anaesthetic by an expert. There is no place for repeated, failed manipulations as this will cause further soft-tissue injury and swelling and increase risk of complications. If the reduction is successful, the fracture position is stabilized by flexion of the elbow above 100° in a collar and cuff support. Closed reduction is not always successful with this fracture so that continuous traction, using the weight of the arm, may be required, at least till the swelling settles. Open reduction and internal fixation is not favoured and is often complicated by prolonged stiffness. Occasionally a fracture is successfully reduced but because of swelling, it cannot be held stable by flexion of the elbow. In such a situation percutaneous pins may be used to fix the fracture and allow the elbow to be rested in lesser degree of flexion.

Any of the three major nerves that course the elbow (median, radial, ulnar) can be injured during the fall. Most nerve injuries are partial and due to neuropraxia. Surgical exploration is hardly ever indicated and spontaneous recovery generally occurs.

Malunion is common and the classical deformity is cubitus varus (Gunstock deformity). As growth is not affected in supracondylar fracture, the deformity is not progressive. Mobility of the elbow is usually excellent and the problem is largely cosmetic. Correction by a humeral osteotomy is effective.

Myositis ossificans not infrequently complicates the injury and results in some permanent loss of elbow motion.

Lateral humeral condyle fracture

This is the most common type 4 injury (Fig. 11.7). It occurs usually after the age of 4 years, at the time of appearance of the capitellar ossification centre. Growth of the lateral side of the humerus will be retarded if malunion occurs. Unlike other fractures in childhood, non-union is a complication of this fracture if significant displacement is left untreated. Therefore, all fractures with more than 2 mm displacement need reduction. Almost always this involves open reduction and internal fixation with fine pins.

Medial epicondyle fracture

This is quite a common injury in children between the ages of 5 and 15 years. The injury is sometimes associated with an elbow dislocation. In fact, the epicondyle is occasionally trapped within the joint, in which case closed reduction is usually unsuccessful. The most obvious sign is extensive bruising on the medial side of the elbow. Diagnosis by X-rays can be difficult in the young child without early ossification of the epicondyle.

The epicondyle is an apophysis and therefore does not contribute significantly to axial growth of the humerus. Isolated injury to the epicondyle

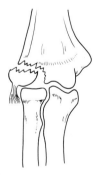

Fig. 11.7 Fracture of the lateral condyle of the humerus with displacement by the pull of the common extensor tendon.

will not usually cause growth deformity of the elbow. Many of these injuries can therefore be treated conservatively with good eventual results. However, fractures that involve the medial epicondyle as part of a medial condylar fracture carry a far more serious prognosis. The differentiation is not difficult in the older child and in them a 'metaphyseal' fragment attached to the epicondyle suggests involvement of the medial epiphysis. The ossific centre of the trochlear epiphysis does not ossify till after the age of 10 years and in children under this age, the medial condylar fracture may not be seen on plain X-rays and the injury may be misdiagnosed as an epicondylar fracture. A widely separated epicondylar fracture and the presence of a haemarthrosis (the medial epicondyle is extra-articular) warn of a medial condylar fracture, in which case an open reduction is necessary.

Pulled elbow

This is a very common elbow injury which occurs typically between the ages of 1–4 years. The injury is usually caused by lifting the child by the arm. What probably happens is a tear of the annular ligament at its attachment to the radius and this allows the ligament to interpose between the radial head and the capitellum when traction is released from the arm. In effect a subluxation of the radial head occurs. The child then refuses to use the arm and holds it protectively in flexion and pronation. Reduction is achieved without an anaesthetic by supination and flexion of the elbow. A click is usually palpable on reduction and with a healthy scream the child is purged of the problem.

Forearm fractures

Fractures of the shafts of the radius and ulna are common fractures in childhood. Unlike similar fractures in adults, the vast majority of these fractures can be managed conservatively but not without difficulty.

Greenstick fractures, particularly those at the junction of the metaphysis and diaphysis, are prone to late deformation and refracture and they require reduction with over-correction by actively completing the fractures. Reduction is easy because the periosteal tube is intact. Complete fractures that are displaced require great skill to treat well. The apparent angular deformity is often due to malrotation and this has to be recognized to achieve a successful reduction. Residual angular deformity is better tolerated in fractures in the distal part of the forearm whilst even small angulation at the proximal and mid-forearm levels will cause loss of rotation. Angulation of more than 10° requires reduction especially in children over the age of 10 years. Fractures in adolescents assume more adult characteristics and more often require operative treatment.

Monteggia fracture–dislocation

This important injury requires awareness to avoid missing the diagnosis. The term is now used to embrace various combinations of a fracture of the ulna with associated dislocation of the proximal radial head. The classical description was of a fracture of the proximal ulna (with anterior angulation) and a consequent anterior dislocation of the radial head. The injury results from a fall on the hand with forceful pronation of the forearm. The anterior variety is most common but the radial head may be displaced posteriorly or laterally depending on the mechanism of injury and the angulation of the ulna fracture. The lateral variety is seen only in children and is more difficult to reduce. Unlike similar injury in adults, Monteggia fracture–dislocation in the child can usually be managed closed.

The diagnosis is not infrequently missed either because the ulna fracture or the radial head dislocation is not recognized. The ulna may not be fractured completely but a reversed bow of the shaft can usually be detected if compared with the opposite limb. X-rays of forearm injury should always include the elbow and wrist to avoid missing dislocations at either end. A line drawn through the long axis of the radius should pass through the capitellum in all views of the elbow. A displacement of this line from capitellum denotes a dislocation of the radius.

Distal radius fracture

Fractures at the wrist level of the radial meta-physis or epiphysis are amongst the most common childhood fractures. There are:

- Buckle fractures
- Complete metaphyseal fractures (usually with avulsion of the ulnar styloid)
- Fractures of the distal radius and ulna
- Type 2 distal radial epiphyseal fractures
- Type 1 distal radial epiphyseal fractures (only in young children)

These fractures, when deformed, are usually displaced and angulated dorsally. They are reduced closed and retained in carefully moulded above-elbow casts with the wrist in pronation and slight flexion for 3 weeks.

Lower limb fractures and dislocations

Pelvic fracture

Children under the age of 10 years, who have little road sense, are most vulnerable to pelvic fractures. Minor fractures with little displacement require no active treatment but a period of bed rest. More severe injuries are commonly associated with visceral damage, massive blood loss, and significant mortality. Unstable pelvic injuries involve disruption of the posterior sacroiliac joint and these injuries are also associated with massive blood loss from retroperitoneal haemorrhage. As this blood loss is internal and into deep structures it may be missed. As these injuries are usually the result of motor-vehicle accidents, head, chest, limb, abdominal and urological damage are often present.

Initial resuscitation should be followed by temporary stabilization of the pelvic ring. This measure alone will reduce blood loss immediately and affect dramatically the likelihood of survival. The beneficial effects of stabilization are probably related to simple reduction of bleeding cancellous bone surfaces and reduction of pelvic volume. Initial stabilization should not be elaborate or time-consuming. The sacroiliac dislocation is reduced and stabilized with external fixation frames. Younger children, under 6 years, with smaller pelves, are better held in hip spicas. De-finitive stabilization of the unstable pelvis is deferred till general control of the patient is achieved. This involves the use of internal fixation devices such as plate, screws or bars. The recent recognition of the need to effect stabilization of the pelvis in massive pelvic injuries is responsible for a marked improvement in survival rate.

Hip dislocation

The child's hip dislocates more easily than the mature hip and accordingly the severity of complications is less. Some 30% of adult hip dislocations are associated with avascular necrosis of the femoral head. The incidence is between 5–10% in the child. The presence of associated acetabular or femoral head fractures will adversely affect the outcome.

Dislocations are generally posterior but occasionally anterior. Reduction should be carried out under general anaesthetic and with muscle relaxation. Posterior dislocations are reduced by traction on a flexed hip. A period of bed rest and traction is enforced for 4 weeks. The outcome of this injury relates directly to the speed with which reduction is carried out. Delay in treatment (more than 12 hours) adversely affects the result.

Fractures of the femoral shaft

These are common fractures and are usually associated with severe trauma, such as a motor-vehicle accident or a fall from a height. It requires considerable force to fracture the largest bone in the body, so that there is usually considerable blood loss into the soft-tissues with extensive soft tissue injury and a high incidence of associated injuries. The patient may be shocked when first seen, but if not, must be treated to prevent shock.

Spiral fractures of the femoral shaft are more common than transverse fractures, are of a torsional type and can occur with much lesser degrees of force.

Sixty per cent of fractures of the femoral shaft involve the middle third of the shaft. The displacement is often considerable, with shortening, angulation and muscular interposition.

Treatment includes:

1. The fracture must be effectively splinted, e.g. a Thomas splint
2. Treatment for present or possible shock must be instituted
3. The patient must be examined for other injuries
4. The fracture is treated definitively

The fracture treatment depends on the age of the patient and the type of the fracture.

Up to 2 years of age, simple vertical suspension of the lower limbs (Bryant's or gallow's traction) for about 6 weeks is sufficient treatment. Above that age limit it is unsafe to elevate the feet so high, and techniques of traction such as the Hamilton-Russell variety (Fig. 11.6) are preferred.

Application of a plaster of Paris hip spica is applicable to many cases, usually after 2 weeks of traction, using a 90°/90° technique to maintain the length of thigh (i.e. both hip and knee flexed to 90°).

Internal fixation is very rarely necessary in a child's femoral shaft fracture and provided varus is avoided, end results are usually good. Mobilization of the knee may, however, be slow due to extensive soft-tissue injury and interplanar adhesion of muscles and ligaments.

Fractures of the tibial spine

These intra-articular fractures deserve special mention as they are, like so many other intra-articular fractures, examples of avulsion of bone by ligamentous attachments.

Such fractures are commonly caused either by heavy blows on the flexed knee acting on the femur alone, or by hyperextension of the knee, with the tibial spine attachment or the cruciate ligament being avulsed.

Most such fractures, which produce an immediate and tense haemarthrosis (which may require aspiration), can be managed by simple retention in a slightly flexed plaster cylinder. Occasionally, however, with a large or severely displaced fragment, open reduction may be necessary.

FURTHER READING

Apley G A 1982 System of orthopaedics and fractures, 6th edn. Butterworths, London
Segelov P M 1986 Manual of emergency orthopaedics, 1st edn. Churchill Livingstone, London

12. Child abuse

E. F. MacMahon

DEFINITION

Child abuse, in its widest sense, means the curtailment of normal development of a child caused by deliberate or neglectful action by an individual, group or culture.

For the purposes of this chapter, it can be defined as a situation in which a child is suffering from serious physical injury inflicted upon him or her by other than accidental means; is suffering harm by reason of neglect, malnutrition or sexual abuse; is going without necessary and basic nurture; or is growing up under conditions which threaten his/her physical and emotional survival.

Historically, child abuse has been culturally condoned, tolerated or denied depending on how a particular society perceived the child population. With the development of child psychology, paediatric medicine and formal education for children, the rights of the child to protection and support during the years of development are now recognized. Abuse of children is accepted as detrimental to the development of their full potential although argument continues as to what parameters constitute abuse.

Child abuse may not be diagnosed because of professional revulsion or reluctance to become involved in the associated complex psychological and legal issues. In addition, a recent Australian survey indicated that local medical practitioners were reluctant to diagnose the problem based on fears of damaging the family and doubts about the clinical evidence. It is important that all those involved in paediatric practice recognize that the problem exists and be alert to indicators and signs to prevent the child from further abuse. As a general rule, consultation with a specialist with expertise in child protection issues is part of the protocol in large centres but in an emergency, or isolated or rural areas, this may not be possible.

Older children may disclose abuse to a medical practitioner while hospitalized or under treatment for organic illness. Physical abuse may be diagnosed on presentation of the first injury at casualty or at the surgery. Repeated infections may point to underlying neglect and frequent attendances at a medical facility may reflect the parents' inability to cope. A vigilant doctor is often in a unique position to diagnose early abuse and institute early intervention which usually favourably affects the prognosis. The importance of early diagnosis is highlighted by the estimation that, if an abused child is not detected at first presentation, the child has a 50% chance of further injury and a 10% chance of death.

A child may be exposed to more than one form of abuse at any one time or over a period of time. Failure to thrive can be an early indicator of neglect which can precede physical abuse. Physically abused children may have injuries to the genital area and sexually abused children may suffer physical injury by way of retaliation if they fail to comply with the abuser's demands. Some degree of emotional abuse inevitably accompanies the other forms of abuse.

Basic knowledge of child development including the range of normal milestones and a rigorous approach to history taking, examination, documentation and referral procedures is essential. The necessity of special investigations will depend on the history and findings. The collection of blood samples, forensic specimens, swabs for sexually transmitted diseases and assessment for other special investigations all involve protocols.

When abuse is suspected, in the absence of specialist attendance, specialist consultation by telephone is advisable or admission to hospital until this is possible.

The general rule is to ensure the protection of the child before therapy. Because of the overlap of the different types of abuse and the possible long-term consequences, a multidisciplinary approach is the most effective one with the proviso that one member of the team accepts responsibility for coordinating casework and follow-up procedures.

CAUSES

There is no one common cause of child abuse. Abuse can occur in any family regardless of class, income, occupation, racial, cultural or religious background. Causes are multifactorial and influenced by the individual personalities of the parent and child as well as social, economic and environmental situations. Predisposing factors may be present in the individual, the family and the environment, and tend to reinforce each other. This illustrates the importance of standard history taking even in the casualty situation when confronted with what seems to be a simple injury in a child.

Societal values and norms concerning violence and force may affect discipline skills and result in injudicious physical punishment. A blanket acceptance of parents' rights to treat children as they see fit can result in rigidity and inability to appreciate what is in the best interests of the child. Fear of spoiling a child may result in inadequate nurturing in the presence of adequate physical care. A summary of causes which may predispose to abuse is shown in Figure 12.1.

Family and social factors which may indicate 'at-risk' children include poverty, a history of violence and poor parent–child bonding. Poverty includes lack of adequate income, poor housing, unemployment, itinerant lifestyles and social isolation with absence of support networks and the opportunity for 'time out' from the stresses associated with child raising.

Marital problems can include an absent husband due to desertion or demands of his employment or may involve conflicts over man-

agement of finance, discipline techniques or different cultural beliefs. There may be a history of domestic violence, a criminal record, or substance, particularly alcohol, abuse. Bonding difficulties may result from the immaturity of parents, poor role models, unrealistic expectations or the experience of abuse in their own childhood. Apparent indifference in a mother may mask underlying depression. Parents with low self-esteem tend to perceive advice as criticism, thus compounding their parenting difficulties. Mental illness accounts for approximately 10% of parents who abuse their children.

There is a higher risk of abuse in children perceived by the parent as different or difficult physically, mentally or emotionally. This includes the premature, the chronically ill, those with congenital abnormalities and the disabled who may require extra care. The healthy infant may be scapegoated as the cause of family problems and perceived as a 'bad baby' because of parental inability to cope with crying, soiling and wetting. The wanted child can become unwanted when he/she fails to fulfil parental fantasy. It is not surprising that the single mother belongs to the high-risk group when all the interacting predisposing factors are considered. A clustering of predisposing factors should lead to a greater alertness to the possibility of abuse and the need for prevention and early intervention.

INCIDENCE AND OUTCOME

Accurate statistics of the incidence of child abuse in Australia are not available because of the lack of a national approach to the problem. There is no uniformity in definition, legislation, reporting procedures and relatively little research.

Statistics from the United States indicate that while child abuse fatalities continue to rise, in most states the number of reported cases per annum has actually decreased. This has been seen to be due to the introduction of state procedures for prioritizing cases because of the great increase in certain at-risk groups. Lack of resources means that some characteristics are no longer being viewed as sufficient indicators of maltreatment, and these include: a child born drug-addicted; homelessness; parental substance

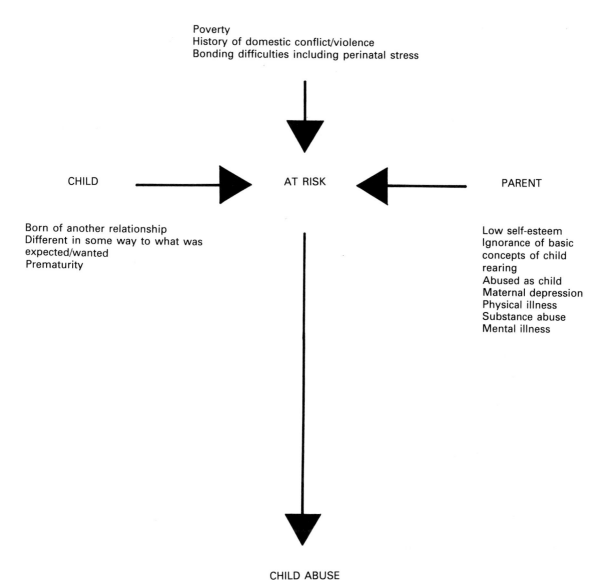

FAMILY/SOCIAL

Poverty
History of domestic conflict/violence
Bonding difficulties including perinatal stress

CHILD → AT RISK ← PARENT

Born of another relationship
Different in some way to what was
expected/wanted
Prematurity

Low self-esteem
Ignorance of basic
concepts of child
rearing
Abused as child
Maternal depression
Physical illness
Substance abuse
Mental illness

CHILD ABUSE

Fig. 12.1 Interacting predisposing factors in child abuse.

abuse; and attempted suicide or drug use by a teenager. While certain circumstances, particularly homelessness, might suggest an abuse situation, one would want to be cautious in applying such a label, though these and similar conditions can signal a family in distress. Of particular concern is the regular use of drugs or alcohol. In summary, each community is tending to define its own concept of abuse and this, as indicated above, is often more a reflection of the availability of resources than the needs of children.

The long-term effects of abuse and costs to the individual and community are reflected in figures which indicate that 85% of children are abused by adults they know and trust and that 44% of all proven drug offenders, 85% of runaways (children who live on the streets) and 85% of teenage prostitutes give a history of child sexual abuse.

Recent Australian studies indicate that even when physical and sexual abuse stops many children continue to show antisocial behaviour, poor school performance and low self-esteem and become social outcasts. As a consequence they have difficulty in forming adult relationships and have parenting difficulties which may involve abuse of their own children. This is the abuse cycle. Generally speaking, abusive parents have difficulty in controlling their impulses, have low self-esteem, poor capacity for empathy with the needs of children and are socially isolated. Nevertheless, it needs to be kept in perspective that most victims of abuse overcome their childhood experiences and become adequate parents. In those who do abuse their own children, good living conditions with effective supports including a non-abusive spouse have been shown to have powerful ameliorating effects.

TYPES OF ABUSE

Neglect and emotional abuse

Neglect is any inadequate or dangerous child-rearing practice which includes failure to provide nurture, adequate nutrition (including fad and bizarre diets), medical care, clothing, shelter or supervision to the extent that the health and development of the child is impaired or put at risk. Such children frequently present as failure to thrive. Neglected children outnumber those who are abused in other ways.

Children may exhibit difficult and disturbed behaviour which may be evidence of emotional abuse. Psychologically destructive patterns of parenting can result in self-inflicted injuries in children and adolescents. Expert evidence is required to prove this diagnosis. Any deliberate self-inflicted injury in childhood requires psychiatric referral.

Neglect and emotional abuse are well-covered in medical texts.

Physical abuse

Physical abuse consists of any non-accidental form of injury or harm inflicted by the caregiver. This form of abuse may take the form of isolated incidents in otherwise supportive parenting or may represent a destructive pattern of parenting, indicative of serious breakdown in the parent–child relationship.

This may present as:

- Bruising
- Head injury, e.g. subdural haematoma
- Fractures and dislocations
- Scalds and burns, including cigarette burns
- Abrasions
- Shaking injuries
- Retinal haemorrhages
- Internal injuries
- Lacerations
- Poisoning

The commonest presentations are bruising, head injuries, burns and fractures, while lacerations and poisoning are relatively uncommon. These children frequently show signs of neglect, including skin lesions, and these should be taken as warning signs.

The most common injuries causing death are multiple rib fractures with laceration of the lung, liver, spleen, mesentery or pancreas with haemothorax and haemoperitoneum. Bizarre forms of physical abuse occur when the caregiver persistently produces symptoms (Munchausen's syndrome) or fabricates symptoms on behalf of the child, causing him/her to be regarded as ill (Munchausen by proxy).

Clinical features

Bruising. Bruising is the commonest presentation of physical abuse but caution must be exercised in inferring abuse on the basis of physical evidence alone. When injury is accidental parents are likely to be cooperative and give a clear history. Abuse must be suspected when the history does not match the type or severity of injury or when details are inconsistent or there is a history of frequent attendance for injury.

It is important to exclude organic causes of bruising in the presence of other physical signs or a history or family history of 'bruising easily'. Blood disorders such as thrombocytopenia, haemophilia or even the more severe conditions such as leukaemia need to be excluded. Because of the aggressive nature and early metastasis of neuroblastoma it may mimic leukaemia or the battered child syndrome with bruising around the eyes. The history is of paramount importance in deciding how intensively to investigate.

The suggested list of tests for the 'easy bruiser' includes:

- Full blood count
- Platelet count
- Prothrombin time
- Activated partial thromboplastin time
- Bleeding time

Referral to a haematologist may be appropriate. Platelet adhesion and aggregation are increasingly being recognized as causes of easy bruising and may be overlooked unless tests for bleeding time/platelet aggregation are included.

The skin is the most common site of haemangiomas which may be considered in the differential diagnosis. Cavernous haemangiomas are deep-seated hamartomas which produce a diffuse irregular swelling and a bluish colouration of the overlying skin (see Ch. 3). Extensive haemangiomas may be associated with thrombocytopenic purpura. The small deep blue-black naevus known as the blue naevus occurs on buttocks, face and hands. Histologically similar is the Mongolian spot which is a blue pigmented area frequently seen in the lumbosacral area in Asians and which usually disappears by puberty.

Attention needs to be given to the age and mobility of the child and the pattern and age of bruises. Suspicion of abuse arises in:

- Precrawling infants if bruising presents in head or eyes
- Leg bruising in children who can only crawl
- Bruising on backs of legs and any parts of the body which do not normally bump against things, e.g. abdomen, chest
- Bruises caused by finger pressure over ribs and on upper arms
- Bruising caused by bite marks — the size of teeth marks will indicate if the bite has been inflicted by an adult

Head injuries. Brain injuries result in the highest mortality/morbidity in abused children.

Non-accidental head injury may be indicated by:

- Patchy loss of hair or haemorrhage below the scalp caused by pulling
- Symptoms of concussion — confusion, double vision, headache, nausea, vomiting
- Subdural haematoma caused by a direct hit or shaking. First indication may be hours after injury and may be drowsiness, coma
- Skull fractures

Fractures. Apart from birth trauma and road accidents, accidental fractures are uncommon in pre-ambulant children. It is essential that the attending doctor consider the possibility of pre-existing bone disease that can predispose the child to fractures or cause bone changes which mimic fractures. Exclusion of organic causes can usually be done by X-ray investigation.

Skull fractures in abused children are more likely to be complex, multiple or depressed with associated intracranial injuries. It is also important to have a high level of suspicion in the case of a pre-ambulatory child who has a femoral fracture with an oblique or spiral pattern.

Fractured limbs may present as pseudo-paralysis — the infant holds the limb inappropriately still. Fractures heal quickly and pain may disappear within a few days. Swelling normally persists for several weeks. Injuries may include:

- Metaphyseal or corner fractures of long bones, caused by twisting and pulling
- Epiphyseal separation — separation of the growth centre at the end of the bone from the rest of the shaft, caused by twisting or pulling
- Periosteal elevation — detachment of periosteum from shaft of bone with associated haemorrhage in periosteum and shaft
- Spiral fractures

Radiology. Because the junction of the cartilage with the shaft of the long bone is one of the weakest areas in the growing child and because these areas are the most vulnerable to the torsion and tension forces that occur when the child is pulled or shaken, epiphyseal separations and adjacent metaphyseal fractures are the commonest lesions. Subperiosteal haemorrhages commonly occur, lifting the periosteum, which then lays down new bone in its new position. Spiral fractures, which are unusual in normal childhood accidents, occur as a result of twisting/shearing forces applied to long bones.

A recent Australian survey of victims of child abuse indicated that in children less than 12 months of age, long bone injury was the most common form of presentation. In 83% of cases, the injuries were multiple. In 14% metaphyseal injury was present and 8% showed periosteal reaction to trauma.

A distressing feature of this survey was a re-injury rate of 44%. Of these re-injured children, 25% occurred in foster homes and 75% occurred on return to biological parents. These figures seriously challenge our present practices of assessment and placement of children after the first abuse incident.

Burns and scalds. Burns and scalds are a common manifestation of abuse and appear to be more premeditated than injuries produced by sudden rage. Buttock, glove and stocking type distribution burns suggest immersion. In cases of nappy rash the buttocks can appear burnt with excoriation but persistent nappy rash can be an indication of neglect as can repeated scalds in an ambulant child.

Other injuries. A variety of more unusual injuries may occur. Hitting and kicking directed to the abdomen can lead to signs/symptoms of intestinal perforation and peritonitis. Cutaneous lesions may present in the shape of recognizable objects such as belts, irons or rope marks. Unexplained neurological features may point to the shaken baby syndrome or undetected skull fractures. Injuries to the mouth may be caused by forced feeding. Even in the absence of swollen lips there may be lacerations or haemorrhages inside the mouth.

Further investigations. Where there is marked bruising or a history of easy bruising, haematological studies are indicated. The urine should be tested for blood in all cases of abdominal injury. Ultrasound may be helpful in assisting diagnosis in abdominal trauma, e.g. duodenal haematoma and pancreatic cyst due to trauma.

A skeletal survey may reveal multiple fractures at different stages of healing. Radionuclide bone scanning can detect early evidence of periosteal injury.

The shaken baby syndrome

The shaken baby syndrome (SBS) is defined as a form of serious physical child abuse involving infants under 2 years of age. The rapid acceleration/deceleration of the head causes characteristic findings affecting three major organ systems — the eyes, the skeletal system and central nervous system. While infants may manifest injury to only one organ system or recover completely it must be remembered that SBS can result in death as well as permanent disabilities such as blindness, developmental delay and motor deficits. A CT scan of the head is a useful diagnostic tool but MRI can detect different ages of fluid collection in injury which may imply several episodes of injury.

MRI is particularly valuable when the origin of neurological injury is uncertain, when the CT scan is normal and retinal haemorrhages raise the suspicion of SBS.

Abused children can be brain injured without visible signs such as bruising. If a baby is shaken it is possible to create sufficient abnormal rotational forces that shearing injuries to the brain can occur and blood vessels between the brain and skull can be split, resulting in haemorrhages.

The most important clinical sign is the detection of retinal haemorrhages. These children usually present in casualty unconscious or with a history of having had a fit or fall from a cot, table or pram. These injuries are inconsistent with any such simple fall and the eye signs may be accompanied by fractured ribs or finger mark bruising over ribs or upper arms which are other indications of the violence of the shaking. However, in the absence of such indicators, ophthalmic examination should always be included as part of the assessment of the possibly abused child.

Sexual abuse

The most widely accepted definition of child sexual abuse (CSA) is that of Schechter and

Roberge in 1976: 'the involvement of dependent, developmentally immature children and adolescents in sexual activities that they are unable to give informed consent to, and that violate the social taboos or family roles'.

This definition encompasses a range of activities which include exhibitionism, fondling of errogenous areas, masturbation, oral sex and vaginal/anal penetration by finger, penis or object. It excludes consensual peer sexual activity and includes child exploitation in pornography and prostitution.

Incest is legally defined as intercourse between biological family members but in practice is taken to include sexual activity between a child and an adult who has assumed a parental role within the family.

Retrospective surveys in the United States, United Kingdom and Australia indicate that 1 in 4 female and 1 in 10 male children have experienced sexual trauma by 12 years of age. The validity of these surveys has been questioned because of variations in definition and methodology. Research problems are compounded by the particular difficulty that sexual abuse does not fall clearly within the domain of one particular discipline. The problem can be met in the disciplines of psychology, sociology, nursing, psychiatry, paediatrics, family medicine, social work, criminal law and education.

Unfortunately this allows for a great diffusion of responsibility and lack of communication between professionals. Nevertheless, CSA is a common problem and the fact that of the reported cases 90% of victims are female and 90% of offenders are male, adds to the complexity and strong emotions involved in this area.

The basis for the conclusion that a child has been physically abused involves the identification of inadequately explained injuries. A diagnosis of neglect rests upon the observation that parental deprivation has led to impaired development in the child. On the other hand, recognition of sexual abuse rarely depends on physical examination and findings. Most sexually abused children do not have physical injuries or any evidence of sexual assault at the time of examination. Recognition of sexual abuse depends on listening to what the child has to say and the child's ac-

count is of paramount importance. Recognition of sexual abuse is also dependent on the listener's willingness to admit the condition exists!

Surveys indicate that less than 2% of CSA reports made by children under 12 years of age are incorrect. Young children do not have a framework of reference to fabricate stories of sexual abuse and good practice can detect the exceptions.

Diagnosis

The diagnosis of sexual abuse is made on the history. The child's disclosure is frequently preceded by behavioural disturbances unusual for that child. It is important to record behaviour prior to disclosure. Non-specific signs may include poor school performance, precocious sexual behaviour or language, excessive masturbation, aggression or withdrawal, sleep and eating disturbances, recurrent enuresis, encopresis, and psychosomatic symptoms such as headache, nausea and abdominal pain. Other behavioural disturbances include running away from home and manifestations of depression including self-inflicted injury or attempted suicide. These all have a variety of causes in children but CSA should be considered in the differential diagnosis.

Possible physical indicators

- Torn, stained clothes in the genital area
- Swelling/redness of the vulva, penis
- Bruises, bleeding from external genitalia, vagina or anus
- Bruises, scratches, bites on breasts, buttocks, lower abdomen/thighs. Finger pressure marks
- Dilated vaginal/anal opening
- Positive test for pregnancy, semen or sexually transmitted diseases

The majority of cases involve digital or genital manipulation and there may be no physical findings.

Guidelines for medical interview/examination

It is important to record the exact words of parent/child. The method of examination should be explained to the child and the examination should proceed in a sensitive, unhurried manner. Children need time to talk, time to trust and time to tell. To this end a child-oriented environment is helpful, as is the presence of the supportive non-offending parent.

It is important to ask non-leading questions and to document multiple incidents, the progression of sexual activity and any detail volunteered by the child which may pinpoint place, time or person.

A general physical examination should be conducted in a good light with the child partially clothed and in the presence of a trusted supporting person, usually the mother. Any trauma should be carefully documented and illustrated and the genital area should be examined last. When no evidence of internal trauma is found, careful inspection of the external urethra, vagina and anus is sufficient. (See below.) Full internal examination is rarely required and should only be done under general anaesthetic in the prepubertal child.

Since physical and sexual assault often go together, a general physical examination is mandatory.

Genital examination. The most useful way to examine a cooperative prepubertal child is in the knee–chest position. This ensures a good view without any instrumentation. Genital examination always includes examination of the anus and the collection of appropriate swabs. Speculum examination in young children should be done only under a general anaesthetic. If there is a history of sexual intercourse, speculum examination is necessary to inspect the cervix and take a Pap smear. Some children object to the knee–chest position and the alternative is the supine position with legs apart and the soles of the feet in apposition in the 'frog leg' position. In this position the child can be distracted with a soft toy and conversation with the mother.

Depending on the history, forensic specimens may need to be taken for semen and blood, cultures including oral specimens may be necessary for sexually transmitted diseases and possibly serology for syphilis and a screening test for HIV virus. The examination and the taking of forensic specimens should be done by an experienced paediatrician or police surgeon. If any doubt exists as to what specimens are appropriate, a pathologist should be consulted.

Positive swabs for gonorrhoea and *Chlamydia* are highly suggestive of sexual abuse. Anal and urethral swabs for *Chlamydia* are painful and rarely positive in the absence of a purulent vaginal discharge. It is therefore hard to justify routine collection. Females with genital human papilloma virus infection should be examined by colposcopy to determine the extent of the infection. If rectal bleeding is present or internal injury suspected, proctoscopy is indicated.

Infection. Non-specific vulvovaginitis and thrush are common in female children and perianal inflammation due to threadworms or poor local hygiene is common in both sexes. It is therefore important to distinguish them from infections which raise the suspicion of sexual abuse.

Children with genital herpes simplex virus (HSV) infection, which can be diagnosed clinically, require a swab for viral culture. HSV-1 infection is less likely to be the result of abuse than HSV-2 infection. Balanitis is common in the uncircumcised penis and varies clinically from mild erythema to multiple erosions which can be mistaken for HSV-2. While venereal warts should raise the suspicion of child sexual abuse, it should be remembered that the human papilloma virus can be transmitted vertically.

Management. Depending on the findings, various regimens of treatment and follow-up investigations may need to be organized. It is essential that reassurance is given to the child and parent(s) to ameliorate the long-term consequences of CSA. Anticipated outcomes frequently verbalized by the parents are that their child will become an abuser, develop a homosexual orientation or a sexually transmitted disease, or be infertile. Reassurance can be undertaken most effectively by a practitioner known or trusted by the family or one with a special interest in this field. Any intrusive and forensic investigation should always be undertaken by someone with expertise in the field.

Parents often have difficulty in dealing with their own feelings of guilt and anger and may experience a grief reaction to what they perceive as the 'loss of innocence' of their child. If the offender is a family member, considerable disruption of family relationships is the rule. The victim may feel blame for the family break-up and may in addition have to bear the brunt of hostility from other family members. The support of non-offending parent(s) is crucial to the victim's prognosis. It is more effective to organize immediate support, counselling and therapy for supportive parents than to embark on long-term psychotherapy for the victim as this is rarely useful.

Prevention

Strategies for the prevention of all forms of child abuse need to be tackled on three levels, primary, secondary and tertiary.

Primary

Primary prevention is a community responsibility and includes reassessment of societal attitudes to violence/pornography and the protection of the rights of the child. The aim is to promote health and to minimize family dysfunction. Examples include education in parenting, life skills programmes, the Protective Behaviours programme, screening programmes for young infants and child care opportunities.

Secondary

Secondary prevention acknowledges that parenting is difficult and stresses are often not met in appropriate ways. This requires support to parents and other caregivers. Education is the responsibility of government, community and volunteer agencies. The essence of 'good enough' parenting requires that parents recognize, or meet the needs of the child or arrange for these needs to be met. Cultural standards may differ from those generally prevalent but abuse or neglect is not present if the basic needs of the child are being met.

Secondary prevention includes the setting up of support groups for teenage parents and the parents of the new, premature or disabled infant.

Tertiary

This is the responsibility of those agencies which have a statuatory responsibility to intervene and protect children from further abuse. Responses include individual and group therapy for abused children and their parents and support groups for the non-abusive parents.

While community priorities will always focus on primary and secondary prevention programmes, medical practitioners will often find themselves consulted about tertiary prevention and need to have an adequate knowledge of community resources.

THE FUTURE

Since the early 60s, when Kempe and others described the battered child syndrome, much more is understood of the dynamics involved in physical abuse and neglect. Because of community education programmes, women are more likely to disclose domestic violence to their family doctor. If doctors openly confront unexplained injury in female patients and children and have a working knowledge of community resources, it is likely that abuse to children in the family can be prevented.

While some community empathy exists with parents who physically abuse their children, the current fatality and re-injury rates do not allow for complacency. The Cleveland Child Abuse Inquiry in the United Kingdom and the McMartin trial in the United States threw doubt on methods of diagnosis and reporting of child sexual abuse and this generated some community outrage and backlash. They also led to reinforcement of the myth that children lie about sexual abuse. The end result of such an attitude is that more children are put at risk and the morale of child protection workers is undermined. Oates, in Australia, has warned of the temptation to defect from the front line of work with victims, in favour of activity in lecturing and needless research.

Perhaps the time has come to remind ourselves of mandatory responsibility, reflected in the words of the original pioneers in the field of child abuse. The words of Drs R. S. and C. H. Kempe are as valid now as they were in the 70s: 'We must not be demoralized or fail to keep pushing forward. Ultimately our children's future and our world's future are one'.

FURTHER READING

Finkelhor D & Associates 1986 Sourcebook on child sexual abuse. Sage Publications, California

Kempe R S, Kempe C H 1978 Child abuse — the developing child. Fontana/Open Books, London

Krishman J, Barbour P, Foster B 1990 Patterns of osseous injuries and psychological factors affecting victims of child abuse. The Australian and New Zealand Journal of Surgery 60: 447–450

Oates K 1985 Child abuse and neglect. What happens eventually? Butterworths, Sydney

13. Sport — physiological and paediatric principles

R. A. MacMahon

Games are a part of childhood and these become formalized as 'sport' at school. Some schools make a fetish of sport and the school heroes are those representing the school, while the 'ugly parent' syndrome of the parents urging on their child regardless of any possible harm is well known.

Sport, when it is regarded as a regular exercise programme, is believed to benefit the child in three main ways, physical, physiological and psychosocial.

PHYSICAL

Regular sport provides an opportunity to learn new skills, increases the sense of well-being, improves cardiopulmonary performance and helps to prevent excess weight gain.

PHYSIOLOGICAL

In general, exercise programmes will increase strength and endurance, the efficiency of the heart and maximal oxygen capacity. However, the physiological limitations imposed by the rate of growth and development at various ages place important limits on the possible training programmes and expectations of young children. Children have a higher metabolic rate than adults, absorb more heat from the environment and generate more heat for a given activity level. They therefore have an increased risk of thermal overload. Prolonged strenuous exercise in hot or humid weather should be avoided and liberal fluids should always be available. Fine coordination reaches its peak between 8 and 10 years so complex motor skills can be learnt and developed in childhood. Speed and endurance can be improved by training, but the ultimate performance will always be greatly influenced by the genotype.

The presence of epiphyses places increased risks on growing bones. Ligaments and tendons may be stronger than the epiphyseal plates and excess load may avulse the plate. Repeated microtrauma or stress injury to immature tissue is of concern and it has been stated that all highly competitive childhood gymnasts who continue in this activity at the national level will develop major bony spinal changes by their early 20s.

Adequate nutrition is important but there is no evidence that any nutrient will enhance athletic performance if taken in increased amounts.

PSYCHOSOCIAL

Sporting activities are an important aspect of social activity and contribute to leisure interests, friendships and self-esteem with achievement. Certainly, children can find a good deal of 'fun' in free play and in properly supervised activity and sports programmes, provided that the enjoyment and activity side is kept as the goal and the winning at all costs aims of some 'ugly' coaches and parents are excluded.

Children, and their parents and coaches, should be taught the difference between aggression and assertiveness in sport. Aggression aims to hurt an opponent either physically or psychologically, whereas assertiveness aims to use physical and psychological skills to the maximum legal limits. On the other hand, vigorous sport is one way of releasing aggression.

Sport can have its negative features. Competitive sport is time consuming with consequent effects on the child's social life, and is always stressful to a degree such that if children are required to compete at high level, appropriate skills training to cope with such stress should be part of the training programme.

MALE/FEMALE DIFFERENCES

There is a good deal of discussion on whether boys and girls should co-compete in sport at school. These discussions are always in general terms, because in school sport, especially in the early years, there are always individual children who are outstanding.

Hormonal influences begin in utero and are responsible for the development of the internal and external genitalia. There is a suggestion that there is an hormonal imprint also produced on the central nervous system. The obvious effect of this hormonal surge is seen after birth in the occasional menstruation of female infants and the presence of prominent Leydig cells in the infant testis. These Leydig cells disappear and only reappear with the onset of puberty. Continuing physical differences are well illustrated by the percentile growth charts in which the male percentiles are of greater magnitude than the female ones.

Other factors of importance are that coordination develops earlier in girls than boys, girls are more flexible but tend to put on fat more readily and the earlier growth spurt of girls means that at the onset of the teen years, girls may, for a short time, be taller and heavier than the boys and have a different social and emotional outlook.

This variable onset of puberty is also important within groups and this is well illustrated by the fact that age teams for contact sports may include tall heavy postpubertal males as well as small immature prepubertal males. This situation is likely to produce both injuries and aversion to sport in the smaller group.

Particular facets of sporting ability determine the competitiveness of boys and girls in a particular sport. For example, the relative strength scores of the shoulders in boys is significantly greater than girls at all ages so that in a sport such as netball, where the players compete for the ball in the air, the boys would always have a great advantage over the girls. This means that if a school team were to be a mixed male/female team, there would be biological discrimination against the girls.

In general, it would seem that there should be ample opportunity for individual boys and girls to co-compete, but it is inappropriate to make this compulsory, as has been done in some school systems.

INJURIES

Common injuries are due to direct trauma, but in children two factors are important in the pattern of injury — overuse and the presence of epiphyses.

Overuse

This is caused by playing an unaccustomed sport or by an intensive training programme and has as underlying factors, microtrauma, chondromalacia, fasciitis, shin splints or stress fractures. These may be due to inappropriate training or playing surfaces, inadequate or faulty equipment, poor technique or skills coaching, training errors or other factors. They present as tendonitis, bursitis, synovitis or stress fractures or cartilage damage. Osteochondritis dissecans may affect the knee, elbow or ankle and stress fractures occur in the tibia, fibula, femur and metatarsals.

The presence of epiphyses

The sites of growth in children's bones are sites of weakness. The growth plate is susceptible to overuse trauma and direct trauma will frequently cause dislocation of the plate rather than bone fracture. There is also a tendency for the growth plate to 'slip', as seen in the well-known slipped epiphysis of the upper end of the femur. In sport, these injuries may present with relatively mild symptoms and signs, so particular care in examination needs to be taken of injuries to the common sites, such as the upper and lower ends of the femur, tibia and radius and the lower ends of fibula and humerus.

Management

Emergency treatment of injuries follows the standard pattern of RICE — rest, ice, compression and elevation. Further treatment depends on a diagnosis of the underlying damage. The treatment of common injuries is discussed in Chapter 11.

CHRONIC KNEE PAIN

This is a common complaint in childhood and adolescence and well illustrates the approach to chronic pain produced by sporting activity.

There are three main causes of chronic knee pain:

- Traction apophysitis (Osgood–Schlatter's disease) — see Ch. 11
- Disorders of the patello-femoral mechanism.
- Osteochondritis dissecans

Disorders of the patello-femoral mechanism

These are common causes of chronic knee pain in childhood. They are due to malalignment of the patella because of knock knee or congenitally tight lateral capsular bands or to excessive laxity of ligaments, especially on the medial side of the knee. All of these conditions may give rise to excessive lateral pressure under the patella and deficient medial pressure. The cartilage of the articular surface of the patella can undergo degenerative changes, known as chondromalacia patellae, and this may also arise due to softening of cartilage during periods of excessive growth in adolescence, especially if there is increased mechanical load due to vigorous participation in sport.

The clinical picture is that of a retropatellar aching pain, worse with prolonged sitting and 'cold starts' but without significant catch, swelling or instability. Reflex inhibition, or in the case

of ligamentous laxity, recurrent lateral dislocation of the patella may give rise to true instability episodes.

Treatment consists of vigorous quadriceps exercises, particularly of the vastus medialis, to obtain realignment of the patella.

Osteochondritis dissecans

The painful knee with this condition is characterized by painful episodic catch, intermittent impaction, locking and instability. There may be minimal physical signs.

This is a condition in which there is a segmental degeneration of an area of articular cartilage and its subchondral bone, usually on the lateral aspect of the medial femoral condyle and this may become partially or completely separated from the condyle. The partial separation gives rise to the episodic catch, while complete separation gives rise to a loose body in the knee joint, which grows larger through synovial fluid nutritional mechanisms.

The loose body gives rise to the more major symptoms of intermittent impaction, locking and instability.

The involved area of the condyle is usually best demonstrated by radiographs of the flexed knee, in an intercondylar view. Arthography or arthroscopy may be required.

Treatment depends on the degree of separation of the fragment. It ranges from a simple limitation of activity, through limitation of weight-bearing, using crutches and slings, to surgical pinning or removal of the fragment.

HEALTH MANAGEMENT AND INJURY PREVENTION

A knowledge of the pattern of injuries of particular sports will allow the physician to give advice on prevention, including whether the child should play that particular sport. Mouth guards and eye shields are essential for certain sports but for a sport such as squash, which has a pattern of eye injury, extra care would be required for the child with eye problems. A child with one eye should be advised not to play it.

Adequate preparation is essential before any vigorous exercise. Warming-up exercises and stretching related to the particular sport should always be a part of this preparation. Inspection of equipment and playing surfaces is the responsibility of those in charge of the sporting event. The rules, equipment and surfaces should be varied according to the age and size of the children involved and basic first aid equipment should be available.

The Australian Sports Medicine Federation, along with other national sports medicine federations, has issued guidelines for the health care of children in sport, with special issues dealing with particular sports. Some parts of the guidelines for medical diseases, from the 'Guidelines for safety in children's sport', are reprinted below with the approval of the Australian Sports Medicine Federation. Complete guidelines are available from sports medicine federations.

Asthma

Asthma is a condition where a variety of trigger factors cause the narrowing of the airways and accumulation of mucus and fluid in the airways, thus preventing the lungs from functioning normally by inhibiting an effective exchange of gases. This results in the typical wheezing respiration of the asthmatic. Importantly, asthma may be manifested only as a cough, undue shortness of breath or poor exercise tolerance, rather than the typical wheeze.

A major difficulty for asthma sufferers is that an asthma attack may be triggered by strenuous physical activity. This is called exercise-induced asthma (EIA) and is extremely common amongst asthma sufferers. Over 80% of asthma sufferers (both adult and children) will wheeze after strenuous exercise.

EIA may start either during, or characteristically, after physical activity. It becomes more severe upon completion of the activity (usually up to 30 minutes after exercise). The intensity and duration of exercise are both important factors in triggering an attack as the rate of ventilation achieved and sustained during exercise determines the severity of the attack of EIA. Usually continuous activities such as running are more likely to produce wheezing than stop-start activities such as football and netball.

Being physically fit can also be of great benefit to those who suffer from EIA because the ventilation required to perform a task will be less and thus the threshold of activity which provokes an attack will be greater.

Asthmatic children should be encouraged to join their peers in all activities but should always be permitted to stop exercising or use their medications when they feel the need. When proper precautions are taken, asthma is not a barrier to participating and competing in sporting activities. Many national sporting champions are asthma sufferers.

Obesity

Many studies show that obesity is not to be simply equated with gluttony — in fact, obese children often eat fewer calories than their lean counterparts. However, there is evidence that obese children do exhibit low levels of spontaneous activity compared to their leaner peers.

Regular moderate activity for about an hour a day can raise the daily energy expenditure by as much as 20% which will make a significant contribution to weight loss. With obese children the emphasis with an exercise programme should be on:

- Enjoyment to ensure the child continues with physical activity, in conjunction with dieting, to control weight
- Regular, preferably daily, moderate exercise of up to 1 hour per day
- An emphasis on total time of activity per day rather than on speed or performance
- Caution with exercise in the heat since obese people tolerate heat poorly and adapt more slowly to changes of temperature
- Allow adequate consumption of fluid during exercise in the heat

Cardiovascular system

Diseases of the cardiovascular system, particularly cardiac disease, are one of the few areas where ill-advised activity can have severe, even fatal, consequences. Having a family history of childhood cardiac deaths or a child's history of a heart murmur requires further medical clarification and clearance. Where serious cardiac conditions are suspected a specialist cardiology assessment, often with complicated testing procedures, may be necessary to define the limitations to be imposed.

Signs and symptoms which should indicate the necessity for further assessment include:

- Undue shortness of breath
- Chest pains with exertion
- Fainting, dizziness or light-headedness with exertion
- Unduly easy fatigue
- Cyanosis of mouth and tongue with exercise

A small number of children and adults do die during exercise from cardiac conditions, but more patients die at rest from similar conditions. More importantly, the majority of those deaths have been preceded by unheeded warning signs.

Sudden death

This can occur at any time at any age and does occur in children playing sport. There are many and varied possible causes, but the supervising physician should be aware of well-recognized risks. These include cardiac problems such as myocarditis, cardiomyopathy, idiopathic subaortic stenosis, anomalous left coronary artery and any evidence of cardiac arrhythmia. Hypertension, often associated with renal disease, is not uncommon in childhood and may also be a factor.

Haemophilia

Because patients with haemophilia have less effective blood clotting than normal, relatively minor trauma can result in relatively large blood loss externally or into muscles, joints or other organs. Such haemorrhages may cause damage to joints as well as muscle wasting and contractures which interfere with muscle and joint function.

The emphasis with sport for haemophiliacs is to minimize the risk of trauma which might result in bleeding. Each individual case deserves separate consideration but heavy contact sports such as football, skate-boarding and boxing should be prohibited.

Drugs in sport

As stated earlier, the prime purpose of sport in childhood is to provide a regular exercise programme. Drugs have been used by some adult athletes in an artificial attempt to improve performance, over and above what can be achieved by a proper training programme and older children who aim at high level competition may become aware that such drugs are available.

All such drugs are now regarded as a method of cheating in a competition and all have side-effects, some of which are potentially dangerous and, in extreme cases, have caused the death of the athlete using them. The drugs used in an attempt to improve performance are stimulants, e.g. amphetamines, anabolic steroids, analgesics, beta blockers and diuretics. Other drugs, such as alcohol and tobacco, impair performance.

Children should be educated on the dangers of drug use in sport from their earliest introduction to competitive sport. As part of this education, they should realise that in high level competitions, such as state championships, they may be subject to random drug testing. Coaches, teachers and parents should be aware that some medications that can be purchased without a prescription from pharmacists and supermarkets may contain drugs which are banned by the International Olympic Committee and can lead to disqualification from many events.

FURTHER READING

Hellstedt J 1988 Kids, parents and sports. The Physician and Sportsmedicine 16: 59–71
Larkins P 1983 Trauma in childrens' sport. Australian Family Physician 12: 359–363
National Health and Medical Research Council of Australia 1987 Children and adolescents in sport. Commonwealth Government Printing Office, Canberra
Reilly T, Watkins J, Borms J 1986 Kinanthropometry lll. Proceedings of the Vlll Commonwealth and International Conference on sport, physical education, dance recreation and health. E and F N Spon, London
Telford R D, Ellis L B, Ashton J J, Rich P A, Woodman L R 1986 Anthropometric, physiological and performance characteristics of 12-year-old boys and girls — should they co-compete. Australian Journal of Science and Medicine in Sport 18: 20–24

14. Major trauma

R. A. MacMahon

Accidents are a major cause of death and illness in childhood and almost as many Australian children aged 1–14 die as a result of accidents than from all other causes.

The two most dangerous locations for children are in a motor vehicle and in the home. Motor-vehicle accidents are the most common cause of major multiple trauma. The initial assessment and management of major trauma is a crucial factor in mortality and morbidity.

It should be remembered that major internal trauma may not be immediately apparent. Triage for major trauma is applied, not only to those obviously seriously injured, but also to those potentially seriously injured, such as those with injuries sustained at speed, in falls from a height and run-over injuries. All such patients need immediate assessment in a trauma room by a competent person.

The assessment of major trauma is complicated by 'battle-field anaesthesia'. Dominique Jean Larrey, Napoleon's surgeon-in-chief, found that soldiers with major trauma often had minimal pain and pain perception in the immediate hours following its infliction and that because of this, in that pre-anaesthesia era, amputations were best performed on the battle-field.

Patients with major internal and life-threatening injuries may have minimal discomfort and show little pain to standard tests immediately following injury, and be thought to have only minor trauma.

A quick orderly routine of assessment is essential in major trauma.

The ABC system is useful.

ABC system of assessment

A Airway — is it patent, is there foreign body obstruction?
Aeration — is respiratory action present, efficient?
— is oxygen needed?
Artificial ventilation — is it needed?

B Bleeding — arrest haemorrhage
Blood pressure — maintain and treat shock
Bones — splint fractures

C Conscious state, head injury
Causative factors still operating, e.g. pneumothorax, hidden bleeding
Control of infection — antibiotics
— tetanus
— gas gangrene

Establishment of a patent airway and adequate ventilation and the arrest of haemorrhage and treatment of shock, are the first essentials.

One person or even one team is not sufficient to manage major trauma adequately. At least two teams are required, an A team and a team to manage the headings listed under B and C. The initial decision to be made is to nominate one person in charge of the resuscitation teams so that there is quick overall assessment of the patient and coordination and direction of the resuscitation efforts.

'A' OR AIRWAY TEAM

The objective of this team is to clear the airway and establish adequate respiration and gas exchange, either by the patient's efforts or by artificial ventilation. The airway may be obstructed by injury to local structures, e.g. by a swollen tongue, by a fractured jaw allowing the tongue to fall backwards, by glottic oedema, by spasm and injury to the vocal cords or by direct injury to the trachea and bronchi, or by thoracic injury.

Foreign material such as grass, dirt, water, teeth, blood and vomitus may fill the mouth and nose or be inhaled. Respiratory effort may be depressed because of a head injury, or may be inefficient because of blood or air in the pleural cavity.

It is often safer to clear the airway, pass an endotracheal tube and use artificial ventilation until the patient is stabilized and then decide if the tube can be removed.

If endotracheal intubation is not possible, a stab cricothyroidotomy through the cricothyroid membrane and insertion of an infant endotracheal tube, or alternatively an emergency tracheostomy (Ch. 16), may be necessary.

Treatment of respiratory or metabolic acidosis is necessary for adequate gaseous exchange (Ch. 2).

'B' OR SHOCK TEAM

Arrest of haemorrhage and treatment of shock should commence with the initial assessment of the patient. Local pressure with pad and bandage will arrest most local haemorrhage but direct pressure or direct clamping or ligation may be necessary for large arterial bleeders. Further loss of blood into the soft tissues will be minimized by splinting of fractures and of limbs with large areas of soft tissue damage.

Multiple fractures or major fractures, e.g. femur or pelvis, can cause major blood loss and are an indication for immediate intravenous therapy.

Shock, or decreased circulating blood volume, is diagnosed by high pulse rate, low blood pressure and poor peripheral circulation with pale, cold extremities.

Note

1. A high pulse rate may be due to many factors.

2. The systolic blood pressure range varies with age so that low values by adult standards may not indicate shock. A systolic blood pressure of 80 mmHg would be normal in infancy.

3. Capillary return in the nail bed requiring more than 2 seconds indicates very poor peripheral circulation.

4. Thoracic injury can be a major factor in shock. The neck veins, if visible, are important indicators of hidden thoracic problems.
Flat neck veins — the patient is hypovolaemic.
Full neck veins — look for — pneumothorax
                — pericardial
                  tamponade
                — myocardial
                  contusion
                — air embolism if
                  there is a
                  penetrating
                  thoracic wound

5. There may be hidden and/or continuing blood loss into:
— thoracic cavity
— abdominal cavity
— soft tissues with multiple or major fractures.

Treatment of shock

This is one of the many situations in which prevention is better than cure. Immediate control of respiration and gaseous exchange, control of haemorrhage, splinting of fractures and replacement of lost circulating blood volume may prevent shock.

The patient who has obviously lost blood but is not yet in shock should be transfused with an amount of blood equal to approximately 1% of the body weight as a preventative measure.

Intravenous lines

Adequate and early intravenous access is essential to the management of shock, both for prevention and treatment. Preferably, there should be a reasonably sized catheter into a reasonably sized vein but a small needle into an available vein helps in emergency treatment.

The site of access is important. If there is major trauma to the abdomen or lower limbs, then the upper limb or neck veins should be used. The internal jugular vein, sitting as it does immediately between and behind the two heads of the sternomastoid muscle just above the clavicle, is a readily available large vein in infants and young children.

Fluid

Fresh whole blood is the ideal replacement for blood loss since the red blood cells of stored blood have less than 70% survival in the circulation. However, re-establishment of the circulation is the prime consideration, so that if blood is not available, plasma or a plasma substitute should be used until it is. Subsequent transfusions can be used to replace haemoglobin. If fresh blood is not available, stored blood can be used but it must be warmed if a large amount is to be given. If there will obviously be a massive transfusion, fresh blood will be necessary, particularly if the total blood volume will be exchanged.

In severe shock there is also loss of interstitial fluid, both from sites of trauma and by transcapillary refill into the vascular compartment, so that replacement of body fluids with a balanced salt solution, such as Ringer's solution or Hartmann's solution, will also be necessary.

Rate

Because shock is a condition in which the circulating blood volume has decreased to the stage at which compensatory mechanisms have failed, fluid replacement should be as rapid as possible with continuous monitoring until the shock has been reversed. This is not a situation in which a preconceived idea of a volume to be given in a certain time, or a volume derived from a formula, should be used. This principle applies also to small infants, though the volume infused rapidly will be very small compared to the volume given to older children. Continuous monitoring by one of the team, with adjustment of the rate and type of infusion as necessary, is required.

Because there is inefficient circulation at the cellular level, there is a lack of supply of oxygen and substrate and a lack of removal of waste products. This may produce organ defects such as the shock lung syndrome or acute tubular necrosis of the kidneys.

Monitoring

Continuous monitoring of the seriously ill patient is essential. This will include the immediate usual measurements such as:

- Temperature
- Pulse
- Respiration
- Blood pressure

but also longer term measurements such as:

- Urine flow
- Head injury chart
- Electrolytes
- Acid–base
- Haematrocrit

and also, where possible:

- Electrocardiogram
- Arterial pressure
- Central venous pressure

Central venous pressure measurements are difficult in infants and children because the subclavian vein is not as readily accessible as it is in adults and the complication rate, e.g. pneumothorax, is much higher.

The haematocrit is unreliable in the bleeding/replacement phase but it stabilizes in 3–4 hours. The trend is more important than the actual values.

'C' SEGMENT

The items in the 'C' segment of the ABC system are essential parts of management, mostly by the B team. In particular, those not engaged in establishing an airway or in treating shock should assess and monitor any head injury and review other systems and organs.

Early and adequate pain relief is an essential part of management.

Central nervous system

A head injury may be part of multiple injuries or may be an apparently isolated injury. Three important factors should be borne in mind in assessing such an injury.

1. Fixed dilated pupils may occur with severe head injury but may also occur from the poor cerebral perfusion of shock from massive blood loss either externally or internally. The former patient should have a bounding pulse, while the latter will be shocked.
2. There is a 3% incidence of cervical spine injuries in patients with head injuries.
3. Associated facial injuries may interfere with the airway.

Assessment of the injury

1. *History.* Sudden deceleration injuries such as sustained in a car accident or a fall from a horse tend to give diffuse brain injury.
2. *Examination of the head.* A laceration is obvious but a depressed fracture or the bogginess over a fracture may be felt but not seen. Blood or fluid from the nose or ear may indicate a basal fracture.
3. *Conscious state.* In adults, this is now usually graduated on the Glasgow coma scale, but this scale depends heavily on the response to verbal commands and stimuli. In infants and young children where knowledge of language is nil or deficient and where the circumstances of injury make an appropriate response to a command unlikely, this scale has marked limitations. Broad general evaluation of the state of consciousness is only possible in this group and the ability to wake up and cry is an important feature. As always, a change in the conscious state is the best guide to deterioration or improvement.
4. *Neurological examination* — particularly limb movements, localizing signs and pupillary signs.
5. *General vital signs.* Pulse rate, blood pressure, respiration and acid–base status are influenced by a head injury and if allowed to

remain abnormal will, in turn, affect the outcome of a head injury.

Note

1. Respiratory management is the most important area of management in head injuries.
2. The patient who talks and deteriorates needs immediate neurosurgical attention.
3. The patient who shows rapid deterioration and signs suggesting an extradural haemorrhage, must have immediate burr-holes, *not* referral to a neurosurgical centre. However, if a surgeon with appropriate experience is not available and the patient is within 1 hour's travel of a neurosurgical centre, then it is probably better to intubate, ventilate and give mannitol, 1 g per kilogram of body weight, rapidly, intravenously, and to then transfer the patient.

Investigation

The main aim of investigations is to diagnose or exclude focal lesions.

Plain X-rays and tomography. These will show skull fractures and cervical spine fractures and dislocations. They also indicate the possible structures involved, e.g. a depressed fracture suggests local brain damage beneath the fracture while one through an air sinus suggests the possibility of a leak of cerebrospinal fluid. A plain X-ray also gives an indication of the force of the injury. Plain X-rays correlate poorly with diffuse underlying brain damage, such as acute general cerebral swelling, shearing injuries of the white matter or traumatic subarachnoid bleeding.

Patients with head injuries must not be left unattended in an X-ray department.

Computerized axial tomography. Where available, this is the method of choice to show the brain matter and intracerebral collections and it will also show shift of the axis of a hemisphere or lobe. CT may be normal when severe generalized irreversible brain damage has occurred and lower brain stem lesions are not seen well by this method.

Angiography. This is needed for direct examination of vascular injuries or to diagnose intracranial collections of fluid or blood if CT is not available. Delayed intracranial haemorrhage can occur after trauma so that reinvestigation will be necessary if there is any suggestion of this.

Magnetic resonance imaging. If available, this is the preferred method of investigating brain stem lesions.

Management

This should be both general and local.

General care includes care of the airway, respiration, acid–base status and treatment of shock. A large nasogastric tube should be passed in the unconscious patient to prevent inhalation of vomitus.

The hydration of head injury patients is controversial but both overhydration and underhydration should be avoided. Diffuse brain swelling will be accentuated by overhydration and by the increased blood flow seen with high carbon dioxide levels. Control of these factors and the use of intravenous mannitol, 0.25–1.0 g/kg as necessary, helps to reduce the swelling but mannitol should not be used until the cerebral problems are diagnosed.

Local care includes debridement and suture of lacerations, care of facial injuries and treatment of depressed fractures and localized intracranial lesions.

Depressed fractures in children are usually isolated lesions and the patient is fully conscious, though rarely the fracture will be compound. The bone may spring back from the initial extent of the depression so that there is more underlying damage than appears likely from the extent of the depression. These fractures usually need to be raised, but if the depression is minimal, surgical intervention is not essential.

Neurosurgical care. Simple head injuries with quick recovery of consciousness need half-hourly monitoring, particularly of the state of consciousness, for 24 hours to detect any deterioration. Acute deterioration suggesting an extradural collection is an indication for immediate burr-holes.

Cases of severe or complicated head injuries should be transferred to a neurosurgical centre,

unless the extent of the injury is such that the outlook is hopeless, but advice should be sought by phone before deciding to refer or not to refer. Transfer patients who have:

- Penetrating or compound injuries
- Deterioration of the state of consciousness
- Severe injuries but who are stable
- Depressed fractures
- Persistent leakage of cerebrospinal fluid
- Infants under 2 years with apparently minor head injury after major trauma

Do *not* transfer patients who have been stabilized but who continue to have:

- Bilateral fixed dilated pupils
- Deep coma and bilateral flaccidity
- Continuous apnoea

Thoracic injuries

Major thoracic trauma in children is usually associated with injuries to other systems such as head and abdominal injuries.

Thoracic trauma is usually classified as closed and penetrating.

Both types can cause injuries to the chest wall, lungs, trachea and bronchi, heart, great vessels and oesophagus and can result in pneumothorax, haemothorax, haemopneumothorax and produce hypoxia and hypotension. The general condition of the patient, the position of the trachea and examination of the chest will generally give an indication of the underlying problem.

Penetrating injuries are not common in childhood but the effects of a penetrating injury can occur in an apparently closed injury because the ends of fractured ribs can cause major lung and vascular injuries.

Multiple fractures of both ends of ribs will produce a 'flail' chest situation with paradoxical respiration, i.e. that segment of the chest wall will collapse inwards with inspiration with consequent interference with aeration.

Fractures of the upper ribs tend to be associated with tracheobronchial and major vessel injuries. Fullness of the neck veins suggests cardiac tamponade, while a widened mediastinum with a left haemothorax suggests aortic transection. Fractures of the lower ribs are associated with injuries to the diaphragm, liver, spleen and kidneys.

In severe thoracic trauma, the thoracic spine may also be injured.

Management

Any airway or shock problems will be immediately treated by the A and B teams (see above). If there is any suggestion of a tension pneumothorax and/or haemothorax, an emergency needling of the chest with, if necessary, insertion of an underwater tube drain, is the first step in management, before any investigations are undertaken. To assess thoracic injury, chest X-rays with supine, erect and lateral views are required. Erect views may be difficult because of the state of the patient, but lateral decubitus views will give similar information and are necessary to diagnose haemothorax. If injury is found serial X-rays will be necessary.

Tube drainage of the thoracic cavity to drain air and blood is often the only active treatment required.

Further investigation and treatment will be required if there is:

1. Mediastinal emphysema, suggesting injury to trachea or bronchii
2. Coughing of blood, suggesting airway injury, pulmonary haemorrhage or aspiration of blood
3. Persistent drainage of large amounts of blood, suggesting injury to major vessels
4. Persistent drainage of large amounts of air suggesting bronchopleural fistula or oesophageal injury

Further investigations may include bronchoscopy, angiography, endoscopy, barium swallow, induced pneumoperitoneum and CT.

For large penetrating wounds or for complicated penetrating or closed injuries a thoracotomy will be required.

Abdominal trauma

Trauma to the abdominal cavity may produce injuries to the gastrointestinal tract, genitourinary system, other major organs and to the lower chest.

The abdominal organ most commonly injured is the kidney but the organ whose injury produces the most serious immediate consequences is the liver.

In the conscious child who can communicate, abdominal trauma is indicated by abdominal pain and tenderness but in the younger child or the unconscious patient, this must be inferred by the presence of abrasions, contusions or fractured lower ribs. Penetrating wounds are, of course, obvious. Major organ trauma can occur in childhood from injuries that seem rather minor, such as a ruptured spleen after jumping down from a high fence.

A specimen of urine should be obtained from any patient with major trauma, particularly to the abdomen or pelvis. If there is gross penile blood, this suggests urethral injury and an urethrogram is required when the patient is stabilized. A specimen of urine is always necessary to detect the presence of blood suggesting urinary tract injury, so that a catheter is passed and if it obstructs in the urethra, it is left in place and a urethrogram performed to show the obstructing lesion. If it passes into the bladder a specimen is taken and examined for red blood cells. If these are present further investigation will be necessary: either a cystogram if there is a suggestion of a ruptured bladder, e.g. fractured pelvis (or CT with contrast if available) or an intravenous pyelogram or nuclear scan if there is upper abdominal trauma.

Profound shock in abdominal trauma is almost always due to a major laceration of the liver, sometimes extending into the vena cava. This degree of shock, with evidence of right-sided upper abdominal injury and an abdominal cavity full of fluid, is diagnostic. There may be fixed dilated pupils, erroneously suggesting major cerebral trauma. Emergency surgery, with preparation for massive blood transfusion, is necessary but it is fundamental to be in a position to clamp the aorta and vena cava immediately on opening the abdomen. On occasions, a preliminary thoracotomy to obtain access to the aorta and vena cava is necessary.

Because of the risk of sepsis in the splenectomized child, splenectomy should be avoided if possible. With adequate monitoring and blood replacement, it is usually possible to avoid surgery in the majority of patients. The state of the spleen is followed with serial nuclear scans. Incomplete tears readily heal but portions of the spleen may have to be excised with more extensive lacerations. If there is gross damage, splenectomy will be necessary.

Shock may not occur or be only mild with renal trauma. Emergency surgery in these situations is rarely required as the bleeding is self-limiting. Renal trauma only needs exploration if there is extracapsular extravasation of dye on an intravenous pyelogram or nuclear scan or CT scan with contrast, indicating rupture of a collecting system into the perirenal space, or if there is no function on that side and a retrograde pyelogram shows a kidney is present, indicating major damage to the renal vessels. Ruptured ureter, bladder or urethra will need early exploration.

Injury to other organs, such as the small bowel or pancreas, may not be easy to diagnose initially. Many cases of perforated bowel will not have free gas in the abdominal cavity on plain X-ray of the abdomen. Repeated clinical assessment, repeated X-rays and repeated other investigations such as serum amylase estimation, will help delineate the need for laparotomy. Abdominal paracentesis is not often helpful. The importance of shoulder tip pain indicating subdiaphragmatic peritoneal irritation must be remembered.

Control of infection

Injuries that breach a surface or viscus will need antitiotic cover and penetrating injuries with devitalized tissue will need prophylaxis against tetanus and gas gangrene.

BURNS

Burns are second only to motor-vehicle accidents as the single major cause of accidental death in children over 1 year of age. The term burn includes injury from a variety of agents, such as hot water, flame and chemicals.

As with all major injuries the initial overall evaluation is the key to management. All clothing and restricting objects should be removed and pain relief given so that there can be adequate assessment.

Emergency treatment of burns should be by liberal washing with cold water until the part is cooled to normal body temperature but not chilled. Nothing else should be applied except possibly a clean covering.

The management and prognosis of a burn depends on the cause, extent and depth, site and associated injury or illness.

Cause

The usual causes are:

- Hot water
- Flame
- Fat
- Chemical
- Electrical
- Explosion

Scalds from hot water, particularly tea, coffee, and cooking water, are the commonest cause of burns in childhood and are most common in boys from 1 to 3 years of age. Flame burns, caused by clothes catching fire, e.g. girl's nightdress, or by children playing around fires or with inflammable liquid, usually produce a deeper burn. Hot fat adheres to the skin and retains heat, so that such burns tend to be deep.

Chemical burns are uncommon in childhood and there are specific emergency applications depending on the type of chemical. Children may get chemicals splashed in the eye and continuous washing with water for 10 minutes is the immediate treatment. It should also be remembered that phenol, common in household disinfectants, can be absorbed from the skin and is neurotoxic. It should be washed from the skin with glycerine, but if this is not available, cold water washing should be used for 5 minutes.

A history of an explosion is important since hot gases may be inhaled causing burns to the airway. Similarly, children trapped in a fire may inhale hot gases, carbon monoxide and toxic products from burnt plastic materials, e.g. hydrochloric acid gas.

Extent and depth

These are key factors in deciding whether the patient should be treated in hospital with intravenous therapy. A particular category is the common extensive burn consisting of erythema with only minor blistering, seen in sunburn of older children and adults. These patients do not need hospital care. However, such a burn in young infants will need hospital care because of fluid loss.

In deeper burns of other types there is marked loss of fluid as oedema or from evaporation and this is proportional to the surface area of skin burnt. If the surface area burnt is extensive, fluid replacement will be necessary. In adults, the rule of nine for surface area is an approximation, i.e. head and neck, 9%; each upper limb, 9%; anterior trunk, 18%; posterior trunk and buttocks, 18%; each lower limb, 18%; and the genitalia, 1%. This rule is easily remembered and can be used as an approximation for children over the age of 9 years (Fig. 14.1).

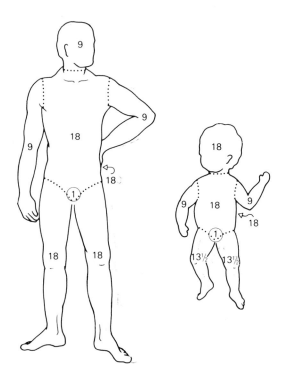

Fig. 14.1 Comparison of the surface area of different parts of the body between an infant of 1 year and an adult.

The infant or young child has a proportionately larger surface area of the head and a proportionately smaller surface area of the lower limbs than the adult. There are special charts depicting the surface area of various parts of the body at different ages and this is the only accurate method of estimating the surface area burnt.

As an aid to memory, a rule of nine can be applied to infants and young children, but it is applied differently because of the difference in proportion of surface area between head and lower limbs. The infant up to 1 year of age has a surface area of the head and neck of 18%, not the adult 9%. The proportion of surface area represented by the upper limbs and trunk are approximately the same at all ages, so the difference is in the lower limbs. The combined surface area of the lower limbs in the infant under 1 year is then not the adult 36%, but 27%, i.e. each lower limb has a surface area of 13.5% instead of 18% (Fig. 14.1).

For each year of age until 9 years, deduct 1% from the surface area of the head and neck and add it to the combined surface area of the lower limbs, so that the adult rule of nine applies above the age of 9 years. The infant and young child who has a burnt surface area greater than 9% should be admitted to hospital and will probably need intravenous therapy.

The depth of the burn is hard to estimate initially in children because of lack of cooperation. In the older child and adult, pin-prick sensation is the most useful method. White or charred areas are obviously deep but it can be difficult to distinguish between deep partial and full-thickness burns. This distinction becomes obvious with time. Electrical burns are usually deep and often involve underlying structures, e.g. tendons and blood vessels. Since in a deep burn there is loss of the whole thickness of the skin and its appendages, skin grafting is necessary in all but the smallest burn.

Site

Burns of particular areas are difficult to manage and even though they involve only a small surface area, warrant admission to hospital. These include:

- Face
- Neck
- Hands and feet
- Flexures
- Perineum
- Circumferential trunk burns
- Inhalational burns

Associated injuries or illness

Patients with associated injuries or illness should be admitted to hospital except with the most minor burns.

Treatment

Treatment of small burns consists of:

- Pain relief
- Cleaning and debridement
- Topical antisepsis
- Sterile bandaging
- Tetanus prophylaxis

Localized deep electrical burns should be considered for immediate excision and grafting, while patients with burns of special sites, e.g. perineum, will be admitted to hospital and treated by exposure and regular cleaning or by the application of silver sulphadiazine cream.

Treatment of extensive burns after pain relief is associated with an extensive use of tubes, including intravenous, urinary, nasogastric, airway and central venous pressure tubes.

Intravenous therapy

Intravenous therapy will be required for infants and young children with more than 9% surface area burnt and for older children with more than 15% burns, particularly if an appreciable area is deep burn. During the first 48 hours after burning, there is loss of fluid, both into the burnt area, which acts as a third fluid space, and from the body via the burnt area. After 48 hours this sequestration and loss ceases and the sequestered fluid is reabsorbed. A diuresis then commences.

It is not possible in the usual clinical situation to accurately measure this loss. The amount of fluid to be replaced is calculated by formulae such as the modified Brooke formula which is:

Amount of fluid = 2 mL × % area burnt × body weight in kg, plus usual maintenance fluid for age and weight, in the first 24 hours.

One half of the replacement fluid is given in the first 8 hours and the other half in the next 16 hours. During the second 24 hours the amount of replacement fluid required is one half that of the first 24 hours, i.e. 1 mL × % area burnt × body weight in kg plus usual maintenance fluid for age and weight.

The replacement fluid is lactated Ringer's solution (Hartmann's solution) with 5% dextrose. There is dispute about the use of colloid in the treatment of burns, particularly in childhood. It is usually not necessary, though concentrated serum albumin may be used in the second 24 hours to maintain plasma colloid osmotic pressure.

This type of formula is merely a method of doing initial calculations but such calculations are very inaccurate so that continual monitoring of vital signs, electrolytes and acid–base status, urine flow and central venous pressure if available, is essential. The most important monitor is urine flow (see below).

Blood is given as indicated by the haemoglobin level and haematocrit.

Urinary catheter

Urine flow is the best estimate of the adequacy of replacement fluid therapy but must be calculated at least on an hourly basis. This means that a urinary catheter is necessary. Urine flow should be at least 0.5–1.0/mL/kg per hour.

Nasogastric tube

Children with very extensive life-threatening burns are at risk from acute gastric dilatation, vomiting and inhalation, so that regular nasogastric aspiration is required.

Airway

Maintenance of an adequate airway and gaseous exchange is a fundamental part of the management of burns as well as of other major trauma. If there has been severe burning of the face and mouth with the usual consequent gross swelling of these areas, or if there has been an explosion or inhalation of hot gases, endotracheal intubation may be required. Rarely, if the upper airway oedema and obstruction interferes with endotracheal intubation, a tracheostomy will be needed. A good rule is, if in doubt, intubate.

Central venous pressure

As discussed previously, this is not readily applicable in infants but is helpful in the older child.

Care of the burn

This consists of debridement and cleaning and the regular application of an antiseptic cream, such as silver sulphadiazine, to prevent infection. This is reapplied as necessary to keep the burn covered and a daily bath allows the covering to be completely renewed.

Death in the first 48 hours after burn is due to shock, which is preventable, and thereafter is due to sepsis and organ failure. Sepsis will also destroy residual epithelium and residual skin appendages and convert a deep partial burn into a full-thickness burn. For these reasons avoidance of sepsis is of fundamental importance.

Systemic antibiotics should only be used for the treatment of cultured organisms, rather than for prophylaxis.

Antitetanus protection should be given to all burnt patients whose burns are such that they require admission to hospital.

Escharotomy

A circumferential non-elastic eschar of a full-thickness burn, with underlying oedema and raised interstitial fluid pressure, will produce venous obstruction, further rise in pressure and finally arterial obstruction.

The clinical pattern in a limb distal to such an eschar is cyanosis, poor capillary return, pallor, loss of sensation and finally loss of the pulse. In the trunk, it can interfere with respiration.

Incision of such eschar down to the fat will prevent distal vascular complications and relieve respiratory splinting. Such incisions need to be extensive.

Grafting

All but the most minor deep burns will require grafting and this is done by harvesting split-skin from unburnt areas on the limbs and trunk.

If the burn is extensive, reharvesting of skin from the same area will be required, so that early grafting, commencing in the first week, is followed by reharvesting at 2–3 weeks. In burns units, bank skin or other forms of covering, e.g. gelatin sheets, are used to cover other parts of the burn pending autografting.

Nutrition

There is a large loss of protein from the burnt area and a large protein requirement for healing. If the child is anorexic, severe wasting can occur and this will worsen the prognosis. Regular nutritional assessment and appropriate feeding, by mouth, by tube or intravenously is an important part of management.

Psychological management

The impact of a major burn in a child can be devastating to the family. Guilt is a major factor and the long illness and cosmetic problems are other major contributory factors. Arrangements for counselling for the family should be an integral part of the management of major burns.

CORROSIVE OESOPHAGEAL STRICTURE

The common corrosive stricture in childhood is caused by caustic soda, which is a common ingredient of strong household cleaning fluids and powders. Such fluids and powders are often stored in low cupboards and are easily accessible to small children.

A history of a child found in a situation which suggests ingestion, means that the mouth should be examined for the presence of anything indicating mucosal burn. If this is found, an oesophagoscopy should be performed to delineate any oesophageal burn. If none is found, then all that is required is reassurance. If a burn is found, then the child is at risk of oesophageal stricture and the most important part of management is to prevent severe stricturing.

Regular dilatations should be commenced as soon as the acute stage has passed and continued until there is no further tendency to restricture. There is disagreement on the use of steroids in the treatment of the acute stage but there is no firm evidence that systemic steroids influence stricture formation. However, injection of steroid into the stricture under endoscopic control, with regular dilatation, seems to allow successful stricture management and may reduce the necessity for oesophageal resection and replacement. There is an increased incidence of early neoplastic change in such strictures.

BIRTH TRAUMA

Birth trauma is responsible for at least 2% of neonatal mortality and for considerable morbidity and lifelong disability. The possibility of birth trauma should be kept in mind in the examination of all neonates but particularly after a difficult delivery.

Apart from bruising, abrasions and lacerations, one of the commonest injuries is a cephalhaematoma. This presents as a swelling over one of the skull bones, usually the parietal, and as the haematoma is subperiostial, the swelling is limited by the bone margins. Such haematomas spontaneously resolve and are uncomplicated but sometimes there is an underlying fracture.

Various types of intracranial haemorrhage occur in the neonate, particularly in the very small premature infant and trauma may play a part in these, though an associated fracture of the skull is uncommon.

The common neonatal fractures are of the clavicle, skull and humerus and the common nerve injuries are of the facial nerve and the brachial plexus. The phrenic nerve is occasionally injured and the spinal cord itself may be damaged, producing signs of a transverse cord lesion which may be misinterpreted as a 'floppy' baby.

Injury to abdominal organs is uncommon but injury to the liver and spleen does occur. Hepatic rupture will produce massive bleeding and shock (see previously).

ACCIDENT PREVENTION

Most accidents are preventable so that the major mortality, morbidity and disability resulting from accidents can also be largely prevented. Such prevention requires education, design and legislation.

Education

Parents and particularly young parents do not appreciate that the home is a more dangerous location than the motor car for children less than 5 years of age. Education on the dangers in the home and on the types and causes of home accidents are the appropriate prophylactic measures. Particular dangers in the home are scalds from tea, coffee or cooking water; burns from open fires, heaters or matches, particularly causing clothing to catch fire; poisoning from medicine left in reach of an agile toddler, or from detergents and cleaning caustics under the kitchen sink; the possibility of falls from steps or stairs; and the possibility of drowning which can occur in very shallow water.

Education of the public in the proper use of a motor car and of safety features such as seat belts is a fundamental aspect of accident prevention. It is also important for parents and teachers to realize that children up to the age of 10 years, because of their immature physical and psychological development, are incapable of coping safely with the complexities of road traffic.

Design and legislation

These are intimately related. Safety design increases cost so that responsible planners and designers are at a disadvantage when the price of their product is compared to that of the cheaper, but less safe product. This is well illustrated by the problem of flameproofing the material from which girls' nightdresses are made. Unless there is a population highly educated in the various safety factors, the price of the garment determines which one is bought so that legislation requiring all garments to be flameproofed is necessary to give effective protection to the population at risk.

Where legislation incorporates basic safety features, then the design of cars, roads, playgrounds and their position, houses, cupboards, electrical equipment and swimming pools must incorporate the appropriate safety features and only then will childhood accidents be reduced.

Medical and paramedical personnel must play an active role in educational programmes and in exerting pressure for design and legislative progress.

FURTHER READING

Articles on childhood injuries 1990 American Journal of Diseases of Children 144: 625–731
Symposium on childhood trauma 1975 The Pediatric Clinics of North America. W B Saunders, Philadelphia, vol 22 no. 2
Teasdale G, Jennett B 1974 Assessment of coma and impaired consciousness. A practical scale. Lancet 2: 81–84

15. Respiratory and cardiac problems in childhood

M. J. Glasson

Symptoms and signs of abnormal function of the lungs, and less often the heart, are common in childhood. The underlying disorder can threaten life, particularly in the neonatal period. When an infant or child becomes unwell and develops episodes of apnoea, tachypnoea, dyspnoea, stridor, wheezing or cyanosis, prompt clinical assessment, investigation and treatment are essential.

DEFINITIONS

Apnoea is absence of breathing and usually has a central cause (reduced 'respiratory drive'). It is common in premature neonates when it is usually brief and self-limiting, but is uncommon at other ages.

Tachypnoea is rapid breathing.

Dyspnoea is difficult breathing.

Respiratory distress is a term commonly used to describe the pattern of respiratory difficulty that occurs in newborns and which includes dyspnoea, tachypnoea, flaring of nostrils, grunting and chest wall retraction on inspiration.

Stridor describes a distinctive harsh noise produced during respiration and usually due to tracheal or laryngeal obstruction. Stridor may be confined to inspiration or rarely to expiration or may occur during both phases of respiration. Stridor in both inspiration and expiration indicates a more severe degree of obstruction than if it occurs in either alone.

Wheezing is a whistling or sighing noise produced during breathing and is often heard only on stethoscopic examination. It signifies partial obstruction of the more peripheral air passages.

Cyanosis is a bluish tinge in the colour of mucous membranes and skin due to the presence of excessive amounts of reduced haemoglobin in the capillaries. Cyanosis associated with little or no respiratory difficulty is likely to have a cardiac cause. When cyanosis is due to respiratory disease there is usually marked dyspnoea. Cardiorespiratory cyanosis occurs when there is an abnormality which permits a right to left shunt of desaturated venous blood. This is commonly associated with congenital abnormalities of the heart or with problems in the change in cardiorespiratory physiology at birth, which have been discussed in Chapter 1.

Rarely it may be caused by non-cardiorespiratory causes, such as depression of respiration because of central nervous system disease or from methaemoglobinaemia.

ASSESSMENT AND INVESTIGATION OF CARDIORESPIRATORY PROBLEMS

An infant or child in severe distress may need immediate oxygen therapy and if there is no obvious improvement, may need intubation or tracheotomy. Acidosis commonly accompanies severe anoxia and prompt treatment of it may be necessary before the condition is stabilized.

Subsequent assessment of the child with severe distress and the initial assessment of those with mild or moderate illness will be made with a full history and thorough physical examination.

History

For the neonate details of the pregnancy may be important, e.g. polyhydramnios suggesting the possibility of oesophageal atresia in an infant who has a choking attack on attempted feeding.

Sometimes, ultrasound examination antenatally may have alerted the clinician to the possibility of an intrathoracic problem in the infant. Marked continuing cyanosis which commenced within hours of birth will suggest transposition of the great arteries whereas difficulty in resuscitation with continuing marked respiratory distress will suggest congenital diaphragmatic hernia.

Particular features in the history may be of prime importance. An acute episode of choking, gagging and coughing suggests inhalation of a foreign body. Even in infants aged less than 6 months, specific enquiry about the possibility of inhalation of a foreign body such as a peanut must always be made when there are acute respiratory symptoms in a previously well child. Severe respiratory obstruction coming on over a few hours with an acute febrile illness suggests acute epiglottis. The slightly older infant or young child with failure to thrive in addition to respiratory symptoms is very likely to have a serious diagnosis.

Physical examination

Physical examination will initially be of the cardiorespiratory system and then will include general examination looking for associated as well as non-associated abnormalities. It should be remembered that even attempted simple inspection of the throat of a child with acute epiglottitis may precipitate total respiratory obstruction.

Physical examination of the circulatory system includes observation of the presence and equality of peripheral pulses, measurement of blood pressure and auscultation of heart sounds. In the respiratory system, the oropharynx must be inspected, the positions of trachea and apex beat noted and the chest auscultated for breath sounds. The cyanosed child whose colour improves following the administration of 100% oxygen is more likely to have a respiratory lesion as opposed to a cardiac problem.

Investigations

Blood gas estimation

Blood gas levels provide an accurate measurement of the adequacy of gaseous exchange in the lung and the state of the acid–base balance within the body (see Ch. 2). This investigation is necessary when there is moderate or severe respiratory difficulty or cyanosis but is not required in acute airways obstruction. Pulse oximetry provides a simple, easy and accurate method of continuous monitoring of · arterial oxygen saturation.

Chest X-ray

A chest X-ray is the only way to differentiate many of the causes of respiratory distress. It is always essential and sometimes may be the only investigation required before treatment is instituted.

If a foreign body in a main bronchus is suspected, both inspiratory and expiratory films should be taken. The affected side will remain comparatively overdistended on the expiratory film because of a ball-valve effect and air-trapping, and the mediastinum will move towards the normal side.

If a cardiac cause is suspected, attention should be paid to the cardiac size and contour and the pulmonary vascularity.

Barium swallow

This is a relatively simple X-ray procedure which is often useful in the diagnosis of conditions such as gastro-oesophageal reflux, H-type tracheo-oesophageal fistula and diaphragmatic hernia. It should, if possible, be carried out with fluoroscopy. There is the risk of morbidity and mortality from inhalation of barium through the larynx or through an H-type tracheo-oesophageal fistula.

Barium studies are absolutely contraindicated for the diagnosis of neonates with possible oesophageal atresia.

'Organ imaging' studies

Ultrasound examination, radioisotope scanning and CT scanning may occasionally be used.

Ultrasound is not suitable for examination of the lungs as the waves do not penetrate air or bone but it is useful for the assessment of pleural effusion. Sector scanning is used in the examination of cardiac abnormalities.

Radioisotope scanning is used to define blood flow to the lungs and is used in specialized centres for cardiac imaging.

CT scanning gives accurate and detailed images of thoracic structures and abnormalities. It is particularly useful for the demonstration of areas of bronchiectasis and in the investigation of mediastinal masses.

Endoscopy

Endoscopic examination of the airways is a specialized diagnostic procedure which can allow precise diagnosis in some instances of airways obstruction. The procedure requires general anaesthesia and a skilled endoscopist equipped with an array of miniature paediatric instruments. An inexperienced operator using inadequate endoscopes is unlikely to identify the true pathology and the procedure may actually put the infant at risk.

Endoscopy is particularly useful in the diagnosis of obstructive lesions of the larynx, trachea and bronchi and in the diagnosis and treatment of the inhaled foreign body.

Flexible fibreoptic endoscopy is likely to be utilized with increasing frequency in paediatrics in the future.

Cardiac investigation

When the clinical features are suggestive of congenital heart disease, an electrocardiogram is required in addition to chest X-ray. Echocardiography and/or the more invasive investigation of diagnostic cardiac catheterization (with or without angiocardiography) are required when the diagnosis remains in doubt.

Respiratory function tests

Spirometry and total body plethysmography can be useful in the diagnosis of a variety of respiratory diseases as well as in the measurement of adequacy of lung function, bronchial reactivity and response to bronchodilators. They are only possible in children above the age of 5 years.

CAUSES OF CARDIORESPIRATORY DISTRESS AND CYANOSIS

NON-CARDIAC CAUSES

In early life

These are almost always the result of congenital abnormalities and they may affect the nasopharynx, the larynx, the trachea, bronchi, lungs or pleural space (Table 15.1). These are almost always diagnosed before the age of 6 months.

The commonest causes are pneumothorax, gastro-oesophageal reflux and laryngomalacia. These and some others will be discussed proceeding in order down the respiratory tract.

Table 15.1 Non-cardiac causes of cardiorespiratory distress in young infants

1. **Oronasopharynx**
   Choanal atresia
   Glossoptosis (e.g. Pierre Robin syndrome)
   Cystic lesions of tongue (e.g. thyroglossal cyst, lymphangioma)

2. **Larynx and subglottis**
   Laryngomalacia (infantile larynx)
   Vocal cord paralysis
   Laryngeal cysts
   Laryngeal stenosis and/or web (congenital or acquired)
   Congenital subglottic stenosis
   Subglottic haemangioma

3. **Trachea and main bronchi**
   Tracheal stenosis
   Bronchial stenosis
   Tracheomalacia
   Bronchomalacia
   Vascular ring

4. **Lung parenchyma**
   Respiratory distress syndrome (hyaline membrane disease)
   Inhalational pneumonia
   (a) Meconium inhalation
   (b) Inhalation via tracheo-oesophageal fistula
   (c) Inhalation due to pharyngeal discoordination
   (d) Inhalation associated with gastro-oesophageal reflux
   Pneumonia — viral, bacterial
   Pulmonary hypoplasia/aplasia
   Congenital diaphragmatic hernia
   Congenital cystic disease of the lung (congenital bronchiolar malformation)
   Congenital lobar emphysema

5. **Pleura**
   Pneumothorax
   Chylothorax
   Pleural effusion

Choanal atresia

Complete obstruction of one or both of the openings of the posterior nasal cavity into the pharynx is a very rare congenital anomaly but it is important to remember this diagnosis because it can be a cause of sudden severe and possibly fatal respiratory obstruction. The atresia may be membranous or bony. Unilateral atresia is more common than bilateral and may not be diagnosed until after the neonatal period when the child first develops a cold or is noted to have a constant glairy discharge from the blocked nostril.

Bilateral choanal atresia is a cause of extreme respiratory obstruction, stridulous breathing and periods of cyanosis because neonates are almost totally dependent upon nasal breathing. These babies will be pink when crying. The diagnosis should be suspected when the symptoms are dramatically relieved by the insertion of an oral airway. Some infants with bilateral atresia present in a less dramatic manner with difficulty in feeding and failure to thrive. The diagnosis is suspected by the inability to pass a catheter through the nose into the pharynx and finally confirmed by endoscopic examination at operation.

It is desirable to obtain a preoperative CT scan to assess the type and thickness of the obstructing plate in the posterior choanal area and help plan treatment. Openings can be created surgically through the atretic segments via the transnasal route or the transpalatal route. Portex tubes are inserted postoperatively for some weeks to maintain patency. Reoperation is quite often necessary because of scar tissue formation.

Pierre Robin syndrome

See Chapter 16.

Lymphangioma

Lymphangiomata arise as the result of abnormality of development of the lymphatic system with failure of coalescence of primitive lymphatics (see Ch. 3). Lymphangiomata occur in almost every part of the body but are most common in the neck. The meaningless term 'cystic hygroma' is often used to describe neck lymphangiomata.

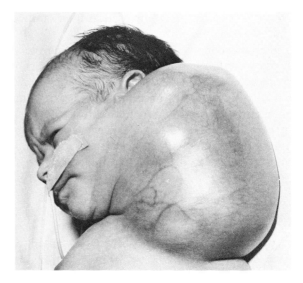

Fig. 15.1 Massive cervical lymphangioma at birth. This lesion was circumscribed and was removed completely.

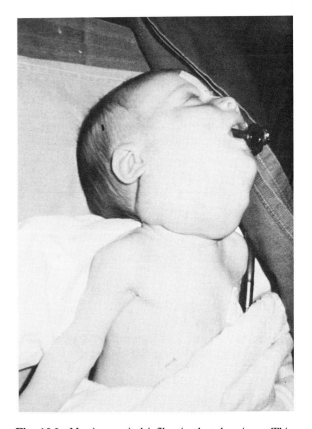

Fig. 15.2 Massive cervical infiltrative lymphangioma. This child required tracheotomy because of involvement of tongue and epiglottis.

Usually, they are circumscribed and produce a clinical swelling but no symptoms (Fig. 15.1).

A rare infiltrative variety may involve the neck and upper air passages massively (Fig. 15.2) and cause respiratory difficulty through airways obstruction. Complete removal of such lymphangioma is impossible and surgical treatment must be directed towards the provision of an adequate airway as well as excision of the mass of the tumour with attention to the final cosmetic appearance. Tracheostomy is sometimes necessary.

Obstructive lesions in the larynx and subglottis

Inspiratory stridor demands investigation especially when it is severe, progressive or associated with other suspicious clinical or radiological abnormalities. Endoscopic examination is necessary for accurate diagnosis of the underlying pathology. Attempts at diagnosis without endoscopic confirmation are merely a clinical guess.

Laryngomalacia is common and causes inspiratory stridor that usually is mild but may be moderate or severe. At endoscopy, there is dramatic collapse of the supraglottic laryngeal structures during inspiration, sometimes called 'flabby larynx'. Laryngomalacia is a self-limiting condition; the stridor begins soon after birth and gradually disappears by 1 to 2 years of age.

Vocal cord paralysis sometimes occurs in the newborn period as a peripheral neuropathy of uncertain cause but it may be associated with congenital heart disease or neurological abnormalities. Recovery commonly occurs over a period of many months.

Occurring unilaterally, vocal cord paralysis usually produces very little clinical disturbance apart from a weak cry. Bilateral vocal cord paralysis causes inspiratory stridor, respiratory difficulty and cyanosis and may be life-threatening. Endoscopy is required to confirm the diagnosis and the treatment is tracheostomy until vocal cord movement returns.

Laryngeal cysts occur in the supraglottic region and are a rare but important cause of airways obstruction in the first few weeks or months of life. Endoscopy under general anaesthesia is required for diagnosis. Treatment consists of marsupialization of the cyst.

Congenital subglottic stenosis is a common condition which usually does not compromise the airway and which causes symptoms (mild stridor) at times of respiratory infection. When severe, significant respiratory difficulty may occur from an early age and necessitate temporary tracheostomy. The size of the airway improves with age and direct surgical attack upon the stenotic area is not required.

Congenital subglottic stenosis is often the underlying abnormality in the child with repeated or atypical attacks of croup.

Subglottic haemangioma is an uncommon cause of stridor in infants but should especially be suspected when cutaneous haemangiomata are present. The diagnosis is made at endoscopy. Most cutaneous haemangiomata do not require active treatment and regress spontaneously with the passage of time. Subglottic haemangioma, however, poses a threat to life through airways obstruction and demands active treatment. Unlike laryngomalacia, the stridor does not start soon after birth but rather at the age of 1 to 2 months.

The preferred treatment is to perform a tracheostomy and irradiate the haemangioma by implanting a radioactive gold grain into its centre. The tracheostomy is necessary only until the haemangioma has diminished in size or has disappeared. Some examples of subglottic haemangioma are suitable for carbon dioxide laser therapy.

Tracheal and/or bronchial stenosis

These occur very rarely as a congenital malformation and sometimes as a complication of tracheal intubation or tracheostomy. A stenotic area may occasionally require endoscopic dilatation; intralumenal stenting is a recent advance. Surgical enlargement is possible but hazardous.

Tracheomalacia

In tracheomalacia, a segment of the trachea is abnormally soft because of abnormalities in the tracheal cartilage and in the posterior membranous trachea. As a result, the tracheal lumen is compromised (especially during expiration) by collapse of the anterior tracheal wall and indrawing of the posterior membranous trachea. The resultant clinical manifestations depend upon the severity of the tracheomalacia and vary from mild symptoms (due predominantly to retention of endobronchial secretions) to severe stridor with or without episodes of respiratory arrest ('reflex apnoea') sometimes with cardiac arrest.

Tracheomalacia very commonly occurs in association with oesophageal atresia and tracheo-oesophageal fistula and should be suspected in children with respiratory symptoms following repair of this lesion. Tracheomalacia can also occur as an isolated anomaly or in association with compression of the trachea by an extramural lesion such as an abnormal artery or a mediastinal mass.

Patients with mild tracheomalacia have little more than a brassy cough and require no treatment. Moderate tracheomalacia predisposes to retention of secretions and the mainstay of treatment is efficient regular chest physiotherapy. Severe tracheomalacia with reduction of tracheal lumen to 20% of normal size, with severe stridor and apnoeic attacks, requires treatment by the operation of tracheopexy (aortopexy).

This operation utilizes the fascial connection between the great vessels and the trachea as a suspensory ligament and results in an increase in the size of the lumen of the trachea at the site of tracheomalacia. Most patients improve with operation.

Vascular ring

Abnormalities in the development of the thoracic vascular arches may result in a persisting (and therefore double) aortic arch, forming a ring which surrounds the oesophagus and trachea producing obstruction in one or both structures. In early infancy, the usual symptom is relentless progressive stridor and often there is failure to thrive. There is danger of sudden unexpected death.

Barium swallow shows a characteristic indentation of the oesophagus even though there are rarely gastrointestinal symptoms.

At endoscopy, pulsatile masses can be seen bulging in the anterior tracheal wall and posterior oesophagus. Aortography is usually necessary to enable the cardiac surgeon to plan treatment. At operation, the vascular ring is divided at its least indispensable point; the severed ends of the arch are usually separated by traction sutures to adjacent structures (aortopexy).

Tracheo-oesophageal fistula

Of the many causes of inhalational pneumonia, tracheo-oesophageal fistula and gastro-oesophageal reflux have surgical implication.

Congenital tracheo-oesophageal fistula is not common but is one of the most important neonatal surgical disorders. More than 90% of cases occur as a lower pouch fistula in association with oesophageal atresia (see Ch. 8). Antenatal polyhydramnios, imperforate anus or the observation of excessive pharyngeal mucus should arouse suspicion of oesophageal atresia and the diagnosis can be confirmed by the inability to pass a large bore orogastric tube.

If oral feeding is introduced (the diagnosis being unsuspected) the infant will choke and develop respiratory difficulty and cyanosis due to aspiration of feeds through the larynx into the lungs. Reflux of gastric content into the lungs through the tracheo-oesophageal fistula can also contribute to respiratory symptoms.

Congenital tracheo-oesophageal fistula in association with a patent oesophagus (H-type fistula) causes respiratory difficulty and cyanosis with feeding. Most cases become symptomatic soon after birth and are diagnosed during the first few weeks or months of life. Barium swallow sometimes confirms the suspected diagnosis but is less reliable than endoscopy and carries the risk of respiratory difficulty from barium inhalation.

Endoscopy permits safe accurate diagnosis and the endoscopist can pass a catheter through the fistula to assist the surgeon in the task of its identification and division.

Gastro-oesophageal reflux

There is a weak physiological sphincter but no anatomical sphincter at the cardio-oesophageal junction and it acts to prevent the upward passage of gastric content into the oesophagus.

Because of the nature of the sphincter, intermittent reflux occurs as a normal phenomenon at all ages. Marked reflux in childhood may present in a variety of ways and is only occasionally associated with any other local abnormality, e.g. sliding hiatus hernia.

Methods of presentation. The most common clinical manifestation of gastro-oesophageal reflux is vomiting. Very many babies have some vomiting from reflux during the first few months of life and require no treatment. The vomiting is effortless and not bile-stained. When there is oesophagitis from acid reflux, there will be failure to thrive and possibly haematemesis and melaena. A minority of patients with significant gastro-oesophageal reflux develop respiratory symptoms due to inhalation. Some of these patients have little or no vomiting. Gastro-oesophageal reflux must therefore always be considered in the differential diagnosis of children with chronic cough, bronchitis and pneumonia and when chest X-ray reveals widespread patchy changes in the lungs suggestive of chronic and repeated inhalation.

Investigation. Barium swallow is a simple but not always reliable method of documentation of the presence of significant gastro-oesophageal reflux. Other diagnostic investigations which are available include oesophageal pH monitoring and radioactive milk scan. The latter test is particularly valuable for those children with respiratory symptoms. Endoscopy is required to assess any associated oesophagitis.

Treatment. Medical treatment of gastro-oesophageal reflux calls for upright posture, thickened feeds and medication (e.g. metoclopramide) to increase gastric emptying. Surgical treatment (fundoplication) is indicated for children with massive gastro-oesophageal reflux who do not respond to medical management. Operation is often necessary when there is significant respiratory disease and for retarded children as these two groups do not respond well to medical management. It is frequently wise to insert a feeding gastrostomy at the time of fundoplication with these children.

Congenital diaphragmatic hernia

Early in embryonic life, the primitive pleural cavities communicate freely with the peritoneal cavity via the pleuroperitoneal canal on each side. The diaphragm develops between the 8th and 10th week of intrauterine life by fusion of the dorsal pleuroperitoneal membrane with the ventral septum transversum, thus obliterating the pleuroperitoneal canals. The common form of congenital diaphragmatic hernia (the posterolateral hernia of Bochdalek) is due to failure of closure of one pleuroperitoneal canal.

Also during the 10th week of embryonic life, the midgut returns from the extraembryonic coelum to the abdominal cavity and undergoes anticlockwise rotation and fixation. If there is a diaphragmatic defect, the intestine passes into the chest. This space-occupying lesion in the thorax, exerting pressure on the developing lung, inhibits lung development.

Other forms of congenital diaphragmatic hernia are eventration, and hernia through the foramen of Morgagni. Eventration of the diaphragm is a condition in which the diaphragm forms but is partly or totally deficient in muscle. Hernia through the foramen of Morgagni is rare and the herniation is anteromedial between the costal and sternal origins of the diaphragm.

Clinical features. The majority of patients with congenital diaphragmatic hernia or severe eventration develop symptoms during the first few hours or days of life. Some are asphyxiated at birth and do not respond to resuscitation. Others have good Apgar scores at birth but soon develop respiratory distress and cyanosis. Occasionally, the symptoms of a Bochdalek's hernia or eventration do not develop for months or rarely years, presumably in the case of Bochdalek's hernia because of blockage of the diaphragmatic defect by the spleen or liver during the interval period.

On physical examination, cyanosis is usually present and responds to the administration of oxygen in all but the most severely affected infants. Palpation of the position of the trachea and the apex beat usually indicates the mediastinal shift away from the affected side, which in the majority of cases is the left. Breath sounds are diminished or absent on that side but bowel sounds are not often audible in the chest. The physical sign of scaphoid abdomen is helpful but its importance has been overemphasized in the clinical diagnosis.

Diagnosis. Antenatal detection of congenital diaphragmatic hernia is occurring with increased frequency using ultrasound examination.

Postnatally, an X-ray to include all of the chest and as much of the abdomen as possible (Fig. 15.3) is usually the only investigation required to confirm the clinical diagnosis. Gas-filled intestinal loops or solid dense structures (e.g. spleen or part of liver) are seen in the chest with no lung visible on the affected side and displacement of the mediastinum and compression of the opposite lung.

Estimation of blood gases and the state of acid–base balance is necessary to objectively assess the

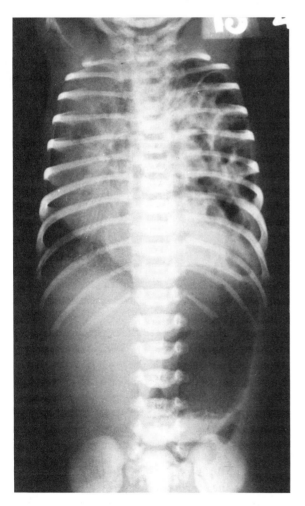

Fig. 15.3 Neonatal left diaphragmatic hernia (Bochdalek). There are bowel loops in the left chest and mediastinum is displaced to the right.

extent of interference to cardiorespiratory function and to help plan treatment, since severely affected infants are hypoxic and acidotic.

Management. As soon as the diagnosis is confirmed, arrangements must be made to transport the infant to a children's unit equipped with the required specialized facilities for definitive treatment. When the diagnosis is suspected antenatally, delivery should be at or close to such an institution.

Endotracheal intubation and intermittent positive pressure ventilation should be instituted as soon as the diagnosis is suspected on the basis of either antenatal ultrasound or postnatal clinical features. With artificial ventilation there is a great risk of the complication of pneumothorax on one or both sides and it is vital to avoid high pressures. Other important measures to be instituted before and during transfer include intermittent aspiration of the stomach via a nasogastric tube (as an attempt to prevent expansion of the intrathoracic intestine) and the administration of 100% oxygen. An intravenous dose of sodium bicarbonate will help combat metabolic acidosis. Cardiotonic agents (e.g. dopamine) and vasodilators (e.g. tolazoline) may be useful when there is evidence of persistent pulmonary hypertension.

Definitive treatment of diaphragmatic hernia consists of operation to replace abdominal viscera within the abdominal cavity and repair the defect in the diaphragm. It is not necessary for this to be undertaken as an urgent procedure. Most surgeons prefer to use an abdominal approach to the operation for neonatal diaphragmatic hernia. The abdominal viscera can be quickly and easily removed from the thorax and the diaphragm repaired after inspection of the ipsilateral lung. Diaphragmatic repair by direct suture is preferred but with large defects it may be necessary to utilize an artificial prosthesis or an abdominal wall muscle flap.

Prognosis. Those patients with congenital diaphragmatic hernia who present after the age of 24 hours have an excellent prognosis. Those who present at an earlier age have a guarded prognosis which is determined predominantly by the severity of the associated pulmonary hypoplasia. When the bowel ascends into the chest long before birth there is gross bilateral pulmonary hypoplasia incompatible with prolonged postnatal survival. Operation should only be offered to those infants who, after resuscitation, have blood gas and ventilatory parameters which suggest adequate lung potential.

Congenital cystic disease of the lung

In congenital cystic disease of the lung (congenital bronchiolar malformation) there is an abnormality of development of the lung parenchyma which results in the formation of one or many cysts within the lung substance. The cyst cavities are lined by ciliated columnar (respiratory) epithelium and the cyst walls contain bronchiolar elements such as smooth muscle. The abnormality is usually confined to one part of one lung, most commonly affecting the lower lobes. The term congenital cystadenomatoid malformation is used for the very rare variant which forms a partly solid mass of gland-like bronchioles and immature alveoli.

Clinical features. Many patients with congenital cystic disease of the lungs are not diagnosed until well beyond the neonatal period when an incidental X-ray is taken or pneumonia develops because of secondary infection within the lesion.

Since the affected part of the lung constitutes a non-aerating space-occupying lesion within the lung, if it is large, the adjacent normal lung and mediastinal structures are compressed and acute respiratory symptoms similar to those with congenital diaphragmatic hernia develop in the newborn period. Chest X-ray (Fig. 15.4) shows an appearance which is easily confused with that seen in diaphragmatic hernia.

Management. Prompt treatment is essential when there is respiratory distress with cyanosis. Intercostal catheterization performed because of the mistaken diagnosis of pneumothorax may rupture a cyst and lead to clinical deterioration from tension pneumothorax. Definitive treatment consists of resection of the affected lobe and the postoperative prognosis is good because the residual lung is usually normal.

Congenital lobar emphysema

Congenital lobar emphysema is caused by weakness and collapse (bronchomalacia) of the

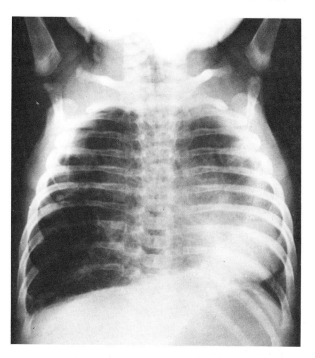

Fig. 15.4 Congenital cystic disease of right lung. The mediastinum is displaced to the left and the grossly abnormal right upper lobe has herniated across the midline.

bronchus to a lobe, creating a ball-valve effect with trapping of air. It almost always involves a single lobe of one lung, most commonly left upper lobe or right middle lobe. In addition, the lobe often has an increase in the number of alveoli ('polyalveolar lobe'). Overall, the affected lobe becomes greatly enlarged but provides a reduced contribution to gaseous exchange.

Clinical features. As with congenital cystic disease of the lungs, some cases of lobar emphysema are not diagnosed until after the neonatal period. Many children who first present after the age of 3 months can be managed expectantly because with increasing age the bronchomalacia becomes less severe and the risk of air-trapping diminishes. Those children who present at an earlier age often have severe respiratory difficulty. Increasing expansion of the affected lobe causes compression of the ipsilateral residual lung, mediastinal displacement to the opposite side, and compression of the contralateral lung.

Diagnosis. Chest X-ray (Fig. 15.5) is often diagnostic. Bronchoscopy is useful in confirming the diagnosis and excluding other pathology.

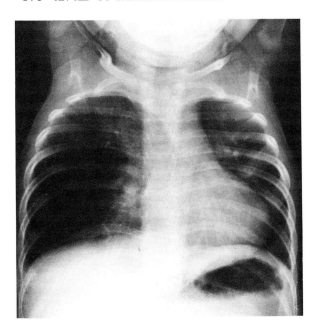

Fig. 15.5 Congenital lobar emphysema, right upper lobe. Chest X-ray shows hyperinflation of the lobe with herniation across the midline and mediastinal shift to the left.

However, it is a hazardous undertaking because of the risk that positive pressure respiration will cause clinical deterioration from further expansion of the abnormal lobe. A surgeon must be present at bronchoscopy and be ready for emergency thoracotomy should the infant's condition deteriorate.

Management. Definitive treatment consists of removal of the affected lobe. It is desirable to allow the child to breathe spontaneously during induction of anaesthesia and to delay positive pressure ventilation until the chest is open. The affected lobe bulges through the wound and its removal is usually easy. The postoperative prognosis is good.

Pneumothorax

Escape of air from the lung into the pleural cavity is a relatively common event in the neonate, but is uncommon in older children.

The causes are:

- The first breaths of life
- Hyaline membrane disease
- Positive pressure respiration
- Obstructive respiratory disease
- Trauma to chest wall or oesophagus
- Staphylococcal pneumonia
- Cystic fibrosis
- Diaphragmatic hernia
- Tracheostomy
- Thoracotomy (postoperative)
- Spontaneous

Birth asphyxia from any cause leads to uneven and incomplete lung expansion so that high transpulmonary pressures are generated with risk of alveolar rupture. This also applies to other obstructive airways disease. The increased use of intermittent positive pressure respiration for babies with prematurity and hyaline membrane disease has produced a parallel increased incidence in pneumothorax as a complication of treatment.

The other conditions are self-explanatory, but on occasions pneumothorax will occur in an otherwise healthy adolescent for no obvious cause.

Clinical features. A small pneumothorax may be asymptomatic and be absorbed spontaneously. A large continuing air leak produces 'tension' with rapid increase in size of the pneumothorax, lung collapse, mediastinal shift and a respiratory emergency situation similar to that already described for diaphragmatic hernia, congenital cystic disease and lobar emphysema.

The major difficulty in the diagnosis of pneumothorax is that it frequently occurs during the course of another serious illness and the sudden deterioration in the infant's condition may be attributed to the original illness. In the older child, pain and dyspnoea are symptoms of the onset, but in the infant, pain is not appreciated by the observer and dyspnoea may already be present. The onset of, or increase in, tachypnoea will be a prominent sign at all ages, unless the patient is on a respirator. Deviation of the trachea to the opposite side, with diminished air entry and hyper-resonance on the affected side, will be found on examination.

Diagnosis. Chest X-ray is the way to establish the diagnosis, but in a patient in acute distress, emergency needle aspiration of a suspected pneumothorax via the second intercostal space in the midclavicular line, is justified.

Management. A small asymptomatic pneumothorax will absorb spontaneously and needs no treatment.

A large pneumothorax must be treated. Some, without 'tension', can be dealt with satisfactorily by needle aspiration. Most cases require intercostal catheterization with the catheter connected to an underwater seal drainage system with suction. This allows the lung to re-expand with resumption of normal gaseous exchange and permits escape to the exterior of air which continues to leak from the lung. With the majority of cases, the air leak closes spontaneously and it is possible to remove the intercostal catheter after a few days.

Older children

Most non-cardiac problems occur after the age of 6 months (Table 15.2). Some will be discussed.

Acute epiglottitis

Acute epiglottitis occurs mainly between the ages of 6 months and 6 years and is a fulminant infection due to *Hemophilus influenzae* type B septicaemia. In a few hours or even less the child becomes progressively more sick with high fever. There is severe respiratory obstruction which initially may not be recognized, the child simply appearing unwell, grey and frequently not swallowing saliva. The older child sits upright, gasping for breath.

Simple inspection of the oropharynx in these patients can occasionally precipitate total obstruction with cardiorespiratory arrest and should therefore be undertaken only when facilities for provision of an artificial airway are readily available. The diagnosis may be apparent without the need for inspection of the oropharynx, which will show a gross cherry red enlargement of the epiglottis.

The treatment of acute epiglottitis is an artificial airway. A nasotracheal tube is the preferred artificial airway, provided an adequately staffed intensive care facility is available. It is wise to insert the tube in an operating theatre environment. Emergency tracheotomy may be required. The antibiotic therapy of choice is chloramphenicol or ampicillin when it is certain that the *Hemophilus* sp. is not ampicillin resistant.

Acute laryngotracheobronchitis (croup)

Acute laryngotracheobronchitis is a more common cause of inflammatory airways obstruction than epiglottitis and also usually occurs in the 6 months to 6 years age group. The infective agent is usually a virus and symptoms characteristically begin in the evening following a mild upper respiratory tract infection. There is a distinctive 'croup' cough or 'bark' and the child, at first, lies quietly without respiratory distress. A minority of patients progress over 24 hours or more to develop respiratory difficulty with stridor and upper airway obstruction due to subglottic oedema and rarely a temporary artificial airway is required.

Inhaled foreign body

The most common cause of the acute onset of respiratory symptoms in later infancy and early childhood is the inhalation of a foreign object, most frequently a peanut. Preferably, peanuts

Table 15.2 Non-cardiac causes of cardiorespiratory distress in older infants and children

1. **Supraglottic**
   Adenotonsillar hypertrophy
   Acute epiglottitis

2. **Subglottic**
   Acute laryngotracheobronchitis (croup)

3. **Trachea and main bronchi**
   Inhaled foreign body
   Tracheal stenosis (congenital or acquired — e.g. postintubation, burns, trauma)
   Tracheomalacia
   Vascular ring
   Mediastinal tumour, e.g. lymphoma, teratoma, foregut duplication, tuberculous lymphadenopathy

4. **Peripheral airways**
   Bronchiolitis
   Asthma

5. **Lung parenchyma**
   Staphylococcal pneumonia
   Inhalational pneumonia (gastro-oesophageal reflux)

6. **Pleural space**
   Pneumothorax
   Chylothorax
   Pleural effusion

7. **Trauma**

should be inaccessible to children under the age of 5 years. A great variety of foreign materials other than peanuts are recovered from the airways of children from time to time including vegetable matter, plastic and metallic objects, pencil tops and grass seeds.

The inhalation of a foreign body is the second most common cause of accidental death at home in children under 5 years of age.

Clinical features. At the moment of aspiration of the foreign body, the child has symptoms of choking, gagging and coughing. Apnoea progressing to cyanosis and cardiac arrest occurs when there is total airway obstruction. Usually the foreign body passes through the larynx into the trachea or a main bronchus and causes cough and wheeze, sometimes with respiratory difficulty. On auscultation, reduced breath sounds may be noted over one lung field.

Sometimes the acute episode is not recognized and chronic respiratory symptoms are the major features.

Investigations. Chest X-ray (Fig. 15.6) is usually abnormal. The foreign body itself can sometimes be visualized; the most common change is overinflation of part or the whole of one lung (caused by ball-valve bronchial obstruction) with air-trapping on the affected side or segment, often with collapse of other areas, and shift of the mediastinum to the opposite side. These signs may only be seen on an expiratory film so that both an inspiratory and an expiratory film should be taken if a foreign body is suspected. Endoscopy is essential both for diagnostic and therapeutic reasons in any child suspected clinically of having an inhaled foreign body.

Treatment. First aid. When a child chokes on a foreign body, nearby adults often invert the child and slap him/her on the back to encourage the object to be ejected. If the child can breathe, speak, make sounds or cough, no attempt should be made to dislodge a foreign body, since any such attempt may increase the degree of obstruction.

If the child is unable to breathe or make a sound he/she should be placed face down over an adult's knee and given four forceful back blows and if this fails, given four rapid chest

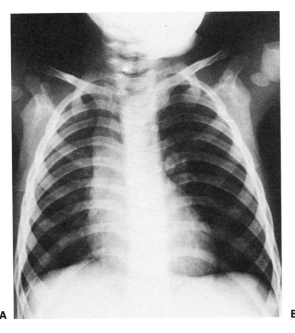 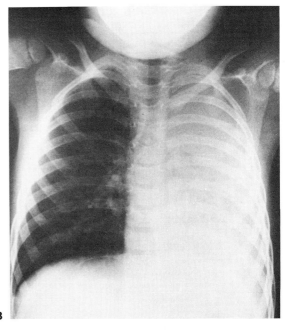

A   B

Fig. 15.6 A: Chest X-ray in expiration shows mediastinum displaced to the right and hyperinflation of the left lung. A foreign body (peanut) was removed from left main bronchus. **B**: Chest X-ray shows collapse of the whole of the left lung and pneumonia. A piece of apple was removed from left main bronchus.

thrusts. These should be repeated if there is no response. The insertion of a large gauge needle through the cricothyroid membrane may be life-saving.

Children who choke on a foreign object should be transported promptly by air or surface transport to a major paediatric unit where all facilities and skilled personnel are available.

Definitive management. Most foreign bodies are successfully removed from the trachea or a large bronchus at endoscopy under general anaesthesia without the need for tracheotomy. A variety of forceps are available for grasping and removing the foreign object. When there has been a significant delay in diagnosis and the foreign body has become impacted, it may be surrounded by granulation tissue. With this situation, repeat endoscopy often must be undertaken 7–10 days later in order to reassess the endobronchial pathology and remove any retained fragments.

Staphyloccocal pneumonia

Staphylococcal pneumonia is a severe condition in children and can have surgical complications of pleural effusion, empyema and pneumothorax. Treatment with an appropriate antimicrobial (usually a penicillinase-resistant antibiotic such as flucloxacillin) given systemically in large doses is essential. Intercostal catheterization is required for drainage of pleural effusion and/or empyema. With advances in antibiotic therapy, the operation of decortication of the lung for empyema has become obsolete.

Staphylococcal pneumonia tends to cause the formation of air spaces within lung substance (pneumatocele). When there is X-ray evidence of this, vigilance is necessary because of the possibility of rupture of one of these air spaces with resultant pneumothorax. This complication will cause a marked clinical deterioration, but usually will be readily controlled by the insertion of an intercostal catheter. Persistent air leak (bronchopleural fistula) sometimes ensues, but usually ceases spontaneously.

Chest trauma

Penetrating injuries of the chest wall are rare in childhood. Children involved in motor-vehicle accidents sometimes sustain blunt trauma to their chest and develop respiratory difficulty due to pulmonary contusion. If the injury results in fracture of a rib, the bone ends may lacerate a blood vessel or the surface of the lung and therefore cause haemothorax or pneumothorax. These respond to simple tube drainage. Occasionally, urgent thoracotomy is required because of damage to major structures signified by continuing haemorrhage or massive bronchopleural fistula.

CARDIAC CAUSES

The embryology of the heart and major vessels is extremely complicated and it is not surprising that congenital heart disease is relatively common (approximately 1 in every 150 live births). Lesions range from those which have no haemodynamic significance (e.g. small ventricular septal defect) through to those which are incompatible with prolonged survival or which are amenable only to experimental surgical treatment including heart transplantation or heart and lung transplantation (e.g. hypoplastic left heart syndrome). Table 15.3 lists some important examples of congenital heart disease.

Table 15.3 Cardiac lesions

1. **Those with a left to right shunt**
   Patent ductus arteriosus
   Aortopulmonary window
   Truncus arteriosus
   Ventricular septal defect
   Atrial septal defect
   Endocardial cushion defect
   Anomalous pulmonary venous drainage
   Cortriatriatum

2. **Obstructive lesions affecting the systemic circulation**
   Coarctation of aorta
   Hypoplasia left heart syndrome
   Aortic stenosis

3. **Obstructive lesions affecting the pulmonary circulation**
   Pulmonary stenosis with intact interventricular septum
   Pulmonary atresia with intact septum
   Pulmonary stenosis plus ventricular septal defect
   Tetralogy of Fallot
   Tricuspid atresia plus hypoplastic right ventricle

4. **Other**
   Transposition of the great vessels
   Transplantation of the great arteries

Clinical features

Common abnormalities such as patent ductus arteriosus, coarctation of aorta and atrial or ventricular septal defects may not produce symptoms but their physical signs are detected at routine examination in early life. If the defects are serious enough to produce symptoms, they are symptoms of cardiac failure or cyanosis.

Low output cardiac failure occurs with the hypoplastic left heart syndrome and obstructive lesions including critical aortic stenosis and coarctation of the aorta and is characterized by pallor, poor peripheral pulses and acidosis due to inadequate tissue perfusion and hypoxia.

Congestive cardiac failure is associated with salt and water retention (signified by hepatomegaly, increasing weight and rarely peripheral oedema) and respiratory difficulty. Factors which contribute to respiratory symptoms include left to right shunting, air-trapping due to airway compression from hypertensive pulmonary arteries, respiratory infection and left ventricular failure.

Cyanosis in congenital heart disease is due to right to left shunting and may be associated with inadequate perfusion of the lungs as in tetralogy of Fallot or normal or excessive pulmonary perfusion as in transposition of the great arteries.

Investigation and treatment

When congenital heart disease becomes symptomatic in early infancy, it is usually possible for the paediatric cardiologist to make an accurate provisional diagnosis of the underlying disorder from the assessment of the physical signs, a chest X-ray, electrocardiogram and echocardiogram. With medical treatment for heart failure (digoxin and diuretics) the clinical condition of many infants improves and it is possible to delay definitive investigation and treatment for months or years.

During the past two decades, there have been dramatic advances in the surgery of congenital heart disease and it is now possible to undertake most corrective heart operations, if necessary, at any age. The mortality from untreated congenital heart disease is highest during the first year of life.

Those patients who have cardiac failure unresponsive to medical therapy or who are severely cyanosed require urgent resuscitation by medical means followed by timely surgical correction or palliation. Advances in echocardiography are now such that many of these operations can be performed without preliminary cardiac catheterization or angiography, although these are still required to define precise anatomy and physiology in some cases.

Surgical treatment

The cardiac surgeon aims to repair the congenital anomaly and produce normal haemodynamics. Cardiopulmonary bypass with hypothermia is usually required for intracardiac correction. Advances in metabolic support of the heart during its arrest using hypothermic and potassium-containing solutions have made a considerable contribution to the safety of this surgery. A preliminary palliative operation without bypass is sometimes undertaken in these patients. Lesions involving great arteries can frequently be repaired without open heart techniques.

Surgery without cardiopulmonary bypass

Persistent ductus arteriosus. This is usually ligated via a left thoracotomy. Division may be preferred when the ductus is widely patent. Spontaneous closure of the ductus can be anticipated in the well neonate. For other neonates, when there is cardiac failure from torrential blood flow through the ductus, pharmacological closure with indomethacin sometimes succeeds. Urgent operation may be necessary and is frequently life-saving for very small premature infants.

Banding of the main pulmonary artery. This operation is a useful palliative procedure when there is cardiac failure due to increased pulmonary blood flow from a left to right shunt at ventricular level, usually due to complex defects not suited for one stage correction. A teflon tape band is placed around the main pulmonary artery in order to reduce the pulmonary blood pressure and flow and reduce the size of the shunt. The child usually improves dramatically, but ultimately with growth, the intraventricular shunt reverses and cyanosis ensues. Banding of the main pulmonary artery is best reserved for those patients whose intracardiac anatomy is not amenable to early total correction.

Resection of coarctation of the aorta. In the usual form of coarctation, there is narrowing of the aorta just distal to the site of the ductus arteriosus. When the coarctation is an isolated anomaly, it is usually possible to control heart failure in the first few months of life with medical treatment and to postpone surgical treatment for some years. When the coarctation is very severe, or there is an associated intracardiac anomaly (most often a large ventricular septal defect with left to right shunt), heart failure in early life is progressive and surgical treatment becomes necessary. Resection and reanastomosis is a standard repair. Alternatively, a flap created from the subclavian artery may be turned down to enlarge the aortic circumference.

Systemic to pulmonary shunts. The creation of an anastomosis between a systemic artery and the pulmonary artery is effective treatment for cyanotic congenital heart defects with diminished pulmonary blood flow. The Blalock shunt (subclavian artery to pulmonary artery) or a shunt of synthetic vascular graft material is favoured.

Systemic to pulmonary shunts are sometimes utilized as a preliminary palliative procedure for potentially correctable disorders such as tetralogy of Fallot, pulmonary atresia and some complicated cases of transposition of the great arteries, where the aorta arises from the right and the pulmonary trunk from the left ventricle. Some children with uncorrectable lesions, such as tricuspid atresia, obtain prolonged, good quality survival from a functioning shunt. Such cases may benefit from a second shunt when the first one becomes relatively ineffective because of the child's growth.

Procedures to improve the admixture of systemic and pulmonary venous blood at atrial level. Transposition of the great vessels with little intracardiac shunt causes severe cyanosis and hypoxia during the first few days of life. Emergency intervention to increase the mixing of the oxygenated pulmonary venous blood and the blood in the systemic circulation is necessary if the infant is to have any hope of survival. This is done by the creation of an atrial septal defect at cardiac catheterization using a balloon catheter (Rashkind procedure).

Open heart surgery

Rapid advances have occurred in the field of paediatric open heart surgery during the past two decades and it is now often possible to repair complex intracardiac defects in neonates of less than 2 kg. For operations to be performed within the heart, it is necessary to have facilities for cardiopulmonary bypass with a machine undertaking the functions of the heart and lungs during operation. Profound hypothermia (18°C) makes it possible to safely cease the circulation for periods of approximately 1 hour and permits the surgeon to perform the delicate intracardiac manoeuvres with precision in a motionless operative field.

The trend in recent years has been towards a policy of definitive repair rather than palliation for patients with congenital heart disease who become symptomatic at a very early age. Furthermore, new operations are being devised and total correction is now possible for many anomalies which were previously considered inoperable and were uniformly fatal.

Abnormalities which produce severe respiratory difficulty and/or cyanosis, and which are considered for total repair in early infancy after failed medical treatment, include ventricular septal defect, aortopulmonary window, truncus arteriosus, total anomalous pulmonary venous drainage, transposition of the great vessels and tetralogy of Fallot.

FURTHER READING

Bailey P V, Tracy T, Connors R H et al 1990 Congenital bronchopulmonary malformations. Journal of Thoracic and Cardiovascular Surgery 99: 597–603

Fonkalsrud E W, Foglia R P, Ament M E et al 1989 Operative treatment for the gastroesophageal reflux syndrome in children. Journal of Pediatric Surgery 24: 525–529

Jordan S C, Scott O 1989 Heart disease in paediatrics. Butterworths, London

16. The face and oropharynx

M. J. Glasson

Disorders of the face, mouth, tongue, tonsils and ear usually produce a visible lesion so that an accurate diagnosis can often be made from thorough clinical examination. A number of important congenital malformations occur in this area, some rare. Injuries and infections are the most commonly acquired problems.

EMBRYOLOGY

The embryology of the head and neck is complicated. The frontonasal process and the maxillary processes develop soon after the second week of embryonic life and surround a cavity which will form the mouth and nose. At the same time, there is a series of hillocks (branchial arches) and valleys (branchial clefts) in the upper body. As embryogenesis proceeds the arches fuse, the first branchial arch forming much of the face whilst the second and third arches form the neck. Part of the base of the first branchial cleft remains open to form the eustachian tube and auditory canal. Branchial arch lesions result from incomplete obliteration of branchial clefts or persistence of branchial structures (e.g. cartilage) that normally disappear.

Congenital abnormalities that result from disturbance of the complex fissuring of the frontonasal process, the maxillary processes and the branchial arches include cleft lip, cleft palate, Pierre Robin syndrome, branchial arch syndromes and preauricular sinuses and tags.

CLEFT LIP AND PALATE

Cleft of the lip and/or palate occurs in from 1 in 700 to 1 in 1000 live births. There is a definite genetic influence. Subsequent siblings of an affected child have a risk of being similarly affected of between 1 in 10 and 1 in 50, depending upon whether there is any other family history. When both parents have a cleft, the risk of involvement in their offspring is between 1 in 2 and 1 in 3.

Diagnosis

The diagnosis is readily made by inspection at birth. The spectrum of abnormality varies as follows:

1. Unilateral incomplete cleft lip
2. Unilateral complete cleft lip
3. Unilateral complete cleft lip with notching of alveolus
4. Unilateral complete cleft lip and palate (Fig. 16.1)
5. Bilateral complete cleft lip and palate (Fig. 16.2)
6. Cleft palate with intact lip
7. Bifid uvula
8. Submucous cleft palate — here the palatal mucosa is intact, but the muscular layers are not; it should be suspected when there is a bifid uvula. The diagnosis may not be appreciated until oronasal escape is noted during phonation

Management

It is important that the nature of the deformity be explained to the parents soon after birth, preferably with the aid of pre- and postoperative photographs of previously treated patients.

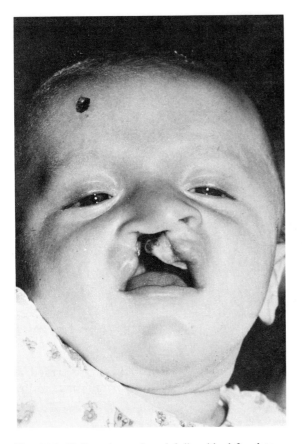

Fig. 16.1 Unilateral complete cleft lip with cleft palate.

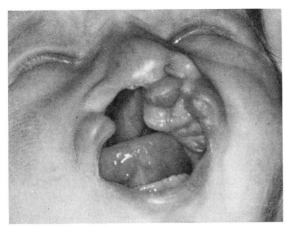

Fig. 16.2 Bilateral cleft lip with complete cleft palate. Note protrusion of premaxilla.

Feeding

The infant with an intact palate experiences no difficulty with sucking and swallowing. Infants with cleft palate can swallow normally but are unable to suck. Breast-feeding is therefore not possible. Feeds can be deposited into the pharynx with an eyedropper or a spoon or by using a soft plastic 'squeeze' bottle. Intragastric tube ('gavage') feeding is not usually required.

Surgical treatment

The aim of treatment is to produce an intact healed lip, alveolus and palate with little or no cosmetic deformity, normal speech and normal dentition. For this to be achieved, it is desirable that treatment take place in a specialized institution by a team which includes a plastic surgeon, ear nose and throat surgeon, orthodontists, speech therapists, psychologists and interested nursing staff.

Infants with bilateral complete cleft lip and palate with protrusion of the premaxilla need early orthodontic attention and should be assessed during the first week of life for preparation of a dental plate to help achieve alveolar realignment.

Operation to repair the lip, the nose and the anterior palate (when involved) is usually undertaken at the age of 2 months provided the infant is thriving. Closure of the lip alone at this procedure is associated with a less satisfactory end result for dentition.

Repair of the palate is performed at the age of 6 to 8 months, well before the onset of speech. The most important part of this operation is to push the soft palate structures as far back as possible to assist in oronasal closure postoperatively.

Secondary operations may be required at a later date (especially if the lip and palate surgery has been performed by an inexperienced operator) to improve the cosmetic appearance of the nose and upper lip and to improve speech when there is considerable nasal air escape. Adenoidectomy must *never* be performed because the adenoids in these patients assist in achieving oronasal closure.

Approximately 20% of children require speech

therapy in the immediate preschool period and early school years and articulation defects may improve with this therapy. Patients with nasality or air escape may require secondary pharyngolasty (palatal lengthening).

Patients with severe defects including deformities of the nose and premaxilla may require maxillary surgery and rhinoplasty during adolescence after completion of the pubertal growth spurt.

Other needs

Orthodontic supervision is required for all patients, especially during the phase of second dentition. Regular assessment by an ear, nose and throat surgeon is also desirable because these patients have an increased risk of otitis media (glue ears) and frequently require myringotomy with insertion of drainage tubes.

PIERRE ROBIN SYNDROME

The combination of cleft palate (with intact lip and alveolus) with micrognathia and glossoptosis (Fig. 16.3) is the Pierre Robin syndrome. The micrognathia causes the tongue to be displaced backwards (and possibly also into the palatal cleft) so that these babies are at great risk of severe airways obstruction. This risk is present for a period of many months until growth of the mandible and other structures ensures a clear airway.

The fundamental aspect of the management of this condition is to be aware that it exists and to examine for it in any infant who has respiratory difficulty at or soon after birth.

The mainstay of treatment is to provide an adequate airway. Nursing in the prone position sometimes suffices, but frequently an artificial airway in the form of a nasopharyngeal tube, an endotracheal tube or a tracheotomy becomes necessary depending upon the severity of the child's airways obstruction. Operation to draw the tongue forwards by attaching it to the lower lip surgically until the risk of airways obstruction has passed is not now used; there is a significant in-

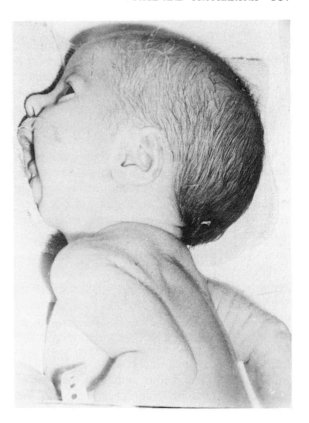

Fig. 16.3 Pierre Robin's syndrome.

cidence of spontaneous separation of the tongue from the lip with concomitant recurrence of respiratory difficulty. Furthermore, later separation may result in the formation of troublesome scar tissue.

The cleft palate in these infants is usually closed surgically at a convenient time during the second year of life.

PREAURICULAR TAGS AND SINUSES

Preauricular tags are relatively common and vary from a simple narrow-based skin tag which will separate spontaneously following simple ligation of the base without anaesthesia, through to large, wide-based, pedunculated lesions which contain cartilage (accessory auricle) and which require formal excision under general anaesthesia.

Preauricular sinuses usually occur on the anterior margin of the helix. Most end blindly (often within cartilage), whilst a few communicate with the external auditory canal. Without treatment, the sinus discharges intermittently and there is a high incidence of secondary infection (usually staphylococcal) with abscess formation. Surgical excision of a preauricular sinus is best undertaken during a quiescent phase. It is sensible to commence antistaphylococcal antibiotic therapy preoperatively if there has been significant intermittent purulent discharge from the sinus. There is a significant incidence of recurrent sinus, partly because of the frequent occurrence of postoperative wound infection and partly because of incomplete removal of the sinus tract.

BRANCHIAL CLEFT AND ARCH SYNDROMES

There are three common presentations of these syndromes:

1. A cystic swelling in the neck
2. A firm subcutaneous nodule in the neck
3. A sinus opening in the neck

Anomalies of the first branchial cleft

Anomalies of the first branchial cleft are much less common than those of the second. They occur along a line from the auditory canal to the angle of the mandible (Fig. 16.4). The most common mode of presentation is as a subcutaneous swelling which commonly becomes secondarily infected with abscess formation.

Anomalies of the second branchial arch

Remnants of the cartilage of the second branchial arch can persist and give rise to a firm subcutaneous lump in the neck, usually overlying the sternomastoid muscle. The treatment is simple surgical excision.

Anomalies of the second branchial cleft

The common second branchial cleft anomaly occurs as a persistence of the entire length of the base of the cleft (branchial fistula). There is a definite familial occurrence. The child is born

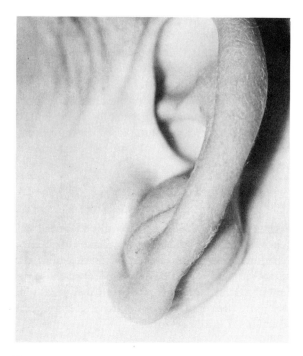

Fig. 16.4 First branchial arch lesion. Note swelling within ear.

with a tiny cutaneous orifice (sometimes bilateral) at the level of the junction of the middle and lower thirds of the anterior border of the sternomastoid muscle. Glairy mucus discharges from the orifice intermittently. A tract lined by squamous or respiratory epithelium leads from the orifice for a variable distance upwards, the common form passing between the carotid vessels to reach the supratonsillar fossa. The persistent discharge is a nuisance and there is a significant incidence of secondary infection. For these reasons, treatment of a branchial fistula is surgical excision of the tract. Operation can be undertaken at a convenient time after the age of 6 months and it is usually possible after making an elliptical incision around the cutaneous orifice to excise the entire fistula through the same incision. Persisting isolated islands of the second branchial cleft give rise to branchial cysts (see Ch. 3).

Ectopic salivary tissue sometimes occurs in the neck and clinically mimics branchial fistulae. At operation, the sinus is usually only a few centimetres long and terminates blindly. Histological examination of the operative specimen reveals the true diagnosis.

SWELLINGS IN THE FACE AND OROPHARYNX

These can usually be differentiated clinically, particularly on the site, colour and consistency. Some swellings that occur in the face and oropharynx occur more commonly in the neck and have been considered in Chapter 3.

Lingual thyroid

A rare anomaly of thyroid development results in the total thyroid mass being situated at the foramen caecum posteriorly in the tongue.

Ranula

A ranula is a retention cyst of a mucous gland in the floor of the mouth. It occurs as a soft swelling, usually on only one side of the floor of the mouth. It may be confused with sublingual lymphangioma which may have a component in the neck. Surgical treatment is usually advised and consists either of complete excision or marsupialization of the lesion into the floor of the mouth. Another cause for a swelling in the floor of the mouth is dermoid cyst (Fig. 16.5).

Swelling of the salivary glands

These are diagnosed by their shape and position.

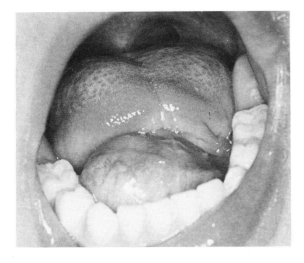

Fig. 16.5 Intraoral dermoid cyst.

Congenital anomalies

These are rare. The parotid gland may be involved in a haemangioma or lymphangioma in the area. Lymphoepithelial cyst of the parotid gland is a recognized entity which probably originates from a remnant of the first branchial arch.

Acquired disorders

Parotid gland. These are almost exclusively of inflammatory origin. Acute viral parotitis (mumps) is common and is usually bilateral. Acute bacterial parotitis is extremely rare.

Recurrent non-specific parotitis is a distinct clinical entity which is common, but is poorly understood. It occurs in children from preschool years to adolescence. There is painful parotid enlargement (unilateral or bilateral) that lasts for several days and which, at the first presentation, is usually diagnosed as mumps. However, the symptoms recur after an interval of weeks or months. There are few or no constitutional symptoms.

The parotid duct orifice is injected and seropurulent fluid is expressed by massaging the gland. Culture of this fluid usually produces a mixture of organisms. The mainstay of treatment is for the child or the parent to massage the gland forwards at frequent intervals in order to encourage drainage from the gland into the mouth. This usually leads to rapid resolution of the parotid swelling. Antibiotic therapy is not usually required.

For the small minority of patients who do not respond to massage, a sialogram should be obtained with the procedure being performed under general anaesthesia in order to enable dilatation of the parotid duct orifice and lavage of the duct system with saline or an antibiotic solution. The sialogram may reveal saccular dilatation of the ducts but sometimes is normal. Following sialography, the episodes of parotid swelling usually occur less frequently; occasional patients require repeat sialography because of continuing symptoms. The pathological basis for recurrent parotitis is poorly understood; symptoms usually abate during adolescence. The phenomenon may have an autoimmune basis. It is important that treatment does not include any form of parotidectomy.

A calculus can occur in the duct of the parotid. If the calculus is in the intraoral part of the gland it can be removed by incision over it. If it is in the gland, a partial parotidectomy will be required.

Submandibular gland. Acute swelling may be sialectasis with a purulent discharge from Wharton's duct. If persistent, the gland is excised.

More commonly, suppurative lymphadenitis of a lymph node within the submandibular gland capsule is the cause of enlargement without infected gland secretions. In draining a submandibular abscess, care is needed to avoid injury of the cervical branch of the facial nerve.

Recurrent swelling of the submandibular gland on one side is commonly due to a calculus in the duct. There is then a history of swelling associated with food and the swelling can often be brought on by a lemon drink. The swelling is seen to occupy the whole of the submandibular gland and the calculus can almost invariably be palpated bimanually in the floor of the mouth. X-ray of the floor of the mouth will confirm the presence of the calculus which is radioopaque in most instances. Treatment is by opening the duct behind the calculus which is removed. If the calculus is within the gland, a total excision of the gland is required.

Neoplasia

Neoplasia of these glands is very rare in childhood but a persistent focal swelling in an older child should be regarded with suspicion.

Jugular phlebectasia

Aneurysmal dilatation of a jugular vein is a rare but important cause of swelling. Phlebectasia of the external jugular vein is usually associated with a haemangiomatous malformation and thus an obvious visible swelling which increases in size when the intrathoracic pressure is raised, for example, during crying. Excision of the varix is usually justified. Aneurysmal dilatation of the internal jugular vein results in visible swelling in the neck only when venous return to the heart is obstructed because of raised intrathoracic pressure (Fig. 16.6). Operation for this innocuous cosmetic problem is hazardous and is not justified.

Macroglossia

Abnormal enlargement of the tongue is not common in childhood. It occasionally occurs as an isolated phenomenon but more often is associated with other anomalies of development. These include lymphangioma (Fig. 16.7), Down syndrome, the Hunter Hurler syndrome, hypothyroidism and Beckwith syndrome. The important features of Beckwith syndrome are exomphalos, macroglossia, visceromegaly and neonatal hypoglycaemia. If hypoglycaemia is undetected and untreated in these babies during the neonatal period, the outcome may be mental retardation.

Tonsils and adenoids

These are prominent parts of the ring of lymphoid tissue in the oropharynx. Their surgical treatment is controversial.

Indications for tonsillectomy

Great difference of opinion exists between clinicians regarding indications for tonsillectomy. Some regard the operation as risky and of doubtful benefit. Others feel that tonsil and adenoid surgery will minimize recurring health problems of different varieties and advocate operation very willingly.

Repeated attacks of tonsillitis with a minimum of three attacks per year over 2 years or six attacks in 1 year are agreed by most authorities to be valid indications for tonsillectomy. Acute tonsillitis can be difficult to diagnose and, if possible, should be distinguished from viral pharyngitis. An exudate on the tonsils with swelling, redness, pain on swallowing and fever are distinguishing features. When tonsillectomy is performed for recurrent tonsillitis it is usual to also undertake

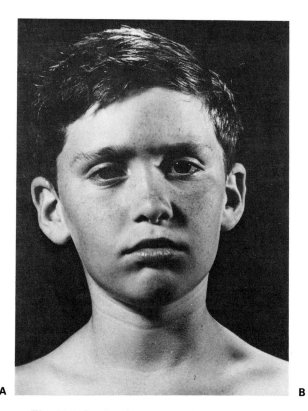
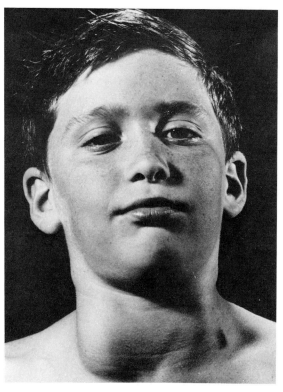

A   B

Fig. 16.6 Jugular phlebectasia. **A:** Child at rest, no obvious abnormality. **B:** Valsalva manoeuvre reveals right neck swelling due to aneurysmal dilatation' of internal jugular vein.

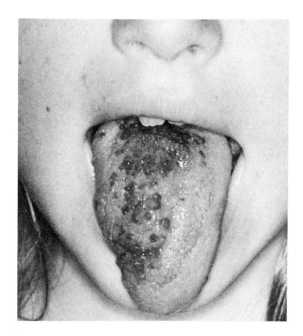

Fig. 16.7 Lymphangioma of tongue.

adenoidectomy unless there is a contraindication for this procedure (e.g. an incompetent palate). It is unusual for tonsillitis to occur during the first 2 years of life so that tonsillectomy for repeated infections is seldom indicated under the age of 3 years.

A small number of older patients (usually teenage) require tonsillectomy for 'chronic tonsillitis'. These patients complain of repeated sore throat, bad breath, bad taste in the mouth and perhaps persistently enlarged regional cervical lymph nodes.

Tonsillectomy has a place in the management of peritonsillar abscess (quinsy). After successful medical treatment in the acute phase there is a valid indication for tonsillectomy during a quiescent phase, especially if there have been previous attacks of tonsillitis. During the acute phase of quinsy with a pointing abscess, tonsillectomy may be preferred over incision and drainage.

Suspicion of neoplasia (usually based upon

macroscopic appearance of the tonsil) is a rare indication for tonsillectomy.

Airways obstruction due to hypertrophy of the tonsils, causing hypoventilation during sleep, noisy breathing and very occasionally cardiac failure, is an important indication for tonsillectomy, sometimes urgent. Anatomical crowding of the oropharynx as seen in patients with Down syndrome and Crouzon's disease predisposes to this. Distinct patterns of obstructive sleep have been recognized. Some patients have restless sleep with frequent change of posture and intermittent episodes of apnoea lasting a few seconds. More severely affected patients have episodes of profound apnoea lasting more than 12 seconds and sometimes associated with cyanosis. It is important to exclude obstruction below the level of the enlarged adenoids and tonsils in these cases whose tonsillectomy should only be undertaken in an institution equipped with paediatric intensive care facilities.

Indications for adenoidectomy

Adenoidectomy is indicated when there is nasal obstruction due to adenoid hypertrophy, persistent nasal or postnasal discharge from infected, enlarged adenoids and when tonsillectomy is being performed for recurrent tonsillitis. Adenoidectomy is unlikely to be beneficial for patients with recurrent ear infection.

Contraindications for tonsil and adenoid surgery

Adenoidectomy is absolutely contraindicated in patients with any form of cleft palate, as it will cause nasal speech due to escape of air through the nose. Relative contraindications include recent upper respiratory tract infection, bleeding diathesis and systemic disorders such as uncontrolled diabetes.

Tonsil and adenoid surgery should never be performed in hospitals which lack the staff and facilities to recognize and manage postoperative complications, especially haemorrhage.

Postoperative management

Regular measurement of pulse rate and examination for haemorrhage is necessary for 12–24 hours. An intravenous infusion should be routine during this period. The patient may experience considerable discomfort during the immediate postoperative period and therefore require sedation. However, narcotic agents should be given with extreme caution and only after thorough assessment by a medical practitioner. The administration of an opiate to a patient who has active bleeding is extremely dangerous.

GLUE EARS

Otitis media with effusion ('glue ears') is common and occurs in approximately 10% of children. There is active secretion of altered mucus into the middle ear behind an intact tympanic membrane. The condition probably occurs as the aftermath of unresolved viral otitis media.

Symptoms

Some patients are asymptomatic and are detected at routine medical examination. The most common symptom is deafness, which may be detected by parents, school teachers or school medical examination. Prolonged slight hearing loss due to glue ears may cause behavioural problems or learning difficulties. The other important symptom of glue ears is frequent earache which usually settles without treatment or with minimal analgesia.

Physical signs

Reduced mobility of the tympanic membrane is the most important physical sign of glue ears and is best assessed with a pneumatic otoscope. The tympanic membrane may also have a yellow appearance with dilated vessels and thickening.

Investigations

Audiometry usually demonstrates a conduction defect of between 20 and 40 dB. Tympanometry reveals little or no ear drum movement.

Treatment

Medical (conservative) treatment in the form of antibiotics, decongestants and antihistaminics may be ineffective. Spontaneous disappearance of the middle ear effusion does take place with time with some patients, but meanwhile the middle ear effusion can have a detrimental effect upon emotional and speech development.

Drainage of the middle ear with insertion of aeration tubes is indicated for children with bilateral glue ears of more than 3 months' duration and with clinically significant hearing loss. The procedure is undertaken under general anaesthesia on a day-stay basis. The tympanic membrane is incised and fluid aspirated from the middle ear. Aerating tubes are inserted through the myringotomy incision to allow sustained middle ear ventilation and prevention of reaccumulation of middle ear effusion.

With tubes in place, it is important to keep the ears dry so that appropriate precautions are necessary when showering, bathing or swimming. Spontaneous tube extrusion eventually occurs and many patients require further tube insertion until eventually the effusion ceases.

TONGUE TIE

Tightness of the lingual fraenum (tongue tie) is common. A white avascular band of tissue on the undersurface of the tongue limits its mobility. The significance of tongue tie is controversial. Some authorities believe that tongue tie does not interfere with speech and resolves spontaneously in due course. Speech pathologists have demonstrated conclusively that the inability to place the tip of the tongue on the roof of the mouth does interfere with the production of certain sounds. Spontaneous resolution does not always occur and tongue tie does interfere with dental hygiene in later life.

Release of severe tongue tie is justified if only to provide unrestricted full movement of the tongue. This is best undertaken under general anaesthesia at or after the age of 6 months. The procedure is undertaken on a day-stay basis and is associated with little or no morbidity.

INJURIES TO THE FACE AND MOUTH

Burns

In early childhood, the most common burn injury is from hot liquids that are accidentally dislodged,

usually by the child. The incident most often occurs in the kitchen with a saucepan, electric jug or container of hot beverage descending onto the child. As a result, the upper part of the body is most frequently involved, but the face often escapes due to reflex evasive action by the child during the incident.

When the face is involved the injury frequently involves superficial skin damage only.

Flame burns occur less commonly than scalds. When a fire occurs within a confined space, such as a house or a locked car, the burn injury frequently involves an extensive area of the body and, inevitably, the face and hands are involved (Fig. 16.8). When there are flame burns of the face and mouth, there frequently are, in addition, burns of the upper airway, including the larynx and supraglottic region. Respiratory difficulties with stridor and intercostal recession should alert the clinician to the presence of an airway injury.

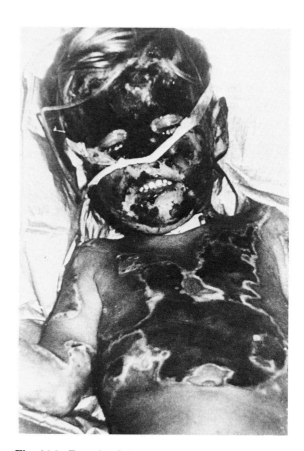

Fig. 16.8 Extensive flame burns with respiratory tract damage. Note tracheotomy.

An artificial airway in the form of an endotracheal tube or tracheostomy will frequently be required for these patients; endoscopic assessment under general anaesthesia is wise as a preliminary.

The principles of management of burns of the face are similar to those for other parts of the body; areas of full thickness burn require excision and split-skin grafting.

Lacerations

Facial lacerations are relatively common in children as a result, for example, of motor-vehicle accidents or falls whilst playing. Suture repair of facial lacerations should always be undertaken utilizing general anaesthesia with sterile conditions. Debridement with or without excision of skin edges is required for contaminated wounds. Accurate apposition of skin edges provides an optimal cosmetic result.

Intraoral soft-tissue injuries result from the child falling on his/her face with a sharp object in his/her mouth or hand. Tears of the soft palate and tongue frequently heal satisfactorily without suture, but where there is a hanging flap of tissue, examination under anaesthesia with suturing may be wise.

Facial fractures

Fractures of the nose

Fractures of the nose occur in bodily contact sports such as football or as a result of direct violence. Laterally directed injuries deflect the nose and cause buckling of the nasal septum. Direct frontal injuries cause splaying of the nasal bones, damage to the nasal septum and frequently considerable bruising and swelling.

Immediate treatment is directed at controlling epistaxis by direct pressure. Reduction under general anaesthesia is required when there is significant nasal deformity.

Fractures of the mandible and maxilla

Fractures of the mandible and maxilla are rare in childhood. Motor-vehicle accidents are the usual cause. Provision of an adequate airway, attention to damaged soft tissues and any associated injuries are important aspects of immediate management. Definitive treatment usually requires the involvement of faciomaxillary and/or dental surgeons. Internal fixation with some form of wiring is frequently required, especially for unstable fractures.

TRACHEOSTOMY

Tracheostomy is the operation which creates a communication between the lumen of the trachea and the exterior. It is a method of providing an artificial airway; the alternative is per oral or per nasal endotracheal intubation.

Indications

Tracheostomy is required for children only rarely. Acute upper airways obstruction due to inflammatory disorders such as acute epiglottitis and acute laryngotracheitis (croup) is best managed with endotracheal intubation in an intensive care facility with adequate numbers of trained medical and nursing staff. Tracheostomy is the alternative when endotracheal intubation is unsuccessful. Diptheria is now a very rare cause of inflammatory airways obstruction but does occur in unimmunized children and tracheostomy remains an essential part of treatment.

Tracheostomy may be required in the management of bilateral vocal cord paralysis, subglottic haemangioma, massive cervical lymphangioma, Pierre Robin syndrome and burns to the airways. For some of these patients, a tracheostomy is required on a long-term or permanent basis. The advent of laser therapy has resulted in avoidance of tracheostomy for patients with laryngeal papillomatosis. Tracheostomy is sometimes performed to assist the provision of ventilatory support in patients who are comatosed from head injury or some other cause. Patients who require prolonged endotracheal intubation for whatever reason are at risk of damage to the larynx and subglottic structures; this is now one of the most common indications for tracheostomy.

Technique

Urgent tracheotomy, performed with any readily available cutting instrument for the moribund patient who has acute airways obstruction, is an operation best avoided but may occasionally be necessary.

Usually, the decision for tracheostomy is made in a controlled situation. When facilities and expertise are available, a preliminary endoscopy may be useful both to confirm the underlying diagnosis and plan management. Tracheostomy is best performed using general anaesthesia and endotracheal intubation.

The patient is positioned with head and neck extended utilizing a sand bag under the shoulders. Although a transverse skin incision may produce a better cosmetic result, a vertical incision is easier and is associated with less risk of damage to the pleura. The dissection is carried down in the midline through fascial planes to expose the trachea. The incision into the trachea should be made at the level of the fourth or fifth tracheal ring. The trachea is best entered by a vertical incision across one or two tracheal cartilages or by incision into the space between two cartilages. Excision of a window of anterior trachea or the creation of an inverted 'U' tracheal flap are procedures to be condemned in children. The final step of the operation is to insert an appropriate tracheostomy tube which may be of metal (with double lumen) or of plastic. The tube is held in place by tapes tied behind the neck; it is important to tie the tapes firmly. It is unwise to place sutures in the skin incision.

Complications

Air which escapes from the trachea around the tracheostomy tube into the soft tissues may track into the mediastinum and subsequently into the pleural space to cause pneumothorax. This is especially likely if the skin wound is closed firmly around the tracheostomy tube or if the tracheostomy is fashioned low in the trachea. Respiratory difficulty may result from obstruction of the tracheostomy tube by secretions and is avoided by efficient and adequate attention to tracheal aspiration. Accidental tube dislodgement is another potential cause of respiratory difficulty in the patient with a tracheostomy. Tracheal stenosis is a potential late complication, especially if the tracheostomy is sited high in the trachea.

FURTHER READING

Beckenhjam E J 1977 Tonsils, adenoids and glue ears — the current state. Medical Journal of Australia 1: 494–496

Benjamin B N 1970 Acute inflammatory airways obstruction in infants and children. Medical Journal of Australia 2: 1254–1257

Healy G B 1981 Acute sinusitis in childhood. New England Journal of Medicine 304: 779–780

Leading Article 1981 Inhaled foreign bodies. British Medical Journal 282: 1649–1650

Ludman H 1981 Throat infections. British Medical Journal 282: 628–631

Paradise J L, Bluestone C D, Bachman R Z et al 1984 Efficacy of tonsillectomy for recurrent throat infection in severely affected children. New England Journal of Medicine 310: 674–683

Stickler G B 1984 The attack on the tympanic membrane Pediatrics 74: 291–292

17. Disorders of the head

P. Upadhyaya

The normal head is symmetrical at birth but there is considerable variation in the general form, depending on racial and familial characteristics. There is a steady increase in size following a well-defined growth percentile chart. The size and shape of the head may be altered by abnormality of the cranium and/or intracranial structures. Delay in diagnosis and treatment of abnormalities of size and shape, or intracranial infections, often leads to serious complications due to underlying brain damage. Commonly encountered surgical conditions are described below.

ABNORMALITIES OF SHAPE

Cephalohaematoma

Birth trauma may produce an eccentric swelling over a part of the head due to a subperiosteal haematoma. This usually overlies the parietal bone. Some infants may have an underlying fracture, but rarely an intracranial injury. Usually the haematoma resolves spontaneously and needle aspiration should be avoided. Rarely, it becomes calcified and presents as a firm, non-tender immobile swelling later in infancy.

Encephalocele

Encephalocele is a congenital deformity of the head caused by protrusion of intracranial tissue through a midline cranial defect, comparable to spina bifida in its embryogenic origin. The mass usually contains meninges, cerebrospinal fluid and cerebral tissue. More than 70% are posteri-

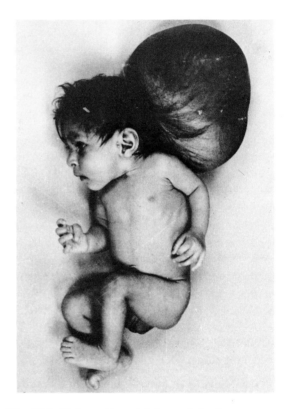

Fig. 17.1 Patient with occipital encephalocele.

orly located and called occipital encephalocele (Fig. 17.1).

The anterior encephaloceles (Fig. 17.2) are found in the region of the forehead, nose and base of the skull. In some Asian countries, e.g. Thailand, frontal encephaloceles are more common. Differential diagnosis includes nasal glioma and dermoid.

The size of the encephalocele sac varies from a small nodule to a size bigger than the head.

197

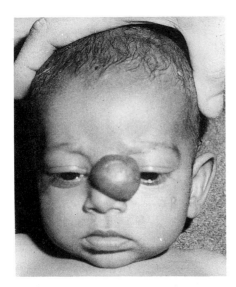

Fig. 17.2 Patient with frontonasal encephalocele.

The overlying skin may be of normal thickness or thinned out and shiny, liable to ulceration and rupture, producing cerebrospinal fluid (CSF) leakage and meningitis. Quite often there is an associated hydrocephalus.

Management

- Physical and neurological examination
- Plain X-ray film of the skull
- CT or MRI scanning
- Air encephalography (in selected cases)
- Surgical repair
- Shunt surgery for hydrocephalus

If the sac is in imminent danger of ulceration and leak, it is excised within 36 hours of birth and the gap repaired with a musculofacial or periosteal flap. The herniated brain tissue is often dysplastic and should be excised. Pushing it into the cranium can produce a fatal rise of intracranial tension.

The anterior encephaloceles require a combined neurosurgical and plastic surgical technique to correct the frontonasal deformity.

Prognosis

Nearly one-third of cases die within the first few weeks. Of the survivors, three-quarters have neurological complications, e.g. cerebellar imbalance, defective vision, spasticity and hydrocephalus.

Craniosynostosis

Craniosynostosis is a condition in which there is a premature fusion (synostosis) of some or all of the cranial sutures. Development of the skull is restricted in the region of synostosis, while compensatory growth occurs at the remaining suture lines. The type of the skull deformity produced depends on the suture lines involved. If untreated the head deformity leads to a severe cosmetic defect and in some cases mental retardation and optic atrophy due to raised intracranial tension. In 10% of cases the sutures of the facial skeleton are also affected producing a craniofacial defect, e.g. Crouzon's syndrome.

The types include sagittal, coronal, metopic and oxycephaly.

Sagittal synostosis

This is the commonest type. Most patients are male. The fused sagittal suture feels like a ridge. Since parietal growth is restricted the biparietal diameter is narrow. Compensatory growth at the coronal and lambdoid sutures produces frontal bossing and occipital prominence. The deformed skull assumes the shape of an upturned boat (scaphocephaly).

Coronal synostosis

Fusion of both coronal sutures produces a shortened head (brachycephaly). Fusion of one coronal suture presents with a flattening of the forehead on the affected side.

Metopic synostosis

Normally the metopic suture helps to produce a broad and rounded forehead. Its premature fusion produces a pointed forehead with the orbits angulating inwards (trigonocephaly). Quite often there is an underlying anomaly of the brain.

Oxycephaly or turricephaly

Fusion of all the cranial sutures produces a tall or tower skull.

Craniofacial deformities

Some patients have craniosynostosis with a severe midface hypoplasia, e.g. Crouzon's syndrome. Fusion of coronal sutures and diminished orbital volume produce exorbitism and divergent strabismus. Hypoplasia of maxillae produces relative prominence of the lower jaw. In Apert's syndrome, besides the craniofacial deformity similar to Crouzon's syndrome, there are other deformities such as syndactyly of the hands and/or feet.

Treatment

The current trend is early surgical treatment of craniosynostosis. Multiple craniectomies are done to restore the normal shape of the skull. With newer surgical techniques, patients with grotesque craniofacial deformities can be given a normal appearance and allowed to lead a normal life.

ABNORMALITIES OF SIZE

Hydrocephalus

Hydrocephalus (water on the head) can be defined as a condition in which an increased volume of CSF is present in an enlarged ventricular system under pressure. It is a pathological state produced by a variety of causes.

The total quantity of CSF present in the intracranial and intraspinal spaces varies from 30 mL in infants to 150 mL in adults. The resting ventricular pressure is 80–100 cm of water. It is estimated that 200–300 mL of CSF is formed every day.

Causes of hydrocephalus

Normally there is a dynamic equilibrium between the amount of CSF produced and the amount absorbed. This equilibrium is disturbed if there is either overproduction or diminished absorption of CSF. In the vast majority of cases there is a pathological obstruction at some point along the pathways of CSF circulation, producing a disturbance of CSF absorption. Depending on the site of obstruction, hydrocephalus can be of two types:

1. *Non-communicating* — when the obstruction is somewhere in the ventricular system so that the dilated ventricles do not communicate with the subarachnoid space
2. *Communicating* — when the ventricles continue to communicate with the subarachnoid space, which itself is the site of obstruction.

Obstructive factors can be divided into three broad groups: congenital, acquired and neoplastic.

Congenital hydrocephalus. This is seen in early infancy. Common abnormalities are aqueductal stenosis, Arnold-Chiari malformation and Dandy-Walker syndrome. In the latter condition a congenital obstruction of the roof foramina produces a cystic dilatation of the fourth ventricle.

Acquired hydrocephalus. Meningitis due to pyogenic bacteria, if not treated adequately, may lead to hydrocephalus. Another cause of post-meningitic hydrocephalus is tuberculosis, which is seen in children 1 to 5 years of age, mostly in developing countries. Intrauterine viral infections and congenital syphilis are other less common causes. Head trauma at birth or later may cause subdural haematoma or haemorrhages in the ventricles and subarachnoid space, producing obstruction in the CSF pathways.

Neoplasms. In 3–4% of cases, hydrocephalus is secondary to intracranial tumours, mostly arising in the posterior cranial fossa and the pineal area. Common types are cerebellar astrocytoma, medulloblastoma and craniopharyngioma.

Pathology

Persistently raised CSF pressure produces dilatation of the ventricles. Initially the thickness of the cerebral cortex is reduced due to opening up of the gyri and, therefore, little cerebral damage occurs. Later, progressive cortical atrophy sets in due to diminished blood supply. Cracks appear in the ependymal lining of the ventricles creating abnormal pathways of CSF dispersal. There is oedema and demyelination of white matter. Neurological signs are due to pressure on cranial nerves, changes in the white matter and compression of the brain stem due to its the caudal displacement.

Clinical picture

This varies with the nature of hydrocephalus, the age of onset and duration of the symptoms. Clinical examination should include examination of the head, neurological examination and assessment of mental development. Clinical presentation varies significantly in infants and children.

Infantile hydrocephalus

This is mostly congenital in nature. Since the cranial sutures are open, enlargement of the head is the first and quite often the only presenting symptom. As the condition advances, the large head forms a marked contrast to a small face and base of the skull. The anterior fontanelle is open and full or bulging. The skin of the scalp is stretched out and the scalp veins are prominent and full, particularly during crying. Cranial bones become thinned out giving a 'crack pot' sign on percussion (MacEwen's sign). Transillumination of the head may be positive at this stage. The eyeballs are rolled down, producing the typical 'setting sun' sign (Fig. 17.3). There may be nystagmus or squint. Fundoscopy may show changes of optic atrophy. Papilloedema is rare.

In longstanding infantile hydrocephalus, milestones are delayed and motor function and language performance are retarded.

Childhood hydrocephalus

This is mostly acquired due to meningitis or tumour. If it commences after the cranial sutures have fused, there are minimal changes in head circumference. In these cases there are overt symptoms of an acute increase in intracranial tension viz., headaches, vomiting and papilloedema.

Abnormal neurological signs depend on the speed and duration of the increased intracranial tension. There may be spastic paresis of lower limbs, sixth cranial nerve palsy, optic atrophy and in acutely developing hydrocephalus, brain stem compression signs.

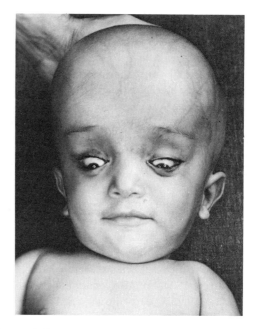

Fig. 17.3 Patient with hydrocephalus. Note the distended veins and the 'setting sun' sign.

Investigations

1. X-rays of the skull with anteroposterior and lateral views will confirm the sutural separation and will show the occasional calcification seen in brain tumours.

2. In infants with an open anterior fontanelle, ultrasound scanning provides an excellent means of visualizing the ventricles and following the progress after shunt surgery.

3. Subdural and/or intraventricular tap may be done to collect fluid for microscopic and biochemical examination and for culture and sensitivity in acquired hydrocephalus.

4. CT scans (Fig. 17.4) will show the nature and severity of ventricular dilatation and presence of basal exudates or tumours of the brain.

5. Invasive techniques such as cerebral angiography and pneumoencephalography are undertaken only in selected cases.

Management

Irrespective of the cause of hydrocephalus, the management is essentially the same: CSF from

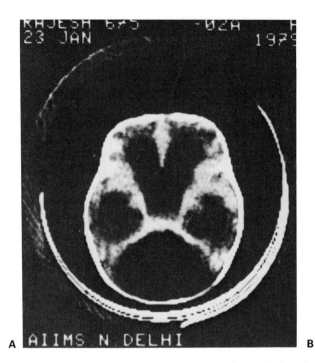
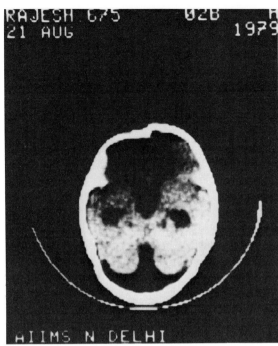

Fig. 17.4 CT scan showing hydrocephalus. **A**: Before shunt surgery, showing dilated ventricles and periventricular lucency. **B**: Seven months after shunt surgery.

the ventricles is diverted to one of the body cavities, viz., right atrium of the heart, peritoneal cavity or the pleura. Currently, the most commonly used procedure is the ventriculoperitoneal shunt (Fig. 17.5). If hydrocephalus is secondary to intracranial masses such as tumours, arachnoid cyst or vascular malformations, the shunting procedure may be combined with or followed by their removal. If the CSF is frankly infected, shunt surgery is absolutely contraindicated. Complications of shunt surgery include shunt blockage and shunt infection.

Conservative management. In borderline early cases, conservative management may be tried with regular ultrasound or CT monitoring of the ventricular size. Commonly used drugs are glycerol and acetazolamide. The latter inhibits carbonic anhydrase and thus may decrease by 50% the formation of CSF.

INTRACRANIAL INFECTIONS

Intracranial infections needing the surgeon's attention are mostly pyogenic, the route of

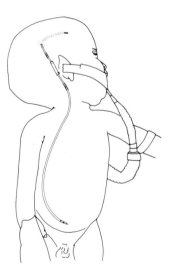

Fig. 17.5 Ventriculoperitoneal shunt.

infection being either haematogenous or direct extension from contiguous sinusitis, mastoiditis or otitis media. Brain, meninges, CSF and cranial bones may be involved separately or in combination. With the advent of CT scanning it has become possible to reach an early diagnosis and also to perform needle aspiration under CT control.

Principles of management include:

- Early diagnosis and precise localization by CT scan
- Prompt drainage of pus
- Appropriate antibiotics, given intravenously
- Treatment of primary source of infection
- Control of intracranial tension and focal seizures

Brain abscess

Brain abscess is an occasional, but serious complication of sinusitis, mastoiditis and otitis media in the paediatric age group. Children with congenital heart disease, particularly tetrology of Fallot, are prone to develop a brain abscess by haematogenous spread of infection. Abscesses arising from infected sinuses and chronic ear infection are seen in the contiguous sites of frontal and temporal lobes, whereas haematogenous abscesses spread in the direction of the middle cerebral artery.

The clinical picture is non-specific initially. Fever is not a constant feature, but there may be some leucocytosis. Sudden onset of hydrocephalus in infants and signs of raised intracranial tension, viz., headache, vomiting, lethargy, irritability, seizures and drowsiness, should arouse the suspicion of brain abscess, particularly if the child has a congenital heart disease or history of sinusitis and chronic middle ear infection. As time passes the level of consciousness diminishes and focal neurological signs may appear.

Diagnosis is made by CT scan with or without contrast. Lumbar puncture is not commonly done. Treatment consists of needle aspiration through a burr-hole. Pus is examined by immediate Gram-staining and cultured for aerobic and anaerobic bacteria as well as for fungi. Appropriate antibiotic therapy is started. Repeated CT scans are done to follow the resolution of the abscess. Rarely, it is necessary to perform craniotomy for a rapidly expanding brain abscess mass.

Subdural empyema

This is a serious condition, more often seen in infants and children than in adults. Infection of the subdural space is often secondary to purulent meningitis, paranasal sinusitis or middle ear infection and sometimes due to haematogenous infection of a subdural haematoma. Pus collection is mostly over the frontoparietal convexities, occasionally extending to the interhemispheric space. Patients present with severe headache, vomiting, signs of sepsis and neck rigidity. Soon focal seizures and deterioration of the level of consciousness occur. Infants have enlargement of the head and a bulging fontanelle.

Management

Diagnosis is made by CT scan and subdural tap. Treatment is by immediate drainage of pus through a needle puncture in infants and through a craniotomy burr-hole in children. Appropriate antibiotics are given intravenously. Steroids are prescribed to combat increased intracranial tension and anticonvulsants to control seizures.

Osteomyelitis of the skull and epidural abscess

Osteomyelitis of the skull is either a complication of a compound fracture or secondary to paranasal sinusitis or middle ear infection. The infection is often due to *Staph. aureus*, but mixed organisms may be present.

The patient presents with a warm, tender swelling over the scalp. If there is an epidural abscess, systemic symptoms such as fever and malaise may also develop. Skull roentgenograms may not show any change in the first 2–3 weeks; later the affected bone has a moth-eaten appearance. However, a CT scan clearly defines the areas of bone destruction and the presence of an accompanying epidural abscess.

Treatment consists of debridement of the wound and removal of infected granulomatous tissue. Infected and dead bone pieces are removed, preserving the pericranium. The epidural abscess is adequately drained and the wound

closed. Operation is followed by long-term antibiotic therapy.

FURTHER READING

Alphen H A M von, Dreissen J J R 1976 Brain abscess and subdural empyema. Journal of Neurology, Neurosurgery and Psychiatry 39: 481–490
Milhorat T H 1982 Hydrocephalus, historical notes, aetiology and clinical diagnosis In: McLaurin R (ed) Pediatric neurosurgery. Surgery of the developing nervous system. Grune & Stratton, New York, p 197–209
Shillit S J, Matson D D 1968 Craniosynostosis: a review of 519 surgical patients. Pediatrics 41: 829–853

18. Body wall defects

P. Upadhyaya

Body wall defects, though of various types and varying degrees of complexity, have common features explicable on the basis of their embryologic development.

Most of them are midline, have a deficiency of skin and muscle, and their associated abnormalities are related to the organs that develop deep to the defect. Thus, posterior body wall defects have an underlying abnormality in the spinal cord or the cranium, while anterior wall defects have associated abnormalities in the sternum, ribs or heart cranially, of the diaphragm and gastrointestinal tract and related organs in the midzone, and of the genitourinary or hindgut system caudally.

EMBRYOLOGY

Early in development, after the amniotic and yolk sac cavities have developed in the morula, a trilaminar embryonic disc forms, consisting of ectoderm, mesoderm and endoderm.

In the 14th day embryo, a longitudinal strip of dorsal ectoderm becomes differentiated to form the neural groove (Fig. 18.1). By the 20th day the margins of the neural plate separate and commence folding over the neural groove.

The process of fusion starts in the cervical region and extends zipper-fashion towards the cranial and caudal ends. The undifferentiated ectoderm and mesoderm then fuse in the midline, dorsal to the fused neural tube. Mesoderm surrounding the neural tube differentiates into dermatomes, myotomes and sclerotomes. Failure of development of the dorsal mesoderm, the part which lies between the neural tube and the surface ectoderm, leads to spina bifida occulta or meningocele. If, however, there is concomitant

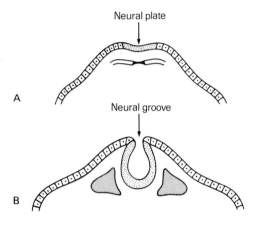

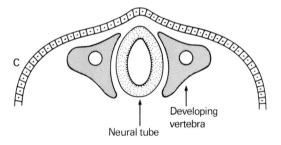

Fig. 18.1 Embryology of spina bifida. **A**: Neurol plate. **B**: Neural groove. **C**: Neural canal.

failure of fusion of the neural tube as well, the result will be myelomeningocele.

The anterior body wall forms by longitudinal and transverse folding of the trilaminar embryonic disc. Four separate embryonic folds, cephalic, caudal and right and left lateral, converge towards the central part of the celomic cavity to form a large umbilical ring. Through this defect, surrounded by amnion, pass the umbilical arteries and veins, vitellointestinal duct and

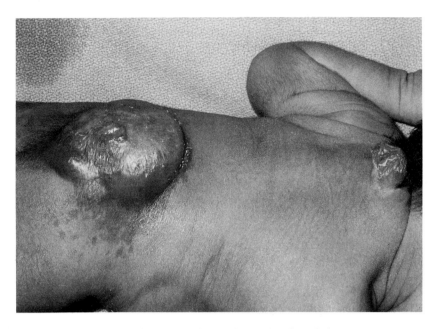

Fig. 18.2 Infant with myelomeningocele. Lumbosacral and cervical myelomeningoceles. Note the neural plate adherent to the centre of the thin shiny sac. The skin at the periphery has capillary haemangioma.

allantois. This is illustrated in Chapter 8 in relation to the development in the embryo of the gastrointestinal tract (see Figs 8.1 and 8.2). Simultaneous mesodermal ingrowth from cranial, caudal and lateral directions completes the anterior abdominal wall, leaving a small deficiency at the site of the umbilical cord. Arrest of this infolding and mesodermal ingrowth results in a variety of midline skin and mesodermal defects with an associated underlying abnormality.

UMBILICAL HERNIA

This is very common and is usually of no significance in itself though it may be associated with other congenital abnormalities or syndromes. Failure of closure of the umbilical ring causes a skin-covered hernia, capped by the umbilical scar. It can be easily reduced. Unlike inguinal hernia, complications are extremely rare. In the majority of cases the hernia closes spontaneously. If it fails to close by the fourth year of life or if it is too large, surgical closure is done preserving the umbilicus.

Other umbilical anomalies

Embryologically, the midgut and the urinary bladder open at the umbilicus via the omphalomesenteric duct and the urachus respectively. Normally these channels shrivel up and disappear, but sometimes the whole or part of the tract persists.

Patent omphalomesenteric duct

This presents as a velvety pink, mucous membrane-lined umbilical opening having a tubular connection to the ileum at the level of a Meckel's diverticulum. The opening may discharge intestinal contents and/or flatus. The condition can be confirmed in doubtful cases by injecting a radioopaque material into the opening at the umbilicus. Surgical treatment consists of excision of the fistulous tract and closure of the fistulous opening. Although not an emergency, the operation should not be delayed, as there is danger of intestinal volvulus and external intussusception through the umbilical opening.

Partial patency of the duct produces omphalomesenteric sinus or omphalomesenteric cyst. Both can be removed extraperitoneally through an infraumbilical incision.

Patent urachus

A moist umbilicus, or urine coming out at the umbilicus, denote a patent urachus. A cystogram (lateral view) and intravenous urogram should be done in every case to rule out associated anomalies such as posterior urethral valves. A urachal cyst can be diagnosed by ultrasound examination. Simple closure of the tract and excision of the cyst are curative.

MAJOR BODY WALL DEFECTS

Major body wall defects in newborn infants have three usual modes of presentation:

1. A midline swelling covered by skin
2. A midline swelling covered by a thin transparent membrane with fluid or an underlying organ visible. This membrane may leak fluid or rupture
3. A midline defect occupied by an underlying viscus

Such a defect occurring in the midline of the back will produce spina bifida. In the anterior body wall, a midline defect produces anomalies such as ectopia cordis in the thoracic region, exomphalos in the mid abdomen and ectopia vesicae in the lower abdomen. Spina bifida is the commonest defect.

SPINA BIFIDA

Spina bifida is the major defect of the posterior body wall. It is caused by a failure of development of the posterior vertebral arches with or without a neural tube defect. Although the spinous processes are missing, the ununited laminae are erroneously referred to as the 'bifid spine'.

Incidence of spina bifida

There is a wide geographical variation in incidence. The overall incidence in the United Kingdom is 3.5 per 1000 births, in the United States is 1 per 1000 births and in Australia it is 0.6 per 1000 births. Pakistanis and North Indians have a higher incidence of 4 to 5 per 1000 births, while Japanese, Jews and Negroes have a very low incidence of 0.1 to 0.3 per 1000 births. Racial variations are not altered in immigrants.

Aetiology

Although the exact aetiology is unknown, it is believed that both genetic and environmental factors play a part. The risk of neural tube malformations increases in subsequent siblings. When the first child is affected, there is a 1 in 20 chance of recurrence in the second child and a 1 in 8 chance in the third child, if the second is also affected. Consanguinity also increases the risk. All these observations indicate the possibility of a polygenic inheritance.

Spina bifida cystica

In spina bifida cystica there is a clinically manifest cystic swelling filled with CSF overlying the spinal defect. It comprises two very different clinical states, myelomeningocele and meningocele.

Myelomeningocele

This is the commonest and by far the most important variety of spina bifida cystica, accounting for 95% of cases. It is commonly lumbosacral, sometimes cervical and rarely thoracic in position (Fig. 18.2). The overlying muscles, spinous processes and posterior vertebral arches of several vertebrae are absent, producing a saucer-like bony defect lined on either side by malformed everted pedicles of the vertebral bodies.

In open myelomeningocele, also called myelocele or rachischisis (Fig. 18.3), the bony defect is occupied by a pink oval plaque with an 'ulcer-like' appearance, which is, in fact, the unfused neural plate with a midline groove through which CSF leaks. Peripheral nerves arising from its ventral aspect course towards the intervertebral foramina. Surrounding the neural plate is a thin

MYELOCELE

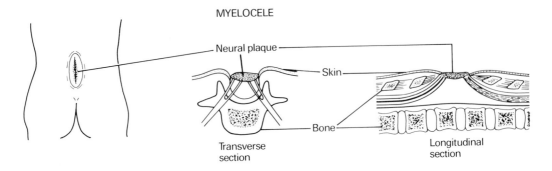

Fig. 18.3 Diagramatic representation of myelocele.

bluish-white membrane representing the fused pia-arachnoid. The dura mater is fused with the surrounding skin which is thinned out and often studded with capillary haemangiomata.

In the case of closed myelomeningocele (Fig. 18.4), the bony defect is covered by a CSF-filled cavity, which invariably contains neural tissue adherent to the fundus or the side wall of the meningeal sac. Unlike a meningocele, the sac is irregular and broad-based. The periphery of the sac is covered by comparatively normal skin, but an irregular area of the fundus is typically lined by thin, shiny, parchment-like scar epithelium. The neural plate is adherent to the dome of the sac and can often be identified on close inspection as a roughened, puckered area. Initially, all myelomeningoceles are open. During intrauterine life or after birth, the epithelial lining at the periphery of the open myelocele grows centrally over the neural plate blocking the leaking central canal in the process. The accumulating CSF distends the sac, lifting the adherent neural plate away from the bony defect.

Extensive spina bifida may have a lumbar kyphosis, making it very difficult to close the skin over the bony protruberance (Fig. 18.5).

Almost all infants with myelomeningocele will have varying grades of motor and sensory loss in the lower limbs and sphincteric incompetence. This is because the malformed denuded spinal cord segment is damaged by intrauterine strains, trauma during delivery or postnatal drying and infection of the neural plate.

In some cases of myelomeningocele, the meningeal sac is surrounded by lipomatous tissue and covered with normal full-thickness skin. These cases have minimal neurological deficit and there is no urgency for surgical repair.

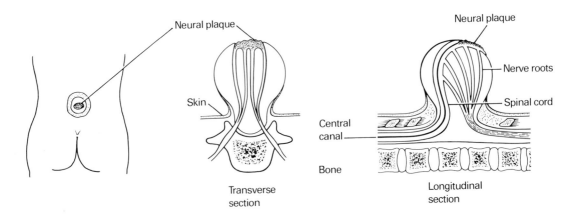

Fig. 18.4 Diagramatic representation of myelomeningocele.

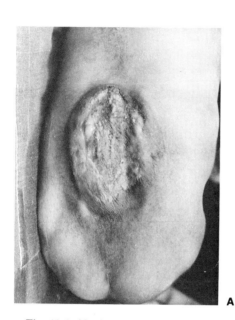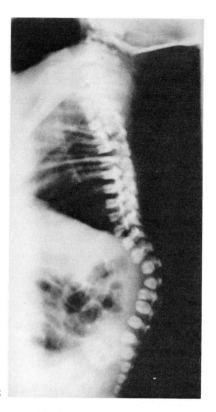

A   **B**

Fig. 18.5 Newborn infant with lumbar myelocele (rachischisis) and kyphosis. **A**: Opened-out neural plate can be seen at the floor of the oval defect. **B**: X-ray showing kyphosis.

Meningocele

This is a comparatively rare condition, constituting only 4–5% of all spina bifida cystica cases (Fig. 18.6). The smooth, regular, usually narrow-necked swelling is covered by full-thickness skin and filled with CSF only. The spinal cord is an-atomically and functionally normal and there is no neurological deficit. The bony defect involves one or two vertebrae only. Treatment consists of excision of the sac and closure of the defect as an elective procedure usually after 3 months of age.

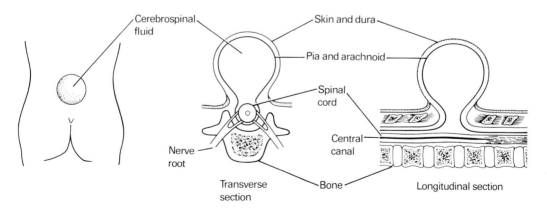

Fig. 18.6 Diagramatic representation of meningocele.

Clinical assessment of the newborn

The newborn infant with spina bifida cystica should be transferred to a paediatric surgical centre as soon as possible. The spinal lesion should be kept covered with a sterile paraffin gauze or a thin plastic film and protected by a circumferential cotton padding and a binder to avoid infection and damage to the exposed neural plate. Management decisions are based on the severity of the lesion, associated abnormalities and the social circumstances. The proposed line of management and prognosis should be discussed with the parents, who should be assisted in making a decision.

Clinical features

Motor loss

In general, high lumbar or thoracolumbar lesions produce spastic paralysis of limbs, while the lumbosacral type manifests as flaccid paraplegia. In the commonly encountered lumbosacral myelomeningocele, the spinal cord function is normal to the L4 level, with flaccid paralysis of the lower segments. Due to the unopposed action of the flexors and adductors of the hip (L1–L3) and the quadriceps muscle (L2–L4), the lower limbs assume a typical posture of flexion at the hips and extension at the knees.

If the integrity of the L5 segment is also preserved the knee becomes flexed by the functioning hamstrings (L5–S1). As the calf muscles (S1–S2) are weak, the foot becomes dorsiflexed due to unopposed action of the extensors of the toes and the peroneal muscles (L5–S1). When the function is normal down to the S2 segment, only the intrinsic muscles of the foot are affected.

If the spinal cord function is lost below T12, there is a total flaccid paralysis of the lower limbs, and consequently no postural deformity. When only the lowermost sacral segments (S4 and S5) are affected, the lower limbs are normal, but the pelvic floor is paralysed, producing a patulous anus and a relaxed perineum.

Sensory loss

Trophic ulcers may develop in the anaesthetic areas of the soles of the feet, heels and over the ischial tuberosities and lower sacrum. Sensory loss also increases the risk of burns and scalds. Constant wetness of the skin due to urinary incontinence further predisposes to its breakdown. The level of sensory loss may not correspond to the level of motor dysfunction.

Bladder and bowel dysfunction

The child dribbles urine. Important clinical signs are:

(a) Compressible urinary bladder
(b) Patulous anus
(c) Perianal anaesthesia

Additional malformations

Hydrocephalus

More than 80% of infants born with myelomeningocele have accompanying hydrocephalus, which is caused by an interconnected anomaly of the hindbrain — the Arnold-Chiari malformation. Nearly three-fourths will need shunt surgery either before or after repair of the spinal lesion (see Ch. 17). If not controlled in time, the progressive hydrocephalus may lead to intellectual deficit, spasticity and optic atrophy, factors which further worsen the prognosis in an already handicapped child.

Skeletal anomalies

Children with extensive thoracolumbar lesions may have a severe underlying kyphosis, making it difficult for the child to sit or to wear urine-collecting bags and orthopaedic appliances. Additional skeletal anomalies, such as hemivertebrae and fusion of adjacent ribs and transverse processes, may be seen presenting as scoliosis or kyphoscoliosis.

Genitourinary anomalies

These have been reported in 20% of cases and include cystic kidneys, horse-shoe kidneys and renal duplications, hypospadias and undescended testes. Hydronephrosis, hydroureter and vesicoureteric reflux may be secondary effects of the neurogenic bladder.

Other anomalies

Cardiac abnormalities, exomphalos, ectopia vesicae and anorectal malformations have also been reported.

Selection of cases for treatment

The aim of treatment is to have an ambulant and continent child (with or without appliances), who is capable of gainful employment and independent living. In 40–50% of infants, a multiplicity of adverse factors prevents attainment of these objectives. A large number die before reaching their first birthday, most of the deaths occurring during the first 3 months of life.

It is generally agreed that active treatment is contraindicated in babies who have:

1. Severe associated anomalies such as congenital cyanotic heart disease or ectopia vesicae
2. Severe paralysis of the lower limbs and sphincteric incompetence
3. Marked hydrocephalus at birth (head circumference more than 2 cm above 90th percentile)
4. Severe kyphosis
5. Meningitis or ventriculitis

Stricter criteria for selection are employed in developing countries where facilities for specialized care are limited.

Treatment

In the absence of adverse factors, early surgery, ideally within 24 hours of birth, is indicated. The aim of the operation is to cover the exposed neural plate with membranes and skin, thereby minimizing the chances of meningitis and preventing further damage to the neural plate.

If the spinal lesion is covered at birth with normal, full-thickness skin, the operation to close the underlying defect can be conveniently postponed for 6–8 months.

During the first hospital admission, radiographs of the spine, skull and hips are taken and a renal ultrasound or an intravenous pyelogram is performed. Ultrasonography and, if available, CT, are performed to make a baseline assessment of ventricular dilatation. A detailed timetable for subsequent visits and a plan of treatment are discussed with the parents.

Subsequent management involves therapy for:

- Hydrocephalus
- Neuropathic bladder
- Faecal incontinence
- Skeletal anomalies
- Home care, education and rehabilitation

Hydrocephalus

Over 80% of infants will develop some degree of hydrocephalus. Frequent measurements of head circumference should detect progressive hydrocephalus, which is confirmed by ultrasound and CT and managed by a timely shunt operation (see Ch. 17). As long as the anterior fontanelle remains open, ultrasonography provides an easy, non-invasive method of serial assessment of ventricular size following shunt surgery.

Neuropathic bladder

Initially the renal function is normal in most infants. As the baby is in nappies, urinary incontinence is not a problem. However, around the age of 2 years, when the child starts walking, incontinence becomes a distressing disability. Subsequently, outflow resistance, often complicated by urinary tract infection leads to raised intravesical pressure, vesicoureteric reflux, hydroureter and hydronephrosis. By the time the child reaches school age, deteriorating renal function becomes the major cause of concern for the treating surgeon. It is, therefore, very important to carry out periodic assessment to detect the earliest signs of deterioration.

The objectives of neuropathic bladder management are to:

1. Preserve renal function
2. Control urinary incontinence

Various modes of managing neuropathic bladder are available. In order to select the appropriate therapy it is necessary to ascertain the anatomical and functional status of the upper urinary tract and to identify the nature of bladder dysfunction in individual cases. Such a comprehensive evaluation should be done before 3 months of age and later on before starting therapy. It includes:

1. Urine examination
2. Renal functions tests — blood urea nitrogen, serum creatinine
3. Radiographic studies — renal ultrasound, intravenous pyelography, voiding cystourethrogram
4. Isotope renography
5. Urodynamic studies to assess bladder and urethral sphincter functions

Recently our approach to management of neuropathic bladder has undergone a radical change. Currently, conservative measures are preferred to surgical procedures for urinary diversion, which is now rarely undertaken.

Clean intermittent catheterization. This is the most effective and widely practised method. It is based on the principle that host resistance is more important in preventing urinary tract infection than small numbers of introduced organisms. It aims to prevent overdistention of the bladder with consequent interference with its blood supply and to regularly remove any residual urine. The method is clean and not sterile. The fundamental aspect of this technique is regular (at least four hourly) and complete bladder emptying, seven days per week. The majority of patients will remain non-infected or only have occasional infections. Some may require long-term prophylaxis with antibiotics if re-infection is a problem.

Drug treatment can be helpful, such as using anticholinergic drugs for the bladder with uncontrolled contractions, cholinergic drugs for the atonic bladder and alpha-adrenergic drugs to increase urethral resistance.

If the bladder has a very small capacity, a bladder augmentation with an isolated segment of intestine may be necessary to increase this capacity. If between-catheterization dribbling is a chronic problem, other forms of treatment may be necessary.

Bladder training. In children with flaccid bladder and in those who have some dribbling between catheterizations, patients should try to void every 2 hours by increasing their intra-abdominal pressures. Crede's manouevre of suprapubic manual compression is not done, particularly in cases with reflux.

Indwelling catheterization. Children with hypertonic bladder and longstanding obstructive uropathy have a serious problem. The bladder is spastic, has a high pressure and reduced capacity. Often there is reflux with hydroureters and hydronephrosis. Indwelling catheterization for several months combined with anticholinergic drugs corrects the ureteric reflux as well as the dilatation of the upper tracts. Following such improvement, intermittent catheterization is carried out.

Urinary incontinence. Most children will be reasonably dry between intermittent catheterizations. Boys who dribble urine can be helped by condom catheters, or penile devices attached to a conduit fixed to the thigh. Occasionally, penile clamps are helpful if not applied too tightly and for too long. Unfortunately, there are no suitable devices for female children and they have to be managed by indwelling catheters.

Surgical treatment. Surgical intervention is done only when conservative measures fail to protect the renal function and keep the child dry. In very young children, when intermittent catheterization is not a practical proposition, cutaneous vesicostomy (tubeless) is a suitable method. It is particularly valuable in children whose urinary tracts are deteriorating due to reflux, hydronephrosis and hydroureters. Other surgical procedures include antireflux operations, augmentation cystoplasty, and urethrotomies. In late cases, cutaneous ureterostomies and antireflux urinary diversion may be required. Implantable artificial sphincters are now being used on a trial basis to attempt to maintain continence.

Faecal incontinence

Bowel dysfunction presents as constipation and/or perineal soiling which may be due to overflow incontinence or inability to control liquid faeces. The majority of children can be satisfactorily managed by diet control, laxatives and occasional suppositories and enemata. Severe constipation and faecal impaction may need colon washouts. Tap-water washouts, if used on a daily basis, can be very effective in maintaining faecal continence.

Skeletal anomalies and orthopaedic management

If cases have been selected properly, most children should be able to walk. One-third will need calipers and braces and the remaining require orthopaedic correction of deformities such as muscle transfers and tendon lengthening and release operations.

The quality of ambulation depends on the level of the spinal lesions and the nature of orthopaedic deformities. Quadriceps femoris is the key muscle for standing. If it is paralysed, satisfactory ambulation is not easily attainable. Cumbersome long calipers with pelvic bands and elbow crutches have to be used, and locomotion is of a very poor quality. It is for this reason that paralysis of the L3 segment or above renders a patient unsuitable for active treatment. Most children prefer to use a wheelchair than cumbersome appliances.

Home care, education and rehabilitation

The home environment should be suitably modified for safety and to facilitate independent activity by the handicapped child.

If the intelligence and level of handicap permit, the child should be encouraged to attend a normal school. A child with more severe physical problems, but of trainable intellectual status, should attend a school for the physically handicapped where occupational therapy befitting the child's capabilities can be provided. For a successful outcome, it is very important to have a team approach for the various aspects of this complex problem.

Spina bifida occulta

In spina bifida occulta there is defective fusion of the posterior vertebral arches, usually of the fifth lumbar and first sacral vertebrae. In a small number of cases there is an accompanying superficial lesion overlying the spinal defect. In a still smaller minority there is an additional intraspinal lesion interfering with the function of the spinal cord and the nerve roots in a variety of ways. As a rule, there is no associated hydrocephalus.

As the name implies, this type of spina bifida is not immediately obvious on inspection or examination, but there is a defective fusion of the posterior arches of L5 and S1 vertebrae (Fig. 18.7). According to clinical presentation it can be divided into four groups:

1. True spina bifida occulta, present in 10–20% of normal individuals as an asymptomatic incidental radiological finding.

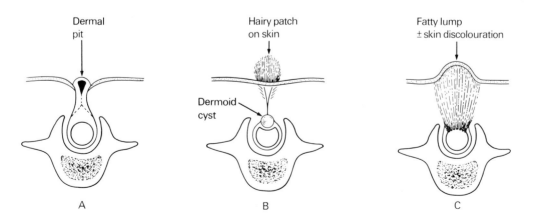

Fig. 18.7 Schematic representation of spina bifida occulta. **A**: Dermal sinus. **B**: Intraspinal cyst pressing on the cord. **C**: Lipomatous mass infiltrating the cord elements.

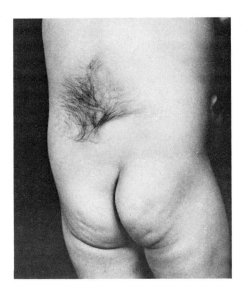

Fig. 18.8 Spina bifida occulta covered by a tuft of hair.

2. Spina bifida occulta with an overlying superficial lesion such as tuft of hair, a capillary haemangioma, a diffuse soft lipoma, a dermal pit or a blind dermal sinus. There are no neurological symptoms. (Fig. 18.8).

3. Spina bifida occulta presenting as meningitis. The overlying dermal sinus may end in a subarachnoid cyst or may go all the way to the spinal theca, providing a passage for bacteria which cause recurrent attacks of meningitis. When the infection has been controlled with antibiotics, the entire sinus tract is excised, including the cyst if present.

4. Spina bifida with neurological symptoms (occult spinal dysraphism). In addition to the superficial lesions described above, there is an underlying intraspinal lesion producing pressure or traction on the cord or the nerves of the cauda equina. The various pathological types include intraspinal lipoma or cyst, dermoid cyst or fibrous bands producing symptoms due to direct pressure or traction.

Neurological symptoms start late, usually between 2 and 5 years, and are slowly progressive. Urinary incontinence or appearance of a limp on one side are the commonest initial changes. The neurological deficit, which is usually asymmetrical, may be of upper motor neurone or lower motor neurone type. CT scan and myelography should be done when symptoms appear. Laminectomy may be necessary to remove intraspinal lesions. A neural deficit may persist, but further damage is prevented by surgery.

ANTERIOR BODY WALL DEFECTS

Anterior body wall defects are mostly abdominal, involving the region of the umbilical cord and a variable extent of the midline, cranially up to the sternum or down to the symphysis pubis. Rarely, the defect is confined to the anterior thoracic wall. These defects include omphalocele, gastroschisis and exstrophy of the bladder or cloaca.

Omphalocele

Omphalocele or exomphalos is a congenital herniation of the bowel and solid viscera through a midline defect surrounded by the attachment of the umbilical cord. If the defect is small, permitting only a small bowel loop into the base of the cord, the condition is called a hernia of the umbilical cord. The size of the omphalocele sac varies from 2 to 20 cm. In larger herniations, most of the abdominal viscera lie outside the abdomen, the capacity of which is inadequate for their bulk replacement (Fig. 18.9). At birth the covering sac is a shiny, avascular, translucent membrane consisting of amnion and Wharton's jelly, structures normally ensheathing the umbilical cord. Within a day or two it becomes opaque, lustreless and necrosed. If not treated properly, there is a danger of rupture and evisceration, and infection and septic complications.

The umbilical cord is attached to the fundus of the sac. The umbilical arteries and vein are seen coursing along the wall of the sac. Malrotation and malfixation of the midgut are universal, while approximately 40% of cases have other associated malformations which include congenital heart disease and abnormalities of the urinary tract. Exomphalos is one of the anomalies constituting the EMG (exomphalos, macroglossia and gigantism) syndrome, also known as the Beckwith-Weidemann syndrome.

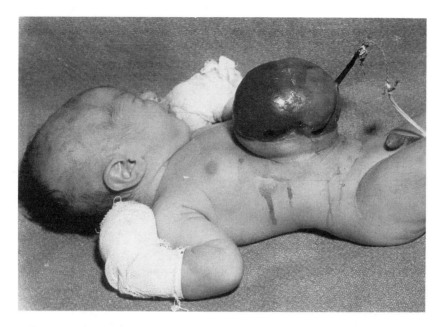

Fig. 18.9 Omphalocele. Infant with a large omphalocele measuring 10 cm in diameter and treated conservatively with Betadine paint. Note the upper half of the sac is occupied by liver. The umbilical cord has already shrivelled up.

Management

During transport the omphalocele is covered with a moist, non-irritant antiseptic dressing (Betadine) to avoid infection and rupture of the sac. Feeds are withheld and the stomach kept empty by nasogastric tube. Hypothermia is prevented by wrapping the infant with sterile cotton pads and a plastic sheet covering.

The aim of treatment is to provide a skin cover without increasing intra-abdominal pressure, which will embarrass respiration and interfere with venous return.

Definitive treatment

It is not possible to achieve primary surgical repair in every case. The mode of treatment and prognosis depend on:

1. Size of the hernial defect
2. The contents of the sac
3. Condition of the sac, e.g. ruptured, infected
4. Gestational age
5. General condition of the infant: hypothermia, sepsis
6. Severity of additional malformations

If the defect is less than 5 cm in diameter, it is possible to excise the sac, reduce the viscera and repair the defect in layers. If primary closure produces tension, the gap between the rectus muscles is bridged by an elliptical piece of Dacron mesh before closing the skin.

When the defect is larger, particularly when part of the liver is lying in the sac, it is not feasible to do a primary repair. In such cases, skin flaps are mobilized and sutured in front of the intact sac. The residual hernial defect is repaired any time after the first birthday. Very large sacs for which even skin closure is not possible need conservative management.

In cases with a ruptured sac the only course open is to remove the remaining sac and the cord and replace it with a Silastic silo, an artificial sac made of Silastic and Teflon in the form of a silo. Every alternate day the capacity of the artificial sac is reduced by placing a row of sutures along its fundus. This manoeuvre gradually increases the space in the abdomen and, in 10–14 days, repair of the defect can be performed. Infection in the line of sutures and inside the silo is a common complication.

Non-operative treatment

Poor-risk cases as well as infants with enormous sacs unsuitable for primary closure are best treated conservatively. This is achieved by hourly application of 1% Betadine or 70% alcohol. Gradual epithelization occurs underneath the eschar which separates in 8–10 weeks. The wound ultimately heals spontaneously, leaving a wide muscle gap, similar to a large incisional hernia, which can be repaired when the child is about 18 months old.

Gastroschisis

Gastroschisis is protrusion of the abdominal viscera, usually the entire midgut loop, through a defect in the anterior abdominal wall at the level of the umbilicus. The defect is small, 1 to 2 cm in diameter, almost always to the right of the umbilicus, which is normally placed, and may in fact be separated from the defect by a narrow bridge of skin (Fig. 18.10). Intrauterine rupture of a hernia of the umbilical cord produces gastroschisis. The herniated intestinal loops become exposed to the effects of the amniotic fluid. Moreover, the narrow opening produces an element of venous congestion in the bowel loops. Both these factors account for the thickened, oedematous and apparently shortened loops of intestine protruding through the defect. This chronic oedema of the gut interferes with bowel function for weeks after surgery. Unlike exomphalos there is a very low incidence of associated malformations.

Management

The immediate needs are:

1. To pass a nasogastric tube for decompression of the upper gastrointestinal tract
2. To cover the exposed intestinal loops in a sterile polythene bag
3. To minimize fluid and heat loss and control infection

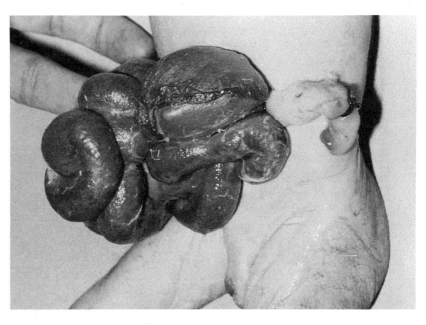

Fig. 18.10 Gastroschisis. The herniated loops of intestine are oedematous and covered with fibrinous matter.

Closure of the defect

Often the bowel can be returned to the abdomen and the defect repaired primarily. If this is not possible a staged approach is used. A Silastic silo is sutured around the exposed loops of intestine as described for ruptured exomphalos. These infants are supported with total parenteral nutrition for several weeks till bowel function returns.

Exstrophy of the urinary bladder

This is a rare anomaly, seen in 1 in 10 000 to 20 000 newborn infants. Boys predominate in a ratio of 5:2. It is caused by failure of fusion of the lateral mesodermal elements of the lower anterior abdominal wall. There is a midline defect bounded by the rectus muscles and the pubic bone on either side. The dorsal urethra and anterior bladder and the bladder neck fail to develop, producing an epispadias and extroversion of the exposed vesical mucosa (see Fig. 6.4).

There are various grades of severity. In minor defects there is epispadias along with exstrophy of the bladder neck, causing urinary incontinence. In severe cases there is wide separation of the pubic bones. The axis of the hip joints is rotated posteriorly producing a typical waddling gait. The gap between the rectus muscles is occupied by the exposed bladder mucosa, everted due to intra-abdominal pressure. Quite often the infant has bilateral inguinal herniae with rectractile or maldescended testes. At times there is a coexisting omphalocele just above the exstrophied bladder.

Cloacal exstrophy (vesico-enteric fissure)

This is a more complex anomaly. Besides all the features of exstrophy of the bladder, there is atresia of the anorectum and colon. The ileum terminates by opening between two halves of the exstrophied bladder. Results of reconstructive surgery are not satisfactory.

Treatment

The aim of treatment is to achieve continence, to preserve renal function and to close the abdominal wall defect. The major problem is to achieve continence without producing back pressure effects on kidneys and ureters. Minor degrees of exstrophy can be corrected by repairing the epispadias and reconstructing the bladder neck and the sphincteric muscle. Larger exstrophies with wider bony gaps are difficult to treat. Two methods are used:

1. A staged primary reconstruction
2. Urinary diversion by ureterosigmoidostomy or colon conduit

Prune belly syndrome (abdominal musculature deficiency syndrome)

A very rare anomaly, mostly seen in boys. There is a developmental failure, to varying degrees, of the abdominal muscles (Fig. 18.11). The more serious aspects of the syndrome are the additional abnormalities of the urogenital system.

The abdomen is rather large and shapeless. The abdominal wall is flabby with no appreciable muscle tone. The skin is lax and wrinkled, giving the 'prune' appearance. Intestinal loops are visible and the abdominal viscera can be easily palpated. There is dilatation of the urinary bladder (megacystic), megaureter and hydronephrosis. There is bilateral cryptorchidism and meatal stenosis.

Prognosis depends on the functional status of the urinary tract and associated anomalies of gastrointestinal, musculoskeletal and cardiovascular systems. The aim of the surgery is to preserve renal function by instituting a free urinary drainage.

MAJOR DEFECTS OF THE ANTERIOR THORACIC WALL

Embryologically, ribs develop from somites. The

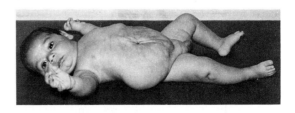

Fig. 18.11 Patient with prune-belly syndrome.

sternum develops from a separate blastema, its mesoderm being arranged as two longitudinal bands separated initially by a midline cleft. The ribs growing ventrally gradually meet the sternal bands and at the same time the sternal elements fuse in the midline forming the sternum.

Sternal clefts

These are rare defects caused by failure of midline fusion or arrest of development. Depending on the extent of mesodermal failure, three types of sternal clefts have been described:

1. *Isolated sternal cleft.* The covering skin is normal and there are no associated underlying anomalies. The heart can be seen pulsating through the U-shaped defect, usually involving the manubrium and upper sternum.
2. *True ectopia cordis.* In addition to the cleft, the newborn infant presents with a heart lying outside the chest wall exposed or covered by a thin translucent membrane. Usually there are associated major cardiac and other malformations incompatible with life in such cases.
3. *Cantrell's pentology.* There is a more extensive mesodermal failure producing a thoracoepigastric ectopia cordis. The five constituents of the syndrome are: bifid lower sternum, epigastric omphalocele, anterior diaphragmatic defect, persistent pericardioperitoneal communications and cardiac anomalies, usually a ventricular septal defect or other bizarre anomalies.

Sternochondral malformations

Depression deformity (pectus excavatum or funnel chest). This is the commonest type of chest deformity. There is a funnel-shaped hollow caused by acute inwards bending of the body of the sternum and the corresponding costal cartilages. The apex of the hollow is the lowest part of the sternum just above the sternoxiphoid junction. Sometimes the deformity is asymmetrical, being deeper on the right side than the left. The abdomen becomes protuberant and there is rounding of the shoulders and stooping of the neck.

These children are usually asymptomatic. Some have a limited capacity for physical work, possibly due to compression of the right atrium and displacement of the heart to the left, producing impaired ventricular filling, manifest during exercise. Rarely, respiratory stridor or dysphagia have been attributed to funnel chest. Indications for surgical correction are:

1. Cosmetic: social embarrassment and mental distress caused by a deep funnel chest deformity
2. Surgical: cardiopulmonary symptoms, displacement of electrocardial axis, diminished capacity for exercise due to compression of intrathoracic structures

Treatment

Basically, the surgical procedure consists of mobilization and elevation of the sternum and its subsequent fixation in the optimal position using a metal strut.

Protrusion deformity (pectus carinatum, pigeon chest)

This is much less common than the depression deformity. It is usually not recognized before 3–4 years of age. In contradistinction to funnel chest, there is prominence of the sternum. The lateral depressions of the costal cartilages may reduce the thoracic capacity and press on the heart.

Treatment

Lateral X-rays of the chest are taken to assess the degree of protrusion and to detect any predisposing intrathoracic causes. Sometimes, spontaneous regression takes place in low protrusions. In less severe cases, therefore, it is advisable to wait. In high protrusion, subpericostal resection of affected ribs is undertaken as in funnel chest.

Chest wall deficiency (Poland's syndrome)

In this syndrome there is unilateral failure of development of the pectoral muscles and deficiency of the underlying second to fourth costal cartilages and ribs producing paradoxical respiration.

The subcutaneous fat, areola and breast tissue are missing on the side of the defect, although a rudimentary nipple is present. Some hypoplasia of the upper limb and deformities of the hand and fingers may coexist.

Treatment

Surgical correction of the chest deficiency is done when the child presents for treatment. Autogenous bone grafts are used to cover the defect.

FURTHER READING

Jeffs D H, Guice S L, Oesh I 1982 The factors in successful exstrophy closure. *Journal of Urology* 127: 974
Martin L W, Torres A M 1985 Omphalocele and gastroschisis. In: Symposium on Pediatric Surgery Part I. Surgical Clinics of North America 65: 5, 1235–1244
Ravitch M M 1971 Congenital deformities of the chest and their treatment. In: Rickham P P, Hecker W Ch, Prevot J (eds) Progress in pediatric surgery 3: 1–12
Reigal D H 1982 Spina bifida. In: McLauren R L (eds) Pediatric neurosurgery. Surgery of the developing nervous system. Grune & Stratton, New York, p 23–48

19. Urinary tract infection and abnormalities of the urinary system

R. A. MacMahon

There are five main patterns of clinical presentation of infants and children with an abnormality of the urinary system:

1. Urinary tract infection
2. Non-specific clinical features
   (a) Pyrexia of unknown origin
   (b) Febrile convulsion
   (c) Diarrhoea and vomiting
   (d) Recurrence of enuresis
   (e) Offensive, cloudy urine
3. A palpable mass
4. Failure to thrive
5. Association with other major abnormalities

The common method of presentation is urinary tract infection. This is usually an easy diagnosis in the adult or older child because they have obvious symptoms such as frequency of urination, burning and scalding. Infants and young children who are in napkins may have these symptoms but because of the napkin it is difficult to associate their symptoms with urination. The possibility of a urinary tract infection should be kept in mind in any infant or child who is ill, even though the symptoms and signs may be non-specific. If there is recurrent low-grade infection there may be no acute symptoms.

A urinary tract infection in infancy or childhood raises the suspicion of an underlying structural abnormality because interference to the free flow of urine allows stagnant urine to remain in the urinary system and this favours the development of infection. It has been stated that stasis is the basis of infection. Probably a third of all girls and one-half of all boys with acute urinary infection will, on investigation, be found to have an underlying abnormality and, of these, approximately one-third will have vesicoureteric reflux.

Occasionally an opinion is expressed that the first urinary infection does not warrant investigation, particularly in girls. This may be true in the parous and/or sexually active female, but is potentially dangerous in the prepubertal child, particularly in infancy. As pointed out above, urinary tract infection frequently presents with non-specific symptoms and signs and may not be diagnosed as a urinary infection. For this reason alone, it will be impossible to know whether this is the first urinary infection or if it is just the first diagnosed infection. The other major problem is that the treating medical practitioner on this occasion has to make an assumption that if a previous urinary tract infection has been diagnosed by another practitioner, then the parents remember this and communicate it. This is an unwarranted assumption.

Physical signs of a urinary abnormality are uncommon. If there is a major obstruction, the proximal dilatation of bladder or kidney may produce a mass, but even a moderately enlarged hydronephrotic kidney may be difficult to palpate in infancy. An obvious congenital abnormality of the external genitalia may suggest the possibility of an underlying problem. If the symptoms and signs do not lead to an investigation of the urinary tract and if diagnosis and, therefore, adequate treatment is delayed, the child may present with renal failure. Rarely, there will be severe hypertension.

Ultrasound examination of the fetus in utero is now such a common practice that many congenital abnormalities of the urinary system are diagnosed before birth.

Because the symptoms and signs are so often non-specific, renal tract abnormalities are usually diagnosed by special investigations.

Special investigations in increasing order of complexity are:

1. Microscopy and culture of the urine
2. Ultrasound
3. Intravenous pyelogram (IVP)
4. Micturating cystourethrogram (MCU)
5. Renal nuclear scan
6. Cystoscopy
7. Retrograde pyelography
8. Angiography
9. CT

The first five of these investigations can be performed without anaesthesia and will usually give all the required information. Cystoscopy, one of the commonest investigations performed in adults, is rarely required in infants and children.

If a urinary problem is suspected, the urine should first be investigated by a standard ward test, but the absence of protein does not mean the absence of infection. Microscopic examination for cells, casts and crystals and culture of a freshly collected specimen is essential to diagnose infection. In infants, a specimen for culture should be collected by suprapubic needle aspiration and, in children over 3 years of age who can usually void on request, by collection of a midstream specimen. If a urinary tract infection is found, treatment of this should be commenced before further investigation. Patients with failure to thrive may have signs of renal decompensation such as metabolic acidosis and a raised serum creatinine level.

Investigation of the urinary system after the detection and initial treatment of a urinary tract infection or of an unexplained metabolic acidosis or renal decompensation is initially by ultrasound examination. This is non-invasive and may indicate the type of lesion and the next most appropriate investigation. Structural detail and drainage are best seen with an IVP, while differential function can be measured by a renal nuclear scan.

As vesicoureteric reflux is the commonest abnormality, an MCU is necessary in most cases to diagnose or exclude it. It must be remembered that, on occasions, an ultrasound or an IVP may appear to be within normal limits but an MCU may show quite marked vesicoureteric reflux. An MCU should not be omitted from the investigation of such patients.

EMBRYOLOGY

During the 4th to 8th weeks of development the nephrogenic mesoderm differentiates in a cranial to caudal direction, forming the pronephros cranially, the mesonephros in the intermediate region and the metanephros or definitive kidney in the caudal region.

At the 4 mm stage of development the Wolffian or mesonephric duct has reached the cloaca, bending at a right angle to enter the cloaca at the level of the first sacral vertebra. At this level the ureteric bud arises from the Wolffian duct and invades the nephrogenic mesoderm which begins to differentiate into a kidney. The ureter elongates and the kidney begins its ascent and rotation. Secondary buds from the ureter and subsequent branches form the collecting tubules and the pelvis and calyces of the kidney. The nephrons arise in the nephrogenic mesenchyme, under the stimulus of the dividing ureteric bud, so that if the ureter is absent, the kidney will not develop.

The caudal ends of the mesonephric ducts, with the origin of the ureters, are absorbed into the developing bladder to form the trigone of the bladder. Vestigial remnants of the mesonephric tubules occur in both sexes, usually associated with the reproductive organs.

The lower urinary tract is not formed from mesoderm like the kidneys and ureter but from endoderm and develops by division of the primitive hindgut and cloaca into a ventral urinary system and a dorsal gut system (See Figs 8.1 and 8.2). The urethra develops from the urogenital sinus (See Ch. 20).

The ureter is incorporated into the developing bladder during the 6th week. Failure of this incorporation, particularly in a duplex system, can cause ectopic ureteric openings. If the incorporation of the ureter into the bladder does not achieve a long oblique intramural course, including fusion of the longitudinal ureteric muscle with the muscle of the bladder wall and trigone, then the sphincter action at the lower end of the ureter may be incomplete and this allows vesicoureteric reflux.

Because of the complex nature of the development of the urinary system, abnormalities are common.

ABNORMALITIES OF THE LOWER URINARY TRACT

Vesicoureteric reflux

This is the commonest abnormality found on investigation in the paediatric age group. It is caused by a failure of the normal sphincteric mechanism at the junction of ureter and bladder to prevent backflow of urine from the bladder when the vesical pressure rises, particularly during micturition. This backwash of urine leads to stasis and a tendency to urinary tract infection and any infection arising in the bladder can be carried to the kidneys by this reflux.

The bladder is a high pressure system while the kidneys and ureters are low pressure systems. There is dispute about whether the pressure wave from the bladder, transmitted to the kidney by marked reflux, can cause harm in itself. In the most severe cases where there is free and open communication between bladder and kidneys, and where the urine actually refluxes into the renal tubules (intrarenal reflux) (Fig. 19.1), it seems likely that this pressure effect contributes to the renal damage.

Vesicoureteric reflux is common in childhood but rare in adults, so that there is a natural tendency for spontaneous resolution of the reflux with time. There is also a familial incidence with 10% of siblings of an affected patient also having reflux.

There are five grades of reflux:

1. Reflux into the ureter but not reaching the pelvis of the kidney
2. Reflux filling the ureter and kidney pelvis but without any distension or dilatation of the system
3. Reflux filling both ureter and pelvicalyceal system of the kidney with distension

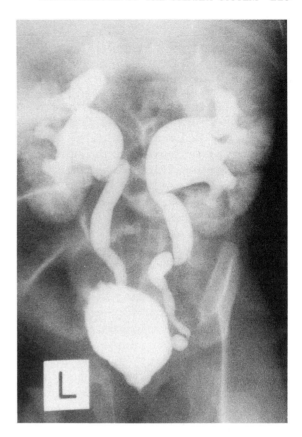

Fig. 19.1 Gross bilateral vesicoureteric reflux with intrarenal reflux.

4. Gross reflux with renal scarring
5. Mild reflux with gross renal scarring and renal insufficiency

The usual method of presentation of vesicoureteric reflux is urinary tract infection. Occasionally, recurrent infections over a number of years that have not been recognized or have been treated empirically without investigation and continuing treatment, may lead to renal deterioration so that the child presents with some degree of renal failure.

Investigation

An infant or child before puberty who has a proven urinary tract infection should be investigated initially by ultrasound and MCU to discover any underlying abnormality, particularly vesicoureteric reflux (Fig. 19.1). It should be remembered that an ultrasound may not necessarily show even marked reflux.

Treatment

Cystitis is common in children, particularly in girls, due to the short urethra and difficulty with vulval hygiene. Reflux may cause renal damage by carrying bladder infection to the kidney, and possibly by pressure effects. Hence the first essential in the management of reflux is to control any tendency to infection. If infections are infrequent and there is only a mild to moderate degree of reflux, and provided infections are diagnosed promptly and treated immediately and efficiently, then upper tract damage should not occur. Often a prophylactic dose of a urinary antibacterial drug, such as nitrofurantoin, taken at night for months or years will control any tendency to infection. The drug used may need to be changed from time to time if resistant organisms develop.

Surgical treatment is not indicated for reflux of grades 1 or 2, but continuing supervision of such children is necessary. Dilatation of the system seen in grade 3 reflux shows some decompensation, so surgical treatment is indicated if the dilatation is marked or persistent or there are recurrent infections. Grade 4 reflux needs early surgery. Grade 5 reflux is the result of unrecognized or untreated reflux and is seen in older children or adults. Surgery for the reflux is not indicated.

Grade 4 reflux is sometimes seen in infants, usually with other major urinary problems. In such cases the renal damage may be due to intrauterine back pressure effects or to dysplasia or a combination of both. Surgical repair is usually required.

Surgical correction of vesicoureteric reflux consists of dissecting the ureters from their abnormally short intramural course through the bladder muscle and making a submucosal track several centimetres in length into which the ureters are placed. With rise of pressure in the bladder as urine collects, there is increasing pressure upon the length of ureter in its submucosal tunnel, so preventing reflux. This is effective in approximately 95% of cases. Recurrent cystitis may still continue even after successful reimplan-

tation of the ureters but should not have any direct effect upon the kidneys. However, the parents need to be warned before surgery that the surgery is not necessarily a cure for recurrent urinary tract infection.

It is also possible to prevent reflux in the uncomplicated case by injecting a Polytef paste beneath the ureteric orifice at cystoscopy.

Bladder diverticula

These are congenital diverticula usually at or adjacent to the site of the ureteric openings. They are related to an abnormality in the development of this area and consist of mucosal protrusions through defects in the muscle coat of the bladder without themselves having a muscle coat. They are found during investigation of the infant or child for urinary tract infection and their size may interfere with the function of the ureter, causing back pressure, or there may be an abnormality of development of the renal unit on that side. The diverticula themselves are easily treated by excision and closure of the muscle opening but if they are small and empty completely when the bladder empties, no treatment is required.

Bladder neck obstruction

This entity is controversial and current thinking is that it almost never occurs in the paediatric age group. Appearances seen on X-rays sometimes suggest that the bladder neck is small but such appearances are almost never associated with any functional obstruction.

Posterior urethral valves

These are abnormal valvular folds of the mucous membrane of the urethra in the region of the verumontanum with consequent back pressure on the posterior urethra, bladder, ureters and kidneys. In the most extreme cases, there is dysplasia of both kidneys and death occurs soon after birth. In mild cases, urinary symptoms may not be noticed until later in childhood or, rarely, in adult life.

The usual presentation is of a male infant with urinary tract infection, poor urinary stream, or

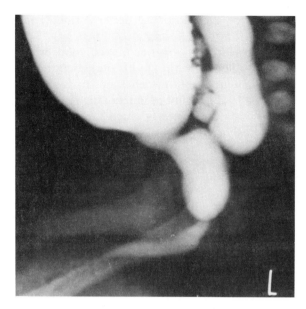

Fig. 19.2 MCU showing marked dilatation of the posterior urethra and back pressure effects on the bladder from posterior urethral values. Reflux can be seen, into a dilated ureter.

renal insufficiency. Investigation, after treatment of the infection and/or renal insufficiency, will show a thick-walled, trabeculated bladder with a grossly dilated posterior urethra, narrowing down to an obstructive lesion at the level of the verumontanum or just below (Fig. 19.2). There may be associated vesicoureteric reflux or obstruction at the ureterovesical junction with back pressure on the kidneys.

Treatment

With appropriate paediatric instruments the valves may be excised per urethra. Long-term management will be necessary because most of these patients will have renal damage, abnormal bladders and may have an intrinsic obstruction at the lower end of the ureters.

Other abnormalities

A variety of major abnormalities may occur in the bladder and upper urethra associated with formation of the anterior body wall (see Ch. 18), or with the division of the hindgut into the urogenital and gut systems. These include absence of the bladder, duplication of the bladder and urethra, abnormal fistula with the gut, a patent urachus or cystic dilatation of the urachus.

ABNORMALITIES OF THE UPPER URINARY TRACT

Obstructive lesions

Ureteral obstructions are common abnormalities. The two common sites of obstruction are at the pelviureteric junction and at the ureterovesical junction.

Pelviureteric obstruction

This form of abnormality is commonly called congenital hydronephrosis. There is an obstruction at the pelviureteric junction usually caused by a narrowing of the lumen. Other unusual causes of obstruction are kinking of this area by a fibrous band, by the valvular effect of a high insertion of the ureter into the renal pelvis, or by a crossing blood vessel. The obstruction is a partial one but the degree of obstruction varies from almost complete obstruction with gross hydronephrosis and minimal remaining renal tissue (Fig. 19.3) to a slight obstruction with pelvic dilatation only. The clinical features of congenital hydronephrosis may be one or more of the following:

1. Palpable mass
2. Intermittent abdominal pain
3. Urinary tract infection
4. Haematuria

If there is marked obstruction with very little flow, then there is considerable retention of urine and a palpable loin mass. In infants this mass will be felt anteriorly in the abdomen. If there is moderate obstruction, then the mass is difficult to feel and may only be felt in periods of diuresis. With prolonged chronic obstruction there is very little pain but if there is acute distension with diuresis, then episodes of pain will be a feature.

Vomiting is associated with severe bouts of pain.

As with any obstructive lesion within the urinary system, there will be stasis of urine and often

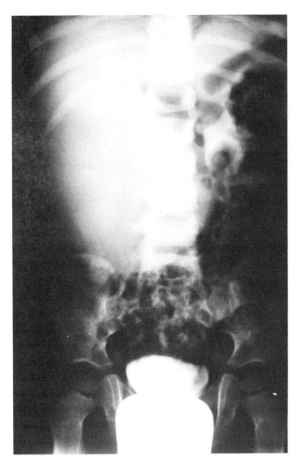

Fig. 19.3 IVP showing a normal kidney and a giant hydronephrosis with dye diluted in retained urine in the pelvicalyceal system.

infection. This infection may have the features of a pyrexia of unknown origin in the infant or may have the localizing features of an apparent pyelonephritis in the older child.

Haematuria is an occasional initial complaint following an injury in the region of the kidney. It is important not to confuse the features of congenital hydronephrosis with those of gross trauma to the kidney in the investigation of these patients.

Investigations. Infection in a hydronephrosis causes rapid renal damage so that investigation and treatment of any infection is the first priority. Ultrasound examination is the investigation of choice as it will demonstrate the large cystic mass. IVP or renal scan shows dilated calyces and pelvis with a nipping at the pelviureteric junction

and delayed excretion. The ureter is usually not seen.

Treatment. Conservation of renal tissue wherever possible is the rule in childhood. Although the kidney architecture seems grossly abnormal, there is a large amount of functioning renal tissue even though the cortex is much thinner than in the normal kidney. Every effort should be made to conserve this tissue. Surgical treatment is required and the obstructing lesion is excised and a long ureteropelvic anastomosis performed. The functional results of this operation are good, though in any kidney with gross distortion of architecture, this gross distortion will always be seen on subsequent investigations.

Ureterovesical obstruction

Obstruction at the ureterovesical junction may be due to stenosis, kinking, or a congenital dilatation of the lower end of the ureter (ureterocele) with a small eccentric opening into the bladder.

The method of presentation in this type of obstruction is almost invariably with urinary tract infection, though if there are renal abnormalities on both sides the patient may occasionally present with renal failure.

Investigation. Ultrasound examination may show both a dilated ureter and kidney but the dilated ureter is sometimes difficult to demonstrate. An IVP may have minimal excretion so that it is difficult to determine the architecture of the renal unit on that side but a renal scan will show differential function (Fig. 19.4). Cystoscopy and retrograde pyelography are often necessary to delineate the anatomy. If a ureterocele is present it will be seen as a space-occupying filling defect in a cystogram (Fig. 19.5).

Treatment. Unilateral disease with evidence of gross renal damage, provided the opposite system is normal, is an indication for excision of the abnormal kidney and ureter. If there is reasonable function on the affected side, the obstructing lesion at the lower end of the ureter can be excised and the ureter reimplanted into the bladder. If there are bilateral abnormalities then every effort should be made to conserve whatever renal tissue is present on either side to delay the onset of renal insufficiency.

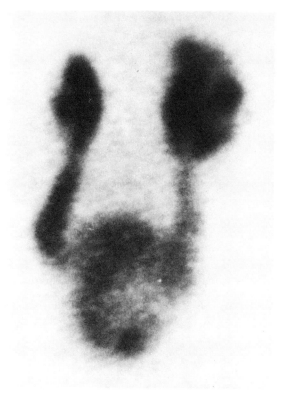

Fig. 19.4 Renal scan with bilateral vesicoureteric obstruction, dilated ureters, hydronephrotic kidneys, one of which has lost most of its renal substance.

Other obstructions

Fibrous bands, valves and diverticula of the ureters occur but are rare. Investigation and treatment follows the pattern outlined above.

Duplication

Duplication of the kidney is found in almost 1% of all autopsies. There are two segments to the kidney with separation of the calyces of the two systems, and a separate ureter for each system. The ureters may be bifid, or Y-shaped, and join together at some point between the renal pelvis and the bladder, or may be completely separate with two separate openings into the bladder. Triplications have also been reported. Duplex systems may be associated with other abnormalities such as cystic dysplasia of one segment or with vesicoureteric reflux (Fig. 19.6). If there is a complete duplication, one ureter may be associated with a cystic dilatation of the lower end of

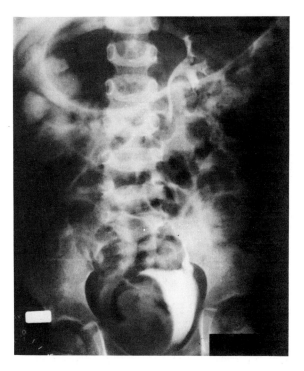

Fig. 19.5 IVP showing a normal left kidney, a hydronephrotic right kidney and a ureterocele producing a filling defect in the bladder.

the ureter (ureterocele) or the ureteric orifice may open in an abnormal situation such as the vagina or urethra in the female or the urethra in the male.

Infection in a duplex system is common if the abnormal opening is obstructed by a ureterocele with back pressure on the affected segment, or if there is a 'yo-yo' effect when the ureters join near the bladder. In this latter situation, urine from one pelvis can pass down its ureter but instead of passing onwards to the bladder, some refluxes up into the ureter of the other segment. In turn, the urine from that segment refluxes back into the ureter and pelvis of the first segment. Rarely, incontinence is associated with an ectopic opening if it opens into the vagina in the female.

Occasionally children with recurrent abdominal or back pain are found to have a duplex system but in the absence of dilatation, obstruction or infection such pain is probably not related to the renal findings.

Cystoscopy will show whether there are two ureteric openings into the bladder and if not, ret-

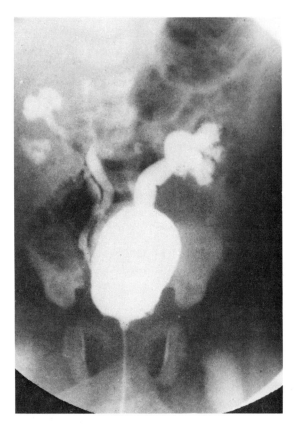

Fig. 19.6   MCU shows bilateral marked reflux and a duplex system on the right side.

Abnormalities of ascent and rotation

Ectopia of the kidney is quite common and rarely there may be bilateral ectopia. The kidney may be anywhere along a line from the upper sacral segments to the renal fossa and it may be felt as an unusually placed mass. Renal pain from an abnormality in such a kidney can be misleading because of its site.

Crossed ectopia is an abnormality in which the kidney lies on the side of the body opposite to the side on which the ureter joins the bladder. Sometimes the ectopic kidney fuses with the normal kidney. Abnormalities of rotation of the kidney are also common and are often associated with other abnormalities. These variations in the position of the kidney, especially horseshoe kidney, may bring the vascular supply and the ureter into such a relationship with the mass of the kidney that some obstruction occurs to the ureter. In this case there will be interference with the flow of urine, with consequent stasis, infection and proximal dilatation.

These abnormalities are diagnosed during investigation of the urinary tract because of urinary tract infection or a palpable renal mass in an unusual site.

rograde pyelography will show the site of union. If there is an ectopic orifice it can be identified by giving an intravenous injection of a dye, such as indigo carmine, which is excreted by the kidneys and which then can be seen issuing from the site of the abnormal orifice, e.g. in the vagina.

Treatment

Severe cystic dysplasia of a segment of the kidney, particularly if associated with a large abnormal ureter and an ectopic ureteric orifice, is an indication for excision of that segment. If there is a caudal join of two ureters draining segments of a kidney with recurrent infection, then excision of the ureter draining the upper segment, with high pelvopelvic anastomosis or ureteropelvic or uretero-ureteral anastomosis, will correct the 'yo-yo' reflux.

Cystic disease of the kidney

There are at least 20 diseases or syndromes associated with different varieties of congenital cystic disease of the kidney, of which multicystic dysplastic disease is the most common. In this type the kidney functions poorly or not at all and may form a large mass that is palpable in the abdomen. Ultrasound examination clearly shows cystic areas in such a mass (Fig. 19.7).

If we exclude liver, spleen, bladder and faeces, the commonest abdominal tumour of a neonate is a cystic dysplastic kidney. Multicystic dysplastic disease is easily diagnosed on ultrasound examination and is unlikely to cause problems so that, theoretically, it could be left in place. However, because it is a mass, because haemorrhage is a possibility and because rarely there is an associated malignancy with a multicystic kidney, it is usually excised. Bilateral multicystic disease oc-

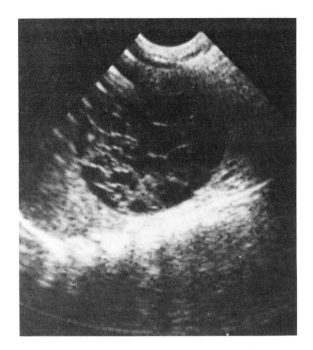

Fig. 19.7 Ultrasound examination shows multiple cysts in a renal mass.

curs and other abnormalities of the opposite kidney, usually hydronephrosis, are common in patients with a unilateral multicystic kidney.

Infantile polycystic disease is another category in which a newborn infant has a distended abdomen due to markedly enlarged, firm kidneys and this enlargement is due to fusiform dilatation of the collecting tubules. This is inherited as an autosomal recessive disease and death in infancy was the rule, but with vigorous renal management it is possible to prolong life to the stage where renal transplantation can be considered. Other forms of renal cystic disease are rarely diagnosed in infancy or childhood.

Renal agenesis, dysplasia and hypoplasia

Renal agenesis is a complete absence of the kid-

ney and there is usually a complete absence of the ureter of that side as well. Unilateral absence of the kidney does not produce a clinical syndrome and is usually found when the urinary tract is being investigated because of some other problem. Ultrasound examination will not demonstrate renal tissue on that side and IVP and renal scan show no function. At cystoscopy, there is a hemitrigone, with absence of the hemitrigone and ureteric orifice on the side of the absent kidney. Further investigations and exploration are unnecessary under these circumstances.

Bilateral renal agenesis can occur and is usually associated with the Potter syndrome, which includes oligohydramnios, large low-set ears, flattened nose and receding chin. The lungs are also hypoplastic, probably because of the lack of amniotic fluid and lung liquid. These infants die in the immediate postnatal period from respiratory failure.

Hypoplasia is the presence of a small but otherwise normal kidney that has reduced function because of its size. Pure hypoplasia is rare but hypoplasia associated with dysplasia (the presence of abnormal structures such as primitive ducts and cartilage in the renal parenchyma) is common. If severe, the kidney functions poorly or not at all so that there is no excretion seen on an IVP or renal scan but a ureteric orifice is seen on that side at cystoscopy. Renal dysplasia is often associated with a hypoplastic or atretic segment of ureter, or with obstruction of the lower urinary tract. A severely dysplastic kidney that is causing no symptoms or signs may be left in situ, or excised.

FURTHER READING

Becker G J 1985 Reflux nephropathy. Australian New Zealand Journal of Medicine 15: 668–676

Gray S W, Skandalakis J E (eds) 1972 Embryology for surgeons. Saunders, Philadelphia

20. Abnormalities of the genitalia. Circumcision

R. A. MacMahon

Abnormalities of the external genitalia are obvious on adequate examination, but may be missed if this examination is not carried out at birth. They are the result of an arrest or failure of development. The common problems are inguinal hernia, hydrocele, the undescended testis, and hypospadias. The pros and cons of circumcision are still debated.

EMBRYOLOGY

The external genitalia are formed from the phallic tubercle and bilateral labioscrotal folds. The initial and intermediate phases of development of the external genitalia are similar in both males and females. In later development, in the female, the phallic tubercle forms a clitoris and the labioscrotal folds form the labia minora and majora, while in the male, the phallus continues to enlarge to form the penis and the labioscrotal folds fuse progressively along the undersurface of the phallus to take the urethral opening to the tip of the penis, while the posterior end of the labioscrotal folds enlarges to form the scrotal sacs. Excess skin encloses the glans of the penis, forming a complete foreskin.

The gonads form from gonadal ridges on the posterior abdominal wall of the developing embryo and these differentiate into the ovaries in the female and testes in the male. This differentiation is under the control of both genetic and hormonal influences (Fig. 20.1).

The indifferent gonad initially stretches from the diaphragm to the pelvis, but by differential development and absorption, towards the end of

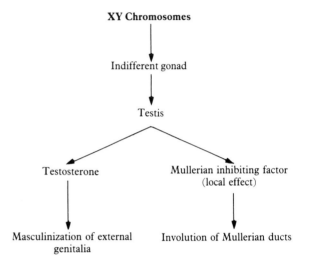

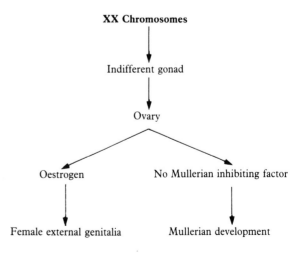

Fig. 20.1 Development of the genitalia, normal sequence.

231

gestation the ovary is at the brim of the pelvis and the testis just within the internal inguinal ring. At this stage, both the ovary and the testis are invested with a layer of peritoneum which almost completely encloses the organ, except where the vessels and ducts enter.

From the 31st to the 35th weeks, the testis migrates from the abdominal cavity to the scrotum, taking with it its connecting fold of peritoneum, the processus vaginalis. This fold should become obliterated at or around the time of birth, but it may not close or may close in varying degrees along its length. It can be seen that this would allow abdominal contents, either fluid, omentum or intestine, to pass down this persistent tract. Depending on the size of the track, this failure of closure will lead to a scrotal hydrocele, an encysted hydrocele of the cord, an inguinal hernia, an inguinoscrotal hernia, or various combinations of these. If the testis does not completely descend it can either be arrested along the line of descent or it may descend to an abnormal ectopic site.

Failure of complete closure of the processus vaginalis and abnormalities of testicular descent are the commonest surgical paediatric problems.

INGUINAL HERNIA

An inguinal hernia is the most important of the common surgical problems met with in infancy. It is due to the persistence of the processus vaginalis, allowing intestine and omentum to descend along it. In females it may contain an ovary and fallopian tube.

Clinical features

The parents or child state that a lump comes and goes in the groin. They may use their own terminology so that it is important to get them to indicate exactly where the lump appears. The lump may be more noticeable late in the day or may only appear with coughing and straining. An older child can be asked to stand and perform the usual manoeuvres of coughing and straining while the groin is examined. If the swelling is in the scrotum it is impossible to get above it.

In infancy, the parents may come with a story highly suggestive of hernia but there is no hernia on examination. In males, a thickened spermatic cord may be felt on that side compared to the opposite side, because of the extra tissue of the hernial sac in the cord. This thickening is most easily found by rolling the spermatic cord on the brim of the pubis. A good history plus a physical sign of a thickened cord is sufficient to diagnose inguinal hernia. In female infants, it may not be possible to feel thickening around the round ligament and a very good history may be the only indication for surgery.

This hernia is more common in boys, occurring in 4–5%, than girls and there will be a patent processus vaginalis on both sides in more than 50% of infants. Bilateral sacs are more common in girls than boys, so that bilateral exploration is advisable in all girls.

Complications

If bowel, usually small bowel, becomes caught in the sac, the inguinal hernia becomes irreducible. Initially there are no other local or general signs but if the blood supply to the loop of bowel is affected there is initially venous congestion leading to further swelling, interruption to the arterial supply and finally strangulation. This produces local inflammatory signs with signs of bowel obstruction.

Incarceration or strangulation may also interrupt the blood supply to the testis so that testicular infarction occurs.

Differential diagnosis

- Hydrocele
- Retractile or undescended testis
- Inguinal lymphadenitis

The clinical features, particularly the exact site of the swelling, will usually be diagnostic. An encysted hydrocele of the cord may be impossible to distinguish from an incarcerated hernia.

Direct inguinal hernia is very rare and is found at operation.

Treatment

The risk of complications is highest in the infant group so that unless there is a strong contraindication, e.g. a very small premature infant with a variety of other problems being treated in hospital, the diagnosis of an infant inguinal hernia is an indication for surgical repair on an early elective list. The operation performed is herniotomy of the sac at the internal ring and as this is a congenital hernial sac, there is almost never any need for herniorrhaphy. The risk of complications is much less in childhood but surgical repair is always necessary. There is no place for the use of a truss in this age group.

If the hernia is irreducible, even if there are no other symptoms or signs, immediate treatment is necessary. The infant should be admitted to hospital, sedated and the foot of the cot raised or 'gallows' traction used to allow gravity to reduce the swelling. When fully sedated, gentle and steady pressure will usually reduce the hernia and the infant is kept in hospital for 24 hours to allow all oedema to settle and a herniotomy to be performed. If it does not reduce, immediate operation is necessary.

If there is any suggestion of strangulation, no attempt should be made to reduce the hernia. The infant should be resuscitated before proceeding to emergency surgery.

HYDROCELE

A hydrocele has the same congenital basis as inguinal hernia but the connection of the processus vaginalis with the abdominal cavity is so small that only abdominal fluid reaches the fundus of the sac and not bowel or omentum. Because the connection is narrow, it is usually possible to get above the swelling, which is smooth and brilliantly transilluminable. The sac fills and empties slowly so that the swelling is most prominent towards the end of the day and may disappear overnight. It is not reducible.

A hydrocele, unless it is extremely large, does not need treatment in infancy. The natural tendency for the processus vaginalis to close in the first years of life will often cure the hydrocele. If it is still present when the child is due to go to school, it is advisable to remove it. The operation is similar to the operation for inguinal hernia in that the processus is ligated at the internal ring, but the fluid-filled tunica vaginalis testis needs to be deroofed to remove the fluid. A formal operation on the tunica is not required.

It may be impossible to distinguish an encysted hydrocele of the cord from an incarcerated inguinal hernia in that both may be irreducible, firm and transilluminable and it is not possible to get above the swelling. If there is real doubt, the swelling should be immediately explored.

THE EMPTY SCROTUM OR HEMISCROTUM

The testis that is not in the scrotum may be: retractile, undescended, malformed or absent.

The clinical problem of the apparently undescended testis noticed by parents or on routine medical examination is a common one. It is commoner in the newborn, being present in 30% of premature infants and 3% of full-term infants, but spontaneous descent of the testis in infancy reduces the neonatal incidence. It remains a common problem, being present in more than 2% of boys after 1 year of age.

Retractile testis

This is a normal variant. The testis has normally descended into the scrotum but there is an active cremasteric reflex which, on stimulation, will pull the testis into the groin. There is often a story that the testis has been seen in the scrotum at times.

If the patient is relaxed and not apprehensive and the skin over the inguinal canal is powdered to stop local stimulation, this type of testis can easily be pushed to the bottom of the scrotum by firm pressure pushing down the line of the inguinal canal. When this pressure is released, the testis will remain in the scrotum if there is no stimulation and can be found again in the bottom of the scrotum on immediate re-examination. This type of 'undescended' testis is normal and will become permanently resident in the scrotum at puberty. Attempts to grasp the bottom of the scrotum to see if there is a resident testis merely pushes a retractile testis towards the groin.

If a palpable testis does not fall into this category it is an undescended testis.

Undescended or malformed testis

This is a common problem, occurring in approximately 2.5% of boys over 1 year of age. Most undescended testes will be palpable along the line of descent or in one of the ectopic sites but 20% will be impalpable because the testis is in the inguinal canal, intra-abdominal, atrophic, dysgenetic or absent.

Approximately 4% of these patients will have only one testis and 0.5% no testes.

Testes arrested in the line of descent

Those arrested in the line of descent frequently have an associated hernia and may have some dysgenesis of the testis itself. Most of these will be between the external inguinal ring and the neck of the scrotum, but some are arrested within the inguinal canal and a small percentage within the abdominal cavity, usually just within the internal inguinal ring. Rarely, if there is an abnormality of development of the epididymis and/or testicular vessels, the testis can be in the region of the lower pole of the kidney, or in the pelvis along the line of the vas.

The testicular vessels are usually short and it is difficult to obtain adequate length of vessels to be able to place the testis into the scrotum without tension.

Laparoscopy

Ectopic testes

These are not in the normal line of descent. The common site is in the superficial inguinal pouch, which is on the external oblique muscle above and lateral to the external inguinal ring. Other sites are: prepenile, in the perineum or thigh adjacent to the scrotum or, rarely, in the opposite scrotum. These testes have an adequate length of vessels to allow placement in the scrotum without tension.

Malformed testes

These may be: atrophic, dysgenetic or absent.

These problems are defined on investigation of an abnormal, undescended or impalpable testis. The atrophic or markedly dysgenetic testis is best excised and a prosthesis inserted at an appropriate time, usually at puberty.

Complications

Infertility. Patients with bilateral undescended testes are infertile, but those treated by bilateral orchidopexy have a paternity rate of 44% compared with a paternity rate of 75% for patients with unilateral undescended testes and for fertile marriages in the population.

Trauma. The testis in the scrotum is mobile and this protects it somewhat from trauma. The undescended testis is relatively fixed and this and its position make it liable to trauma.

Torsion. The undescended testis, particularly the one arrested in the line of descent with a complete investment by a hernial sac, is liable to undergo torsion. The diagnosis of torsion of a testis in the inguinal canal or in the abdomen is difficult.

Malignancy. There is an increased risk of malignancy in the undescended testis and this has been variously estimated at from 4 to 10 times that of the descended testis. Whether orchidopexy lessens this risk is debated but there is no firm evidence that early orchidopexy has a favourable effect. At least orchidopexy places the testis in a position in which it can be easily examined for possible malignant change. It should also be remembered that up to 20% of malignancies in such patients occur in the normally descended testis. There is evidence that the abnormal gonocytes, from which germ-cell tumours arise, are present from birth, and may be identifiable on biopsy as carcinoma-in-situ. Even with this increased risk, testicular malignancy in the patient with undescended testis is rare.

Treatment   *After 1 yr*

Age. The ideal age for the treatment of the undescended testis is debated. To allow adequate development of the testis, particularly spermatogonia, the testis must be resident in the scrotum well before puberty and there is general agreement that it should be in the scrotum before school age. Some evidence has been found that ultramicroscopic changes can be found in the undescended testis within the first year of life and this has been used as an argument for orchidopexy within the first year. On the other hand, it is well known that some testes spontaneously descend within the first year, and there is also evidence that some undescended testes are the result of developmental abnormalities, so that the microscopic changes are present from birth. Further, early surgery carries more risks than later surgery.

For want of definitive information on which to base a firm statement on the best age for treatment, it seems that the age when they are out of napkins is appropriate, thus avoiding the extra risks of irritation and infection of the surgical wounds. /

Hormone therapy. This has little place in the treatment of the true undescended testis. In the fat child in whom it is difficult to decide whether the testes are retractile or undescended, injections of chorionic gonadotrophin, 500–1000 international units twice per week for 4 weeks, will bring the retractile testis into the scrotum. As the effects of the injections wear off, the testes tend to return to their previous position.

Gonadotrophin stimulation therapy is also used for the patient with bilateral impalpable testes. This stimulation will produce a rise in the testosterone level in patients with testicular tissue, but no change in those without such tissue. In these latter patients, exploration is not indicated.

Surgery. The treatment of the undescended testis is surgical exploration to define the type and site of the testis and, if possible, to dissect the vas and vessels as far as necessary to allow placement of the testis in the scrotum without tension in the cord. This may require extensive retroperitoneal dissection. If there is some tension, fixation of the testis to the scrotum will be needed.

Orchiectomy is indicated if the testis is dysgenetic and also if there is a high intra-abdominal testis with a contralateral normally descended testis.

Bilateral intra-abdominal testes are treated by staged orchidopexies; or by division of the testicular vessels with reliance on the blood supply from the vessel to the vas; or by division of the testicular vessels and microsurgical anastomosis

of them to vessels in the groin. Biopsy may be indicated to delineate any evidence of carcinoma-in-situ.

THE RED SWOLLEN SCROTUM OR HEMISCROTUM

This is an important entity in childhood, since it raises the possibility of torsion of the testis. The common adult cause of this clinical presentation, epididymoorchitis, is very uncommon in childhood, except in infancy and particularly in infants with other major malformations.

Differential diagnosis

Torsion of the testis

This is a volvulus of the testis on the spermatic cord with interference to the blood supply of the testis. In the neonate, because of the laxity of the tissues, the tunica vaginalis testis and the testis may undergo torsion within the scrotum. This is called an extravaginal torsion. In children the torsion is intravaginal. In these cases the testis hangs free in the cavity of the tunica vaginalis testis, due to a lack of mesentery-like effect of the normal longitudinal attachment of the tunica along the posterior aspect of the testis.

Clinical features. These features are different in the neonate and the older child.

In the neonate this is an intrauterine torsion and the infant is born with what appears to be a bruise or haemorrhage of the scrotum. The scrotum is swollen and the testis is difficult to feel. There are usually no signs of acute inflammation. The swelling and bruising gradually disappear leaving an atrophic testis.

In the older child the common presentation is that of an acute inflammatory lesion of the hemiscrotum with pain, swelling, redness and tenderness. The onset may be sudden during activity, such as bike-riding, and may cause a reflex type of vomiting.

This is an epididymoorchitis type of presentation but epididymoorchitis is uncommon in this age group. Therefore, apparent epididymoorchitis in childhood should be regarded as torsion of the testis until proved otherwise.

Occasionally the onset is less acute, with recurrent bouts of scrotal pain leading to a more acute episode. In all cases there is an inflammatory hydrocele and this makes it difficult to feel the testis, which is initially acutely tender but later is insensitive.

Epididymoorchitis

This is uncommon in this age group and may be associated with an acute urinary tract infection or with an abnormality of the urinary tract allowing reflux of urine along the vas. It is more likely if there is an obvious abnormality of the development of this region, such as a high imperforate anus. Recent urethral instrumentation predisposes to this type of infection.

The clinical signs are indistinguishable from torsion and exploration is usually necessary to exclude torsion.

Torsion of an appendix of the testis or epididymis

These are tiny pedunculated polyps, either attached to the upper end of the testis or to the upper end of the epididymis. The appendix testis is also known as the hydatid of Morgagni and is a remnant of the upper end of the Müllerian or paramesonephric duct.

Because they are pedunculated they may undergo torsion and produce a clinical syndrome similar to, but not as acute as, torsion of the testis. An inflammatory hydrocele may make it difficult to palpate the testis but the testis itself is not tender and the torted appendix may be felt as a local, acutely tender nodule. The signs and symptoms will gradually settle within a few weeks without treatment but surgical excision of the nodule relieves symptoms within a few days.

Idiopathic scrotal oedema

This is an allergic type of condition of the scrotal skin with increased temperature, redness, mild tenderness and oedematous swelling. The signs are not confined to the hemiscrotum but include the whole scrotum and spread to the surrounding skin. The testis is normal. This condition will settle spontaneously but antihistamine therapy is helpful.

Diagnosis

This is made on the history and physical examination. Special investigations are rarely helpful, though the finding of pus in the urine would suggest epididymoorchitis.

Radioisotope scanning will show no blood supply to the testis if there is complete interruption to the blood supply and may show increased flow with epididymoorchitis.

Treatment

Emergency surgery with exploration of the testis and detorsion is mandatory if a torsion of the testis is diagnosed or suspected. Surgical excision of a torted appendix of testis or epididymis is the treatment of choice, though they may be treated conservatively.

CIRCUMCISION

Circumcision is an operation to remove the foreskin, the double fold of skin that circumferentially covers the glans penis at birth. It has been part of initiation ceremonies of various peoples and tribal groups throughout the ages and may be part of religious ceremonies.

The foreskin is firmly adherent to the glans at birth and gradually becomes detached from it, so that by 3 years of age 90% of foreskins are retractable. This means that 10% are still not retractable at this age. Normal hygiene with soap and water is all that is required and the foreskin should only be retracted for cleaning if it can be done easily. Occasionally, a lump of smegma will collect between the glans and the foreskin and if it cannot be immediately extruded, it will present as a firm whitish nodule. This will discharge spontaneously in time and is part of the natural separation of foreskin and glans.

In Western society the request for circumcision of an infant is usually for a 'social' reason — that the father or other brothers are circumcised, that it is more hygienic or that it improves the cosmetic appearance.

Medical indications for circumcision are uncommon. They include: recurrent balanitis, phimosis, paraphimosis, as part of a hypospadias repair or previous inadequate circumcision.

Recurrent balanitis, or infection beneath the foreskin, may be mild or severe. Episodes of mild redness of the tip of the foreskin are not uncommon in young boys and usually settle rapidly with the application of a protective cream. These are not an indication for circumcision. Recurrent attacks of acute inflammation with spreading infection and pus beneath the foreskin are an indication for an interval circumcision between attacks.

Phimosis or stricture of the opening in the foreskin is uncommon. It is diagnosed by a thin urinary stream with ballooning of the foreskin and not by the apparent size of the opening, which often appears very small in infancy. Phimosis is rarely congenital and usually occurs following a poorly performed previous circumcision or by repeated trauma and infection from ill-advised efforts to retract the foreskin.

If an inadequate amount of foreskin is removed at circumcision, such that the circular scar of the excision is left distal to the base of the glans, the contraction of the scar will produce a thick firm phimosis that will require a recircumcision. If the mother has been told that the foreskin must be retracted and repeated attempts are made to retract a tight adherent foreskin, with cracking, fissuring and infection of the tip of the foreskin, then phimosis can occur, necessitating circumcision.

Paraphimosis is a condition in which a tight foreskin has been retracted proximal to the base of the glans penis and cannot be returned to its usual position because of this tightness. This causes a circumferential constriction of the distal penis with consequent venous engorgement and swelling of the penis distal to the obstruction. Manual reduction under anaesthesia is usually possible though occasionally a dorsal slit of the prepuce and constricting band is necessary. Circumcision is advisable following such an episode and, while it may be done at the time of reduction, it is usually advisable to perform it as an interval procedure.

Hypospadias repair involves the use of the hooded foreskin as a pedicle flap.

A previously inadequate circumcision is a relative indication for recircumcision. If there is a scar distal to the glans with phimosis, it will be necessary, but if there is merely an excess amount of residual skin, it is doubtful if this is a real indication for further surgery.

Since circumcision is an elective operation, it should only be performed when the infant is in good health and there are no contraindications.

Contraindications

- General disease, e.g. upper respiratory tract infection, bleeding disorder
- Local sepsis
- Dermatitis of the genitalia, e.g. ammoniacal dermatitis
- Hypospadias
- Neuropathic bladder — the foreskin protects the glans
- Ambiguous genitalia — until definitive treatment is planned

The ethics of performing circumcision because of parental request but without medical indication are debatable. The risk of complications, though small, is an argument against circumcision.

Complications

- Haemorrhage
- Local infection — this may cause septicaemia
- Irritation and ulceration of the unprotected glans, sometimes causing meatal stenosis
- Removal of too much skin — the 'ring-bark' effect; occasionally skin grafting is necessary
- Urethral fistula
- Mutilation of the glans
- Death from complications of the above or from anaesthesia

If circumcision is performed as a formal surgical procedure in an operating theatre with appropriate facilities, and anaesthesia and surgery are performed by appropriately trained or supervised anaesthetists and surgeons, then the risk of complications is small. If it is performed as a so-called minor procedure in inadequate circumstances by inadequately trained personnel, then the risks are markedly increased.

Technique of circumcision

There are three main techniques: formal excision, crushing the foreskin and excision, and the use of bell-type instruments, either metal or plastic.

Formal excision of the foreskin with glans and penis under direct vision and with tying of any vessels that bleed or may bleed, and with formal suturing of the two cut edges of the base of the foreskin, is a safe and effective method but takes more time than other methods.

Crushing the foreskin, after separating it from the glans, is done with a large pair of semiblunt forceps, such as bone-cutting forceps. This obliterates the vessels, and the foreskin distal to the crush line is excised, usually without bleeding. The incision line then retracts behind the glans and a dressing is applied. This is a quick method but needs good judgement on the site of application of the crushing forceps, otherwise too much or too little foreskin may be removed.

Bell-type instruments have a bell-shaped hollow metal or plastic dome that fits over the glans and protects it. A separate ring is then applied to encircle the foreskin and crush the foreskin between the ring and the lip of the bell. The excess foreskin is then excised.

Postoperative care

It is important that the epithelium of the glans penis be protected from minor trauma until it has thickened. Napkins soaked with urine and covered with faeces are the main cause of trauma and infection so that exposure of the glans for as much of the day as possible and a covering layer of cream to protect the glans are helpful.

Malignancy

There are conflicting reports in the literature on the relationship of circumcision to the incidence of cervical cancer in the female and penile cancer in the male. No definite conclusions can be drawn, as yet, on these relationships.

HYPOSPADIAS

Hypospadias is a condition in which the external urethral meatus is situated on the under surface

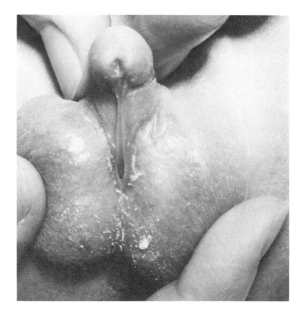

Fig. 20.2 Hypospadias showing a penoscrotal urethral opening and chordee.

of the penis in a position proximal to its normal site at the tip of the penis (Fig. 20.2). It is classified by the position of the opening such that the hypospadias may be glandular, coronal, penile, scrotal or perineal. Any of the more major forms of hypospadias may be associated with some type of intersex abnormality. There are frequently short blind pits at, or proximal to, the site of the normal opening and these may be confusing when trying to decide which is the external urethral meatus. The urethral meatus is always the most proximal opening.

As this is a failure of development of the terminal part of the urethra with the associated corpus spongiosum and skin, there is a deficiency of tissue on the inferior surface of the penis, with associated inferior angulation called chordee and there may be some stenosis of the meatus. The prepuce also fails to form inferiorly so that the foreskin forms a hood on the dorsal surface of the penis. This condition occurs in approximately 1 in 250 boys and it can be transmitted according to Mendelian principles (see Ch. 22).

Associated abnormalities are common, especially undescended testis, but other abnormalities of the urinary system may be present in 10 to 20% of cases. Usually these are of a minor nature.

Treatment

Treatment is required if there is stenosis of the meatus, chordee or the position of the meatus is markedly abnormal. Hypospadias of the glandular type does not need treatment, but hypospadias of the shaft of the penis proximal to the corona will certainly need treatment.

The coronal type is the most difficult group in which to decide if treatment is necessary. Any interference with function rather than the cosmetic appearance is the deciding factor. If the urinary stream goes persistently downwards and is difficult to direct, or if there is a bend on erection, then surgical correction will be required.

There are more than 150 operations described for the correction of hypospadias and from this it can be seen that no one operation is completely satisfactory. The repair may be done as a one or two stage procedure, but the basic principle is to use the hooded foreskin as an already existing pedicle skin flap that will be swung onto the ventral surface of the penis, to provide the extra skin necessary for the repair. This flap covers the defect produced when the area distal to the meatus is dissected and the fibrous tissue excised to allow the penis to straighten. It is also used to form a tube to take the opening to the tip of the penis. These operations should be performed when the child is out of napkins but before he goes to school.

EPISPADIAS

Epispadias is a condition in which the opening of the urethra is on the dorsum of the penis, instead of at the tip of the glans. The embryology of this condition is obscure. The abnormalities are the reverse of that in hypospadias in that there is a rather short, dorsally angulated penis and the opening may be anywhere along the dorsum of the shaft of the penis or at the base of the penis. Openings at the base of the penis are often associated with abnormalities of the bladder sphincters (Fig. 20.3).

FUSED LABIA

Adhesion of the posterior ends of the labia minora in infancy and early childhood is quite

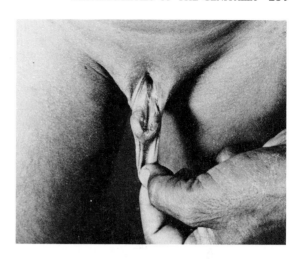

Fig. 20.3 Epispadias showing the urethral opening at the anterior abdominal wall and a dorsal groove in the penis.

common, due to the extremely fragile skin of the labial mucosa and the tendency to chronic irritation and minor infection in this area. This is not true fusion of the labia and is of no consequence. There is a tendency to retention of urine in the vagina and an increased risk of infection because of this. Treatment is simple in that the application of an oestrogen cream for several days will usually change the character of the mucosa and allow the labia to separate. Surgical separation is almost never required. Reapplication of the oestrogen cream may be necessary from time to time if there is a tendency to recurrence but this tendency disappears with time.

INTERSEX

There is no clear definition of an intersex state. In the paediatric age group it is usually taken to be a condition in which there is doubt as to whether the external genitalia are obviously male or female on examination. This definition excludes some of the abnormalities of the sex chromosomes, such as XO or Turner's syndrome, and XXY or Klinefelter's syndrome, because the appearance of the external genitalia and the decision about the sex in which the patient will be reared is not usually in doubt.

Intersex states are rare but the problems posed by them are compounded manyfold by late recognition. The intersex state identified at birth, immediately investigated and an appropriate sex assigned, while obviously needing major adaptation on the part of parents, friends, and relatives and major support from medical advisers, will be much less of a problem than the case in which there is delayed diagnosis or procrastination in investigation and appropriate assignment of sex. Change of sex under these circumstances, while possible, always has major consequences for the family and after the first few years of life, may have irreparable consequences for the individual.

It can be seen from Figure 20.1 that anything that interferes with the development of the male external genitalia will leave indeterminate type of genitalia which could be either male or female, whereas action by excess androgens on the intermediate development of the female external genitalia can cause masculinization.

Intersex states usually present clinically in the newborn period or at puberty.

Infancy

- Ambiguous genitalia
  - Hypospadias with no palpable gonads
  - Hypospadias with one palpable gonad
  - Micropenis with no palpable gonads
- Oedema of the hands and feet — indicating a chromosomal abnormality

Puberty

- Amenorrhoea
- Inappropriate hormonal effect

Chromosomal or internal genital organ abnormalities may or may not be part of the syndrome.

A basic fact of differentiation needs to be kept in mind when considering the various intersex states. Jost found experimentally in rabbits that removal or ablation of the fetal ovary did not interfere with the development of the female genital system but removal or ablation of the fetal testis during an early critical period prevented the differentiation of male structures and resulted in female development of the ducts, urogenital sinus and the external genitalia.

The type of problem that can be caused by abnormal development of the gonads is illustrated by a condition called mixed gonadal dysgenesis.

In this there is an abnormal sex chromosome constitution and mosaicism, such that one gonad is acted upon by XO chromosomes and the other by XY chromosomes causing different development between the two sides. The gonad on the side with XO chromosomes does not develop and remains a streak gonad, with a fallopian tube and a unicornuate uterus on that side because of failure of production of Müllerian inhibiting substance. The gonad on the opposite side becomes a testis because of the XY chromosome but such laterality is rarely complete, so that this testis does not have completely normal function. A vagina is present and the phallus may appear as an enlarged clitoris or a small penis with marked hypospadias.

The diagnosis and treatment of the intersex state is a highly specialized form of management involving paediatrician, paediatric surgeon, paediatric endocrinologist and paediatric psychiatrist. The important factor is the initial diagnosis, and a high index of suspicion and immediate investigation are the most important factors in management.

The newborn infant with ambiguous genitalia or the apparent male child with hypospadias and impalpable testes should be immediately investigated before a random assignment of sex is made.

Congenital adrenal hyperplasia

Congenital adrenal hyperplasia is the commonest form of intersex state. It is due to a recessive inheritance defect of one of the enzymes involved in the pathway of conversion of progesterone to cortisol and the usual defect is the 21-hydroxylase defect. Excess androgen is produced with consequent virilization of the external genitalia of female infants.

Because of the failure to produce cortisol, there is a degree of salt loss that may be severe. If these patients are presumed to be male at birth, they may not be diagnosed for years or may present with episodes of apparent gastroenteritis with vomiting and diarrhoea, salt loss, dehydration and shock due to loss of sodium and water.

With early diagnosis and treatment, such infants can be raised as normal females, though needing both cortisone and salt replacement. Surgical treatment is needed to correct the abnormalities of the external genitalia.

FURTHER READING

Depue R H 1984 Maternal and gestational factors affecting the risk of cryptorchidism and inguinal hernia. International Journal of Epidemiology 13: 311–318

Editorial 1979 The case against neonatal circumcision. British Medical Journal 1: 1163–1164

Elder J S 1987 Cryptorchidism: isolated and associated with other genitourinary defects. Pediatric Clinics of North America 34: 1033–1053

Giwercman A, Muller J, Skakkebaek N E 1988 Cryptorchidism and testicular neoplasia. Hormone Research 30: 157–163

Jost A 1953 Problems of fetal endocrinology. The gonadal and hypophyseal hormones. Recent Progress in Hormone Research 8: 379–418

Osborn L M, Metcalf T J, Manani E M 1981 Hygienic care in uncircumcised infants. Paediatrics 67: 365–367

Pagon R A 1987 Diagnostic approach to the newborn with ambiguous genitalia. Pediatric Clinics of North America 34: 1019–1031

21. Ethics in paediatric surgery

K. C. Pringle

It is only relatively recently that the public, in general, has recognized the fact that there are very few (if any) certainties in medicine. Until recently, the average patient felt 'the doctor knows best' and, in general, trusted him to do his best. (The male pronoun is used advisedly in this historical context: this approach to medical ethics could be termed paternalistic.) Now, largely because of the success of modern medicine, there are often options available and it is sometimes necessary to offer patients (or the parents of patients) a series of options, each with its own advantages and disadvantages. All too often, it is apparent that the patients (or their parents) are not able to make a selection of the best treatment or management, but are rather forced to attempt to choose the option that is least likely to produce harm. In many cases, the doctor is not in a position to advise the patient (or parents) as to the best choice, but should rather restrain himself (or herself) to outlining the choices available as accurately as possible in order to allow the patient (or parents) to make their own choice.

Just what a doctor should do when the patient (or parents) abrogates this responsibility and asks the doctor to make the choice for them is an area of persistent debate. Solutions vary from suggesting that the doctor force the patient (or parents) to make a decision (any decision), to the concept that the doctor should (paternalistically) make the decision for the patient in their best interest. The first option has overtones of coercion, and the second option overtones of excessive submissiveness on the part of the doctor. It is also interesting to note that while a paternalistic ap-proach to patient care was the norm 30 to 40 years ago, a paternalistic approach is now no longer considered appropriate in the modern clinical situation. The best choice would seem to be somewhere between these two extremes, that is, to guide the patient (or parents) into a position where they feel they can make a decision. Unfortunately, this is not always possible. Out of such clinical problems has arisen the relatively modern field of biomedical ethics. This field is really an offshoot of the broader discipline of philosophy.

Although not all authorities would agree, it is probably best to distinguish between medical ethics (which mainly deals with the relationships between members of the medical profession) and biomedical ethics, which is more concerned with fundamental moral problems and the relationship between doctor and patient.

In general, biomedical ethicists subscribe to one of two main theories of ethics:

1. Utilitarian theories, which gauge the worth of actions by their ends and consequences
2. Deontological theories (derived from the Greek word for duty, deon), which are founded on the premise that the concept of duty is independent of the concept of good

Both ethical theories provide a framework of principles within which it is possible to determine morally appropriate actions.

In both there are a series of subservient principles:

- Autonomy (derived from the Greek word for self-rule; which is central to discussions about informed consent)
- Non-maleficence (above all, or first, do no harm)
- Beneficence (which implies a duty to provide positive benefits whenever the opportunity presents)
- The principle of justice (which has to do with fairness of distribution of benefits and burdens in society)

In general, utilitarians do not hold any principle (other than the concept of utility) as a supreme principle. Deontologists, on the other hand, may well do so. They believe that right actions are not determined solely by the production of non-moral 'good'. This is in contrast to the utilitarian concept that in all circumstances one ought to produce the greatest possible value over disvalue for all persons affected.

Many clinical situations in neonatal surgery raise important ethical issues. These centre around two main themes, first, 'what is in the child's best interest?' (with an important subsidiary question being, 'who should decide what is in the child's best interest?'), and the problem of the just allocation of scarce resources. Major ethical problems are less common outside the neonatal nursery, but these still occasionally arise. Parental refusal to give consent to medically indicated treatment raises important ethical issues that should be addressed.

The reader is warned at this point that if clear 'black and white' answers to any of these questions are hoped for, then this chapter should be skipped over, and some oracle should be sought. The fact is that there are no absolute answers to any of the questions raised in this chapter. In each of the areas to be discussed, there are shades of grey and almost no answer to the questions raised is categorically 'right' or 'wrong'. Many people could argue either side of any given question, logically, and with equal fervour. Some of the questions raised will be illustrated by case histories. All of these case histories are based on fact, although in all the cases some of the details have been altered to preserve patient confidentiality.

ISSUES IN THE NEONATAL INTENSIVE CARE UNIT

What should be done for (or to) a newborn with major congenital anomalies who will require multiple operations? How much weight should be placed on predicted intelligence or the presence (or absence) of a normal complement of chromosomes? If there is to be a decision for treatment or no treatment, who should make that decision? Should the state have any role in this decision?

Case 1

A baby boy was born at term. He weighed 2.8 kg, his Apgar scores were 3 at 1 minute and 8 at 2 minutes. On examination, he was found to have a thoracolumbar spina bifida, with kyphosis, and severe talipes equinovarus. He was paraplegic, and had a severe degree of hydrocephalus. The head could be transilluminated, and on ultrasound the thickest cortical mantle was 5 mm. In addition, he was found to have an imperforate anus. The clinical assessment was that this patient would need immediate major surgery to close his back. He would also need to have a colostomy, and a ventriculoperitoneal shunt performed. If he survived, he would require surgery on his feet, and major spinal surgery to allow him to sit upright. He would be confined to a wheelchair. The chances of this child having normal intelligence would be negligible.

Should treatment by initiated? It could be argued that this child appeared to be headed for a miserable existence. His prospects for gainful employment are minimal. He would be faced with three major operations as a neonate, and a series of major painful operations on his back and legs as he grew older. Complications from one or more of these operations are almost inevitable, increasing the morbidity. Some would argue that this amount of probable pain and suffering is excessive, and this patient would be better off if no treatment were to be initiated and that 'nature be allowed to take its course'. On the other hand, there are those who would argue that life itself is the primary consideration and the quality of that life and the suffering endured are of secondary importance and should not enter into the decision-making process.

It is worth noting that while in the past there has been an air of urgency about these decisions, with the parents instructed to arrive at their decision within 24 hours, there is no real justification for this approach. With modern antibiotics and surgical techniques, there is almost no necessity for urgent surgery. The pros and cons of the decision should probably be weighed by the family and their advisors over several days. In the meantime, the infant could be kept comfortable with no real threat of an adverse effect on the outcome if the decision is made for active treatment. The vexed question of how the infant should be managed if the decision is for no active treatment will be left till later in this chapter.

How should chromosomal analysis affect decisions for treatment? While few would advise active treatment for a child with a major fatal chromosomal anomaly such as trisomy 13 or trisomy 18, the child with trisomy 21 and a treatable congenital anomaly is an entirely different story.

Case 2: 'Baby Doe'

Baby Doe was born in Indiana on 15 April 1982. He had trisomy 21 (Down syndrome) and an oesophageal atresia and tracheo-oesophageal fistula, together with a possible coarctation of the aorta. His parents refused treatment, and he died on the sixth day of life. However, some individuals objected to the parents' decision and filed an application to the courts to override the parents' decision. The case eventually went to the State Court of Appeals, who agreed to hear the case (long after the baby had died) and who ultimately upheld the parents' decision.

Enter the US Federal Government, who issued a series of regulations (that were all contested) mandating life-saving interventions for all newborns regardless of handicap. Failure to provide life-saving treatments to handicapped newborns (even if it could be argued that such treatment was not in the child's best interests) risked the withdrawal of all Federal funds to the institution concerned. To one who was involved in the treatment of newborn patients in the United States at that time, it appeared that the most important result of this series of regulations was to increase the number of severely handicapped infants who survived to 'graduate' from the neonatal nurseries.

The most iniquitous feature of the 'Baby Doe regulations' was that although the Federal Government forced the parents and the neonatal nurseries to treat these infants, no funding was supplied to provide this medical care, nor to provide for the ancillary support services that these infants would require if their outcome was to be optimized. Many commentators have suggested that this intervention by the state was ill-advised and detrimental to a large number of newborn babies. This includes both those whose suffering was unnecessarily prolonged (as was the case in the infant mentioned in Case 1), as well as those whose entry to a neonatal intensive care unit was delayed or prevented because the bed was occupied by one of these children. In this instance, it appears that the state (the Federal Government of the United States) both over-stepped its authority and simultaneously abrogated its responsibility to the handicapped newborns and their parents.

This case does raise important questions as to who should decide such difficult questions. It is, in fact, impossible to pass practical legislation in this area. Each case is different, and what is vitally important to one set of parents may seem trivial or irrelevant to another pair. The Baby Doe regulations appear to have unequivocally demonstrated that the state has little or no role to play in management decisions affecting babies with major congenital anomalies, except, perhaps, to lay down the broadest possible guidelines.

Given that the state has a limited role in deciding the management of a neonate with major congenital anomalies, who should make these decisions? What rights should the parents have in this area? What weight should be given to consideration of the effect that the new addition to the family will have on the siblings and the marriage relationship itself?

Case 3

A baby boy was born at term to an impoverished family living in a small town. He was the sixth child in the family. All of the other children were normal and healthy. At birth, the child was found to have a small sacral myelomeningocele, and a mild talipes equinovarus of his left foot. The head was of normal size. There was an obvious neurological deficit of the S4 and S5 and coccygeal segments. The baby was transferred to a major paediatric surgical centre, and the father, travelling by private car, arrived several hours after the baby. An ultrasound of the baby's head revealed an Arnold-Chiari malformation with minimal hydrocephalus. The father was told that the child would be minimally handicapped, but would be incontinent of urine and faeces. He was warned that ventriculoperitoneal shunting and urinary diversion (ileal loop) may be required. He was told that the child would probably have normal intelligence. He was given a comprehensive booklet that clearly explained the implications of spina bifida and was told to take that to his wife (still in the home-town hospital) and to return the following day with a decision as to whether or not the child should be treated.

The father returned the following day and requested that no treatment be instituted and that the baby should be demand fed and left to die of meningitis when the back lesion became infected. He gave the following reasons:

1. He was employed as an unskilled worker in a low-paid job. While all medical expenses would be paid by the Handicapped Children's Foundation, no compensation would be available for travelling expenses or time lost from work. This would force the family into debt, with no prospect of relief.

2. The marital relationship was under considerable stress, and the parents felt that the addition of a handicapped infant to the family would almost certainly be the final stress pushing them to divorce. This would certainly be detrimental to the rest of the family.

The parents were offered the option of putting the child up for adoption. They refused, pointing out that while it was considered socially acceptable for a single mother to place a child for adoption, it certainly was not socially acceptable (especially in a small town) for a couple to do so. The parents stated that if it were to become known that their child had been placed for adoption, then they would be ostracized. Again, in such circumstances, divorce was considered to be almost inevitable. The parents were not prepared to move, citing the lack of any work skills on the part of the father and the very slim chance that he would be able to obtain work.

This case raised considerable controversy within the institution involved. However, it illustrates very clearly the fact that if one respects parental autonomy, then this may well result in the parents choosing an option that causes considerable distress to the members of the team responsible for the care of an infant. It is, therefore, vital to remember that if a series of options are to be offered to a family, then the options offered should not include anything that is considered to be unethical by the members of the treating team.

If resources are limited, should one initiate treatment, knowing that by doing so, other infants will probably be disadvantaged in that they will not have access to treatment because of the limited space in the neonatal intensive care unit? Should one knowingly tie up space in the neonatal intensive care unit for a prolonged period?

Case 4

A baby was born at 38 weeks' gestation with a gastroschisis. No other anomalies were found. The defect was quite small, and there appeared to be only a small amount of thick-walled intestine protruding through the defect. Initially, this was thought to be a good sign, suggesting that although there was probably an intestinal atresia, there would probably be a reasonable amount of small bowel. However, a plain X-ray of this baby's abdomen at 6 hours of age revealed gas in the stomach and dilated duodenum, with no gas beyond the first loop of jejunum. This suggested a high small bowel atresia. A barium enema filled the colon only as far as the mid transverse colon and it appeared that the colon at this point was attached to the mass protruding from the defect. These findings suggested that the bulk of the intestine had been lost, when the blood supply was cut off at the edge of the defect. It was clear that there was a severe degree of 'short gut syndrome' and that it was likely that survival would only be possible with the help of prolonged parenteral nutrition, probably lasting months or years.

Is an exploratory laparotomy justifiable? If the preoperative assessment proves to be correct, should a jejunocolic anastomosis be performed? Should parenteral nutrition be instituted? In general, laparotomy does not commit the team to treatment, although it does make it more difficult to alter course if the decision is taken not to perform a jejunocolic anastomosis. If an anastomosis is not performed, then a jejunostomy would probably be required, since it would generally be considered unacceptable to leave the infant with an atresia and spend a short life on a nasogastric tube. If the laparotomy confirms the preoperative investigations, and reveals only 10–15 cm of jejunum and a microcolon beginning at the mid transverse colon, then this child has only a slim chance of survival, and that survival will be utterly dependent on whether the child can tolerate long-term central venous nutrition without developing cholestatic jaundice. The critical decision, therefore, is the decision as to whether to institute central venous nutrition (CVN). A decision to institute CVN is a decision to maintain the child in hospital for at least 2 to 3 months, before CVN can be established at home with all the stress that it entails for the family. This will mean that a bed that could be used for other infants will be occupied by this baby for at least as long. CVN is, of course, much more expensive than enteral feeding.

It must be remembered, however, that this infant is in every other respect entirely normal, and may ultimately be able to lead an entirely normal life, although it will probably be several years before it can eat a normal diet. Weighed against this possibility is the expense of months or years of home CVN, and the drain that this will have on the hospital's resources, which could be used to treat a number of other patients.

EUTHANASIA

If the decision is made not to repair a major congenital defect in a newborn child, how is that child to be managed?

It is generally agreed that not all children should be treated to the fullest possible extent, since for some children (for example, a child with a high thoracic myelomeningocele with severe hydrocephalus and a severe kyphosis) aggressive treatment will only result in subjecting the child to multiple surgical procedures (with all their attendant morbidity) with very little hope of a reasonable quality of life. In such cases, active, aggressive treatment will only prolong the child's suffering. The conventional approach to such a child would be to provide adequate fluid (by the intravenous route if required) and any necessary pain relief, but not to give antibiotics for any infection and to allow 'nature to take its course'. Whether this is, in fact, the best option has been hotly debated for many years. In general, most would prefer to draw a fine but distinct line between actively killing such a child, and allowing it do die. Some have argued that withholding treatment for all such poor prognosis infants will result in the loss of the few who would do well, or their survival with worse handicaps than they would have had if they had full active treatment.

If treatment is to be withheld and the child allowed to die, would it not be more humane to kill the child with an overdose of some drug? Shelp has argued for this approach with disturbing conviction. Others have argued that allowing active euthanasia of children (who cannot speak for themselves) may possibly lead to a general downgrading of the status of children. While active euthanasia may be beneficial to an individual suffering child, concern has been expressed that allowing such an approach may adversely affect the treatment of other infants not so severely affected, to the detriment of the whole of society. Clearly, this issue is unlikely to be resolved in the near future.

REFUSAL OF TREATMENT

What should be the doctor's response if the parents refuse appropriate treatment? How, for instance, should one respond if the parents of a child with suspected appendicitis refuse permission for appendicectomy? In the United States, in most jurisdictions, this would be regarded as a form of child abuse, and under the mandatory reporting laws in most States, the physician would be required to petition the local children's court for a 'Care and Protection Order'. Certainly, one should attempt to persuade the parents that the appropriate treatment should be carried out, even if they are reluctant to give their consent. In an early case, it may even be appropriate to allow the parents the benefit of some prolonged observation. However, if the child has a perforated appendix and generalized peritonitis then, in the face of continued parental refusal to give permission for appropriate surgery, the doctor should adopt a paternalistic attitude and apply to the appropriate courts for permission to override the parents' wishes.

FUTURE DIRECTIONS

Finally, it must be pointed out that ethics is a field that changes from society to society, and also changes with time. The Hippocratic Oath bound the doctor to support his teacher and his sons for no charge. It also bound him to never give a deadly drug or suggest its use, to refrain from procuring an abortion, to refrain from sexual relations with patients, and, in addition, demanded that on no account should a doctor divulge confidential information about a patient. However, the Hippocratic physician was paternalistic, directing his patients to do what he thought was in their best interest. The overriding consideration was the principle of beneficence for an individual patient. Informed consent was centuries away.

In modern biomedical ethics, the pendulum has, perhaps, swung too far in the opposite direction. Patients are demanding their rights to autonomy and justice, and are often loath to acknowledge the duties of beneficence and non-maleficence towards others. Paternalism has become an outmoded and currently unacceptable medical ethic. The field of biomedical ethics can, however, be expected to continue to change due both to the pressures of a changing society's perspective of the role of the physician, and because of the changing availability of alternative treatments. Already these changes are occurring. There are currently major debates taking place over issues in fetal therapy, and there is currently a very brisk debate (in the United States, especially) about the use of fetal tissue for such things as the treatment of Parkinson's disease and diabetes. Other similar issues will almost certainly need to be discussed as medical technology continues to advance.

FURTHER READING

Beauchamp T L, Childress J F 1983 Principles of biomedical ethics, 2nd edn. Oxford University Press, New York
Pless J E 1983 The story of Baby Doe. New England Journal of Medicine 309: 664
Shelp E E 1986 Born to die? Deciding the fate of critically ill newborns. The Free Press, New York

22. Congenital malformations: teratogenesis, genetics and principles of management

L. J. Cussen

The management of malformations is one of the most important aspects of paediatric surgery. The frequency of malformations has not increased significantly in recent years, but as other diseases are eliminated or controlled, an increasing percentage of infants and children referred to paediatric surgeons are suffering from congenital malformations. In highly industrialized countries, over half of all paediatric surgical patients have malformations, and this pattern is becoming more apparent in developing countries.

The clinician who is caring for a malformed baby needs to have the information to answer questions that are usually asked by the parents.

What is wrong with our baby?

Why did it happen?

How will it affect our baby and our family?

What can or should be done about it?

Will it happen again if we have more children?

WHAT IS WRONG WITH OUR BABY?

To answer this question it is necessary to have a clear concept of the definition, nomenclature and classification of malformations.

Definitions

The following definitions are the recommendations of a conference convened by Dr R. L. Christiansen in 1975.

Malformation: A primary structural defect that results from a localized error of morphogenesis, e.g. cleft lip.

Deformation: An alteration in shape and/or structure of a previously normally formed part, e.g. torticollis.

Anomalad: A malformation together with its subsequently derived structural changes, e.g. Robin anomalad (comprising the primary malformation of a hypoplastic mandible and the secondary structural defect of glossoptosis with cleft palate).

Malformation syndrome: Recognized patterns of malformation presumably having the same aetiology and currently not interpreted as the consequence of a single localized error in morphogenesis, e.g. Down syndrome.

Association of malformations: A recognized pattern of malformations which currently is not considered to constitute a syndrome or an anomalad, e.g. oesophageal atresia, tracheo-oesophageal fistula, vertebral defects, anal atresia and renal defects.

Nomenclature

Single malformations are best named by a description of the abnormality, together with the anatomical site, e.g. club foot, or else by a classical term that is widely known, e.g. hypospadias.

Multiple malformations may be named in a variety of ways. The most appropriate name for a group of malformations is based on the cause, e.g. congenital rubella syndrome, but as the causes of most malformations are not known, other methods of nomenclature must be used. Some names are descriptive of either the whole pattern of malformation, e.g. cloacal exstrophy, in which opened-out bladder and intestine take the place of the lower anterior abdominal wall and the patient has anorectal agenesis, exomphalos and genital abnormalities, or else of some prominent feature or features of the pattern, e.g. prune belly syndrome, in which there is hypoplasia of the muscles of the anterior abdominal wall, dysplasia of the urinary tract and undescended testes.

Other malformations are named after the author or authors of the first report of the condition, e.g. Down syndrome, or of a definitive report, e.g. Hirschsprung's disease. There is a move to discontinue the use of an eponym when the cause of a syndrome is discovered and also to discontinue the possessive use of eponyms, but many names, such as Down syndrome (trisomy 21) and Hirschsprung's disease, are entrenched by long usage.

Classification

It is difficult to classify malformations adequately with our present knowledge. One system of classification is given in Table 22.1.

WHY DID IT HAPPEN?

The knowledge that malformations are relatively common in newborn children may help the parents of an abnormal child to realize that they have not been singled out for misfortune.

The causes of most malformations are un-

Table 22.1 Classification of malformations

Malformation	Classification
1. Single	
Known aetiology	By cause, e.g. phocomelia due to thalidomide
Unknown aetiology	By anatomic site, e.g. ventricular septal defect.
2. Multiple	
Syndromes	
(a) Known aetiology	By cause, e.g. congenital rubella syndrome.
(b) Unknown aetiology	By anatomic site, e.g. oculo-auriculo-vertebral syndrome.
Anomalads	By anatomic site, e.g. cleft lip and palate anomalad
Association of malformations	By anatomic site, e.g. association of vertebral defects, anal atresia, tracheo-oesophageal fistula, oesophageal atresia and renal defects.

known, but a knowledge of background factors helps understanding and preliminary counselling. These factors are:

1. Incidence and prevalence of malformations
2. Causes (if known) or associated features which may be:
   (a) Predisposing factors
     (i) Parental age
     (ii) Parental consanguinity
     (iii) Race
     (iv) Geographic location and social stratum
     (v) Maternal disease
     (vi) Multiple pregnancy
     (vii) Season of birth
     (viii) Birth rank
     (ix) Sex of infant
   (b) Precipitating factors
     (i) Teratogens
     (ii) Chromosomal anomalies
     (iii) Genetic anomalies
     (iv) Unknown

Incidence and prevalence

The frequency of malformations may be expressed as incidence or as prevalence. Incidence is the number of new cases of a condition in a given population in a specified time. Prevalence is the ratio of the number of cases of a condition at any time in a given population to the size of the population at that time.

The incidence and prevalence of malformations are not known accurately in most regions, but from surveys in various communities it has been estimated that from 1–15% of all liveborn children have one or more congenital malformations. The lower figures have been obtained mostly from retrospective surveys of newborn infants while the higher figures have been obtained mainly from prospective studies with long-term follow-up of the subjects in the population.

The incidence and prevalence of malformations seem to vary from one community to another, presumably because of different aetiological factors, and this variability is certainly true of some specific malformations, e.g. myelomeningocele, cleft lip.

Representative figures, given in Table 22.2, for

Table 22.2 Incidence of malformations of different systems

System	Incidence of malformations in liveborn children
Musculoskeletal	1:70
Cardiovascular	1:125
Genitourinary	1:140*
Gastrointestinal	1:170
Central nervous	1:190
Respiratory	1:230
Other	1:40
All systems	1:14

* If vesicoureteric reflux, usually due to a malformation of the vesicoureteric junction and present in more than 1% of all children, is included, the incidence of genitourinary malformations would be greater than 1:60.

the incidence of malformations of different systems are from a prospective survey of over 50 000 liveborn children, organized by the National Institute of Neurological and Communicative Disorders and Stroke, USA.

Figures from the same survey for the incidence of specific malformations of interest to paediatric surgeons are given in Table 22.3. Some of these figures are at variance with those from other published surveys.

Causes and associated features

Information about the known causes of malformations is necessary to reassure parents that their child's malformation is not due to something that they have done or failed to do, e.g. a drug taken or not taken by the mother during the pregnancy. Malformations result from interference with normal processes of development. This interference may be due to deficiency or excess of an endogenous factor involved in normal development, or alternatively, may be due to an exogenous agent or teratogen acting on the embryo or fetus.

Our knowledge of the causes of human malformations is limited, but we can recognize two groups of factors that are aetiologically important and these may be termed predisposing and precipitating factors.

Table 22.3 Approximate incidence in liveborn children of some common malformations

Malformation	Incidence
Inguinal hernia	1:70
Polydactyly	1:140*
Hypospadias	1:140 (male infants only)
Club foot	1:260
Ventricular septal defect	1:290
Pyloric stenosis	1:330
Syndactyly	1:400
Megaureter-hydronephrosis	1:530
Congenital dislocation of hip	1:560
Funnel chest	1:560
Hydrocephalus	1:670
Pulmonic valve stenosis	1:900
Cleft lip, with or without cleft palate	1:1000
Hypoplasia of all or part of a limb	1:1000
Patent ductus arteriosus	1:1100
Myelomeningocele	1:1100[+]
Coarctation of aorta	1:1400
Cystic kidneys	1:1500
Cleft palate without cleft lip	1:1700
Craniosynostosis	1:2000
Anal atresia	1:2000
Malrotation of intestines	1:2000
Exomphalos	1:2500
Aortic stenosis	1:3100
Transposition of great vessels	1:3300
Fallot's tetrad	1:3300
Posterolateral diaphragmatic hernia	1:3300
Hirschsprung's disease	1:3300
Oesophageal atresia with tracheo-oesophageal fistula	1:5000
Biliary atresia	1:6000
Duodenal atresia	1:7000

These figures may vary significantly from one ethnic group to another and from one geographic location to another.
* Polydactyly occurs in about 1:100 liveborn black American children and in about 1:1000 liveborn white American children.
[+] The incidence of myelomeningocele varies from about 1:240 liveborn children in Wales to about 1:3000 liveborn children in Japan.

Predisposing factors

These, as the name implies, predispose the embryo or fetus to the development of a malformation but do not actually cause the malformation.

Parental age. Very young mothers or mothers aged more than 35 years have an increased risk of having children with malformations, e.g. neural tube defects or Down syndrome respectively. Children born to fathers aged more than 40 years have an increased risk of certain genetically determined malformations, e.g. achondroplasia.

Parental consanguinity. This increases the risk to the child of autosomal recessive malformations such as infantile polycystic kidneys.

Race. Some malformations are more common in certain ethnic groups than in others, e.g. cleft lip is found more frequently in Japanese (1.7 per 1000) than in white (0.9 per 1000) or black (0.4 per 1000) American children.

Geographic location and social stratum. The incidence of myelomeningocele in offspring of Irish parents is greater when the children are born in Great Britain than when they are born in the United States. Myelomeningocele is more common in infants born to parents of poorer social strata than in infants born to well-to-do parents.

Maternal diseases. Some maternal diseases can increase the risk of malformation in a child, e.g. children born to mothers with untreated phenylketonuria have a very high risk of microcephaly compared with children of mothers who do not have phenylketonuria.

Multiple pregnancy. Some, but not all, surveys indicate a small increase in the incidence of malformations in children of multiple, as compared with singleton, pregnancies.

Season of birth. Certain malformations have a seasonal distribution, e.g. congenital dislocation of the hip is more common in infants born in winter than in infants born in other seasons.

Birth rank. First-born children are more prone to have pyloric stenosis, myelomeningocele, congenital dislocation of the hip or hypospadias than are later-born children.

Sex of child. Boys are more likely to have some malformations, e.g. inguinal hernia, Hirschsprung's disease, than are girls. On the other hand, congenital dislocation of the hip and cleft palate without cleft lip are more common in girls than in boys.

Precipitating factors

These actually lead to the development of malformations. As an approximation, 10% of malformations are caused by an exogenous agent or teratogen, 5% are due to a chromosomal anomaly, 20% are due to abnormal genes and in 65% of cases, the cause is not known. Chromosomal anomalies and abnormal genes are really mechanisms rather than causes of malformation, but for the purposes of this discussion they can be considered as precipitating factors.

Teratogens. Normal human development follows a regular pattern and we can distinguish three main periods of development of the embryo and fetus from the point of view of teratogenic activity.

The first period, *from 0 to 17 days*, is characterized by proliferation of cells and implantation of the blastocyst. Teratogens acting at this time tend to cause death (presumably if all cells are damaged) or have no effect (presumably if only a few cells are damaged and replaced by proliferation of the undamaged, non-specialized cells).

During the second period, *from 17 days to 7 weeks*, all the main organs and tissues are forming, and as would be expected, the embryo is highly susceptible to teratogenic agents. Exposure to teratogens at this stage may result in malformations or, if there is severe damage to the embryo, in death.

The third period, *from 8 to 40 weeks*, is a time of general growth of all organs and tissues. Teratogens acting on the fetus during this phase may cause retardation of growth, but do not commonly cause malformations, except in organs or systems that are still forming, e.g. external genitalia.

It is important to note that a teratogen may act to induce malformation of an organ before its earliest stage of development by acting primarily on an even earlier stage of development of the embryo, with secondary effects on the development of the specific organ. It is therefore usually impossible to determine the earliest stage at

Table 22.4 Teratologic termination periods for some malformations

Malformation	Teratologic termination period
Myelomeningocele	End of 4th week
Tracheo-oesophageal fistula	5th week
Duplex ureter	End of 5th week
Polydactyly	End of 6th week
Cleft lip	7th week
Thyroglossal cyst	7th week
Ventricular septal defect	End of 7th week
Anal atresia	End of 7th week
Syndactyly	End of 8th week
Branchial cyst/sinus	End of 8th week
Cleft palate	End of 9th week
Posterolateral diaphragmatic hernia	End of 10th week
Hypospadias	End of 13th week

Table 22.5 Human teratogens

Agent	Major malformation(s)
1. Deficiency	
Normal starvation	Myelomeningocele, hydrocephalus
Maternal iodine deficiency	Goitre
2. Physical	
Ionizing radiation	Microcephaly
3. Chemical	
Androgens	Virilization of female fetus
Cyclophosphamide	Syndactyly
Diethylstilboestrol	Virilization of female fetus
Ethanol	Microcephaly, cleft lip or palate
Folic acid antagonists	Hydrocephaly, cleft palate
Hydantoins	Microcephaly, cleft lip, congenital heart disease
Isotretinoin	Cleft palate
Lithium	Ebstein's anomaly of tricuspid valve
Maternal diabetes mellitus	Caudal regression syndrome
Maternal phenylketonuria	Microcephaly
Maternal tobacco smoking	Cleft lip, cleft palate
Methyl mercury	Microcephaly
Progesterones	Virilization of female fetus
Thalidomide	Phocomelia, congenital heart disease, oesophageal atresia, duodenal atresia
Trimethadione	Anomalies of central nervous system
Valproic acid	Myelomeningocele
Warfarin	Nasal hypoplasia
4. Animate	
Cytomegalovirus	Microcephaly
Herpes virus hominis, type 2	Microcephaly, microphthalmia
Rubella virus (wild)	Microcephaly, patent ductus arteriosus, cataracts
Varicella zoster virus	Limb reduction defects
Venezuelan equine phalitis virus	Hydranencephaly, micro phthalmia
Treponema	
Treponema pallidum	*Hydrocephaly*
Toxoplasma gondii	*Microcephaly, hydrocephaly microphthalmia*

which a teratogen can have acted in causing a particular malformation, but the latest gestational age at which a teratogen can act to cause the malformation can often be determined and is known as the teratologic termination period for that malformation.

Teratologic termination periods for some malformations of interest to paediatric surgeons are given in Table 22.4.

Knowledge of teratologic termination periods can be useful in reassuring parents that some event during pregnancy was not related to the development of a malformation in their child. A list of human teratogens is given in Table 22.5. It should not be assumed, however, that exposure of a human embryo to any of these agents will necessarily result in a malformation, nor that agents not listed in Table 22.5 are necessarily harmless.

Chromosomal anomalies. Chromosomal anomalies are changes in the normal chromosomal complement, or karyotype, of cells, and several mechanisms are involved in their pathogenesis.

Non-disjunction (Fig. 22.1) is due to failure of chromosomes to divide equally between daughter cells at mitosis or meiosis, so that a daughter cell has a greater or lesser number of chromosomes than normal, e.g. regular Down syndrome (trisomy 21).

Translocation (Figs 22.2 and 22.3) is the transfer of part of one chromosome to another

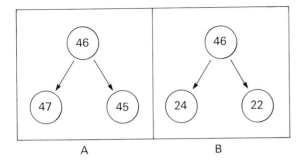

Fig. 22.1 Non-disjunction. Failure of chromosomes to divide equally between daughter cells at mitosis or meiosis so that a daughter cell has a greater or lesser number of chromosomes than normal. Number of chromosomes shown in each cell. **A**: Mitosis. **B**: Meiosis.

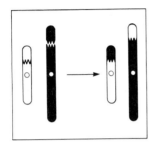

Fig. 22.2 Reciprocal translocation. Interchange of material between two chromosomes.

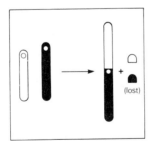

Fig. 22.3 Translocation with centric fusion. One-way transfer of material from one chromosome to another.

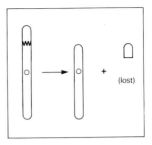

Fig. 22.4 Deletion — loss of part of a chromosome.

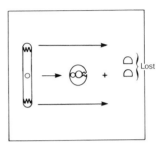

Fig. 22.5 Deletion with formation of a 'ring' by fusion of two sites of breakage of a chromosome.

Deletion (Figs 22.4 and 22.5) is the loss of part of a chromosome. This may follow a chromosomal break, and the deleted material is lost at the next mitotic division, e.g. 'cat-cry' syndrome, with loss of part of the short arm of chromosome number 5. Deletion of chromosomal material from the two ends of a chromosome may lead to formation of a ring (Fig. 22.5).

Another variety of chromosomal anomaly is *inversion* of part of a chromosome which will alter the sequence of nucleic acid and may lead to altered expression of one or more genes.

The addition, loss or alteration of position of such large amounts of genetic material would be expected to interfere with normal development of the embryo and fetus and so cause malformations. In fact, autosomal anomalies are almost always associated with multiple malformations, and anomalies involving sex chromosomes are often, but not always, associated with malformations. Anomalies of sex chromosomes are 2 to 3 times more frequent than those involving autosomes.

Occasionally, chromosomal anomalies may be familial. Clinically, normal individuals may have

chromosome, e.g. translocation Down syndrome. This transfer may be reciprocal, i.e. an interchange of material between two chromosomes (Fig. 22.2), or may involve a one-way transfer from one chromosome to another by centric fusion (so-called robertsonian translocation) (Fig.22.3). A translocation may or may not involve loss of chromosomal material.

a balanced chromosomal translocation, where part or all of one chromosome is transferred to another chromosome. The total amount of chromosomal material in each cell therefore remains the same, but at meiosis, the abnormal chromosome will move to one or other of the resulting cells which will therefore contain excessive or deficient amounts of chromosomal material and on fertilization, the resultant fetus will have an unbalanced chromosomal pattern, with associated malformations and possibly intrauterine death. A pedigree with multiple spontaneous abortions, therefore, may indicate an underlying balanced translocation in one or other parent.

Any of the chromosomal anomalies usually involves all cells of the patient, but in some cases, two or more cell lines may be present, each of which has a different karyotype, and this condition is termed chromosomal mosaicism.

The presence of mosaicism will often modify the typical clinical appearance, or phenotype, of the patient and if one of the cell lines has a normal karyotype, there may be few or no clinical features of the syndrome. While these patients may, therefore, be clinically normal or near normal, it is possible that they may transmit the chromosomal anomaly to their children, depending on the karyotype of the parental germ cells.

The incidence of malformation syndromes associated with some of the commoner chromosomal anomalies is given in Table 22.6.

Genetic anomalies. Malformations that are genetically determined may be transmitted in a dominant or recessive fashion and the abnormal gene may be on an autosome or on a sex chromosome.

In general it may be said that:

1. Genetically determined diseases transmitted in an autosomal dominant manner tend to be less severe clinically than diseases transmitted in an autosomal recessive manner.

2. At present a metabolic defect cannot be demonstrated for most genetically determined malformations but, as biochemical testing for heterozygotes becomes more sophisticated, the distinction between dominant and recessive disease will necessarily become less distinct.

Table 22.6 Incidence of common chromosomal anomalies in liveborn children*

Syndrome	Usual karyotype	Approximate incidence in liveborn infants
Klinefelter	47,XXY	1:500 (males)
Down	47, XX or XY, + 21	1:660
Turner	45, X	1:2500
Edwards	47, XX or XY, + 18	1:3000
Patau	47, XX or XY, +13	1:5000

* Overall, most embryos with chromosomal anomalies are spontaneously aborted, so that, at the time of conception, the incidence of many of these syndromes is much higher than the figures in this table would indicate e.g. Down syndrome is present in about 1:200 and Turner syndrome in about 1:50.

3. The clinical manifestation of the effects of abnormal genes may be modified by a number of factors, e.g. penetrance and expressivity. Discussion of these factors is beyond the scope of this book but further information can be obtained from the additional reading list.

Polygenic inheritance. Relatives of patients with certain malformations, including pyloric stenosis, cleft lip, cleft palate, club foot, myelomeningocele or congenital dislocation of the hip, have an increased risk of having the same malformation, and the closer the blood relationship, the greater the risk. The risk of recurrence of such malformations increases with the number of affected first-degree relatives. However, the pattern of recurrence in close relatives is not that seen in conditions due to mutations involving a single gene and it has been suggested that these malformations are partly or completely determined by the combined effect of several genes, a process termed polygenic inheritance. If there is a sex difference in the incidence of such a malformation, relatives of a patient of the less frequently affected sex have a greater risk of having the malformation than relatives of a patient of the more frequently affected sex.

Interaction between genes and environment. It is artificial to adhere too strictly to a separation between genetic and environmental factors in the pathogenesis of a given disease, as even those conditions that are ascribed to a mutant gene, e.g. galactosaemia and phenylketonuria, may require environmental factors to induce disease, e.g. galactose and phenylalanine respectively.

Conversely, a given teratogen, e.g. thalidomide, will only induce the specific malformation of phocomelia in those species (man, rabbit) that are genetically susceptible to the action of the teratogen. Even within a single species, individuals may be unduly susceptible or resistant to a given teratogen. This difference in susceptibility to malformation has been shown to have a genetic basis in some species, e.g. cleft palate induced in mice by exposure to hydrocortisone, and a similar genetic susceptibility may explain the variable development of malformations in human embryos exposed to a given teratogen under apparently comparable circumstances.

Unknown. In approximately 65% of malformations the cause is not known. These malformations may be due to the interaction of genetic and environmental factors, but at present we have no clear idea of what these genetic and environmental factors may be, or of their respective roles in inducing malformations.

HOW WILL IT AFFECT OUR BABY AND FAMILY?

The effect of a malformation on a baby will, of course, depend on the type of malformation, on any associated features and on the availability of treatment, e.g. duodenal atresia can be readily treated by surgery in a baby with trisomy 21, but is only one factor in determining the long-term prognosis for the child.

An accurate diagnosis is most important when answering the question, 'How will this malformation affect our baby?'. Many of the problems that arise in advising parents about the probable outcome of a malformation in their baby come from a mistaken diagnosis or from failure to recognize associated malformations or clinical features, e.g. the management of a baby with a cleft palate but no other abnormality will differ from that of a baby with a cleft palate as part of the Robin anomalad and the prognosis of both of these babies will differ markedly from the prognosis of a baby who has a cleft palate as part of the trisomy 13 syndrome.

It is therefore important to obtain a comprehensive history, and especially an adequate family history, to carry out a thorough physical examination and to perform any necessary investigations before giving an assessment of the prognosis. Particular attention should be given to the possibility of mental handicap, which is found in association with a number of malformation syndromes. If, as often happens, doubt exists about the diagnosis or prognosis, a consultation should be sought with a clinical geneticist. This may lead to some delay in giving parents the information they are seeking, but delay is preferable to giving wrong advice.

On the other hand, one of the main complaints of parents of malformed children is that they are not told the child's diagnosis and prognosis early enough. In practice, it is usually reasonable to tell the parents immediately of your suspicions about the presence of a malformation, explain that confirmation is necessary and keep them informed as the results of consultations and investigations become available. Parents will need to know about any risks or possible complications of surgery, about any handicap, physical or mental, which may remain after surgical repair of a malformation and about what effects such a handicap may have on the child's education, social relations and prospects of employment.

Parents may be concerned not only with how a malformation may affect the baby, but also with how the presence of a malformed baby will affect the family, and in discussing this with the parents it may be helpful to use the concept of the 'clinical burden' of a malformation. The clinical burden may be defined as the total adverse effect of the malformation on the patient, the family and the community, and includes death, surgical procedures or medical treatment, survival with a handicap, and the possibility of occurrence of the malformation in others. For example, the 'clinical burden' of anal atresia is greater than that of duodenal atresia, although the life-threatening intestinal obstruction common to both lesions can be repaired with a very low mortality rate, because residual defects in function are more frequent after repair of anal atresia than after repair of duodenal atresia. Similarly, the 'clinical burden' of a newborn baby dying with the infantile type of polycystic kidneys is greater than that of a newborn infant dying with bilateral cystic dysplastic kidneys, because the former is an hereditary disease with a 1 in 4 chance of recurrence in future siblings, while the latter is a sporadic disease with only about a 4% chance of recurrence.

Another example is that many surviving children with myelomeningocele will have multiple severe handicaps including incontinence, variable impairment of locomotion and often some degree of mental handicap. Caring for such a child will obviously place restrictions on many normal family activities and so will constitute a 'clinical burden' to the family.

WHAT CAN BE DONE ABOUT IT?

This involves care of both the patient and the family.

Care of the patient

The first decision for the surgeon is whether operative repair of the malformation is technically possible, as some malformations, e.g. anencephaly, are irreparable. If the malformation can be repaired, the next decision is whether or not the patient can survive. An infant may have several malformations, some reparable and others not, or may have some other potentially lethal condition such as severe cerebral hypoxic damage. If survival is not possible, then only supportive treatment can be offered.

Occasionally, difficult moral and ethical decisions may arise when there is a conflict between the two desirable aims of prolonging life and preventing suffering. In such a case, prolongation of life for a comparatively short time by a complex surgical procedure may only increase the patient's suffering. Decisions about treatment in these situations are never easy and the welfare of the patient should be the primary consideration in formulating any plan of management. To reach a decision, the surgeon should obtain whatever assistance is available from medical and nursing colleagues, theologians, philosophers and even lawyers, as recent judicial decisions in some countries have established legal requirements for the management of certain malformations. The surgeon should then discuss with the parents the various options for management and the likely outcome for each and recommend one option, but be prepared to accept the decision of the parents if they choose another option.

If the surgeon considers that the parents' decision is not in the best interests of the patient, he or she should point this out to the parents and advise them to obtain a second opinion. If a decision is made not to attempt surgical repair of a malformation, then the infant should be treated in the same way as any normal baby and given feedings, warmth and normal nursing care, with any drugs necessary to alleviate pain. Investigations or painful procedures should be avoided. The infant will usually remain in hospital, but some may go home, depending on the wishes of the parents and their ability to cope with the situation. Decisions to avoid surgical treatment need not be irrevocable and the plan of management may be modified at a later stage, depending on the infant's condition and progress.

In the long-term care of the patient with a residual handicap, it is most important that the child obtains the maximum benefit from his or her residual capabilities and that there is no further loss of function, e.g. because of contractures of limbs induced by lack of adequate physiotherapy and orthopaedic care, of tissue damage caused by infection, or of mental handicap due to lack of stimulation.

Care of the family

In most cultures, handicapped individuals are not readily accepted and, faced with a baby who is less than perfect, the parents may be inclined to reject their child and may feel rejected themselves. The surgeon should help the parents to accept their baby by demonstrating and stressing the normal features of the infant and should also try to convey acceptance of the mother and father as worthwhile individuals.

Care of the family will include helping the parents and siblings to cope with any problems arising from the malformation and its treatment, advising them realistically of the prognosis, both immediate and long-term, and counselling them about the risk of recurrence of the malformation in any future children. It is important to discuss the diagnosis, prognosis and any problems likely to arise from the malformation and its treatment as soon as possible.

However, it should be remembered that the discovery that their child is malformed will be a great shock to parents and hence they may not comprehend much of the information that they are given at an initial consultation. Further interviews are therefore necessary to repeat and reinforce the initial advice, to allow the parents to seek further details and to express their hopes and fears about the future of their child.

Such advice will include information about the work involved in caring for a child with a temporary or permanent handicap, how the home may be modified or altered to alleviate this workload and what facilities for support are available in the community, e.g. parents' organizations, visiting nurses, special schools and day-care centres. Other problems may arise with siblings whose needs are not met because of the time and effort required to cope with the malformed child, or who can be subjected to teasing by their peers. These problems may frequently be averted by alerting the parents to potential sources of trouble. It is also necessary to avoid overprotecting the handicapped child and to maintain as normal a pattern of family activity as possible.

WILL IT HAPPEN AGAIN IF WE HAVE MORE CHILDREN?

All parents of malformed children should be counselled about the risk of recurrence of the malformation in future children. The ideal genetic counsellor is a clinical geneticist, but all clinicians should be familiar with the basic concepts of genetic counselling. Vague or possibly misleading statements, made in an attempt to give reassurance, must be avoided.

As stated previously, it is most important to make a correct diagnosis of the type of malfor-

mation, bearing in mind that a particular set of clinical features (the phenotype of the patient) may not always be the result of the same genetic constitution, or genotype. For example, microcephaly may be an autosomal recessive condition, or may be a consequence of untreated maternal phenylketonuria, or may follow maternal exposure to physical agents (e.g. ionizing radiation), chemical agents (diphenylhydantoin) or animate agents (e.g. rubella virus). The risk of recurrence of microcephaly in future children would therefore be 25% in the autosomal recessive type, over 80% in untreated maternal phenylketonuria, negligible if due to exposure to physical or chemical agents and exposure did not occur in a subsequent pregnancy and virtually negligible if due to infection with rubella virus, regardless of maternal exposure to the virus during a subsequent pregnancy. Recognition of various malformations and of their possible causes is based mostly on clinical experience, although there are a number of books and at least one comprehensive computer program which deal with the subject.

It is most important to obtain a complete family pedigree for each patient, with particular attention to the relevant malformation or pattern of malformations. This will include specific information about all children of both parents, whether living or dead, about any stillbirths or spontaneous abortions and about the parents themselves and their immediate relatives. For example, hydrocephalus without myelomeningocele in a male child may be sporadic, in which case the risk of recurrence in future children is less than 5%. However, if a maternal great-uncle had died in infancy with the same condition, then it may very well be X-linked recessive hydrocephalus, with a recurrence risk of 50% in future male children. Another example is that of a malformed infant born to a mother who has had recurrent spontaneous abortions. This type of pedigree is suggestive of a balanced translocation in the karyotype of one of the parents, usually the mother, with a high likelihood of recurrence of the malformation in future pregnancies, and it would be essential to determine the karyotype of both parents to exclude this possibility.

It seems probable that genetic probes will be used with increasing frequency to improve accuracy in diagnosis of individual malformations. This technique is only available for a few conditions (e.g. the autosomal dominant, or adult, type of polycystic kidneys) at present, but many more genetic probes will undoubtedly be discovered in the near future.

Calculation of the risk of recurrence of a specific malformation can become more difficult if one or other of the parents of an affected child remarries. In the case of an autosomal dominant condition, this usually does not constitute a problem, because the parent with the abnormal gene will nearly always have clinical features of the disease and so can be readily identified. In the case of an X-linked recessive disease, the carrier status of the mother can often be determined by laboratory tests in conjunction with pedigree analysis.

In autosomal recessive conditions, however, the risk of recurrence will depend upon the likelihood that the parent's new partner is heterozygous for the relevant abnormal gene. If the carrier status of the new partner cannot be determined by laboratory tests, the risk of occurrence can be calculated from the frequency of the particular disease in the population. If an autosomal recessive disease is found in 1 in 10 000 persons in a population, and since autosomal recessive diseases are found, on average, in 1 in 4 children when both parents are heterozygotes, then both parents will be heterozygous for the relevant gene in 1 in 2500 families (1 in 10 000/4). The frequency of the relevant gene in individuals in the community will therefore be 1 in 50 (the square root of 1 in 2500). Since the original parent is an obligatory heterozygote for the abnormal gene, the risk of a child of the new union being affected will be 1 in 50 (the risk that the new partner will be heterozygous for the gene) times 1 in 4 (the risk of an autosomal recessive disease with both parents being heterozygous for the gene), i.e. 1 in 200.

When all relevant information has been obtained, the parents can be given information about the risks of occurrence and of recurrence of the malformation and should be helped to appreciate the significance of these risks. The risks may be explained in terms of the laws of probability, but many parents can better comprehend the analogy of tossing a coin. Most parents find that a risk of more than 10% is too high, but some will not accept a risk of 1%, while others are relatively unconcerned about a risk of 25%. It can sometimes be helpful to express the risk in terms of the likelihood that a future child will not have the malformation in question, e.g. 99% likely. The risk of recurrence of a given malformation is, of course, additional to the general risk of any child having an unspecific malformation. Risks of recurrence should be given not only to parents of children with genetically determined malformations, but also to those children with malformations due to chromosomal anomalies or teratogens, or to an unknown cause, as, even when the cause is not known, it is usually possible to give an empirical risk of recurrence.

The parents should also be advised about the various options open to them, including adoption as an alternative to future pregnancies. Repeated discussions will be necessary to clarify any points that are still unclear. The parents should not be directed to follow a particular course of action, but should make up their own minds on the basis of the information given them by the counsellor.

Detailed information about genetic counselling is beyond the scope of this book, but it is helpful to have an idea of the empirical recurrence risks for some common malformations (Table 22.7)

Table 22.7 Approximate recurrence risk of common malformations

Malformation	Risk with one affected first-degree relative
Cleft lip with or without cleft palate	1/25
Male index patient	1/40
Female index patient	1/15
Cleft palate without cleft lip	1/50
Club foot	1/35
Congenital dislocation of the hip	1/25
Congenital heart disease (type unspecified)	1/25
Myelomeningocele	'Local risk'* ×8
Pyloric stenosis	
Male index patient	1/30
Female index patient	1/15

* 'Local risk' is the incidence of myelomeningocele in the newborn in the country or region where the parents live.

It should be noted that these recurrence risks apply only to isolated malformations and not to malformations occurring as part of a syndrome.

Examples of isolated malformations of which some, but not necessarily all, cases are inherited in an autosomal recessive manner, with a recurrence risk of 1 in 4, are:

- Adrenogenital syndrome
- Amelia, phocomelia
- Cataract
- Craniosynostosis
- Diaphragmatic hernia
- Hydrocephaly
- Hypospadias
- Microcephaly
- Micrognathia
- Polycystic kidneys (infantile type)
- Polydactyly
- Robin anomalad
- Umbilical hernia

Malformations of which some, but not necessarily all, cases are inherited in an autosomal dominant manner, with a recurrence risk of 1 in 2, include:

- Amelia, phocomelia
- Anal atresia
- Branchial cyst
- Cataract
- Cleft lip
- Craniosynostosis
- Duplex kidney and ureter
- Exomphalos
- Funnel chest
- Hydronephrosis
- Hypospadias
- Inguinal hernia
- Osteocartilaginous exostosis (multiple)
- Patent ductus arteriosus
- Polycystic kidneys (adult type)
- Polydactyly
- Robin anomaled
- Syndactyly

Malformations of which some, but not necessarily all, cases are inherited in an X-linked recessive manner, with a recurrence risk of 1 in 2 in males, include:

- Anal atresia
- Cataract
- Cleft palate
- Hydrocephaly
- Androgen insensitivity syndrome

As you can see from above, it is possible for a given malformation to be genetically determined in more than one way, e.g. amelia/phocomelia may be transmitted as an autosomal recessive or as an autosomal dominant trait.

FURTHER READING

Beckman D A, Brent R L 1986 Mechanisms of known environmental teratogens: drugs and chemicals. Clinics in Perinatology, 13: 649–687

Christiansen R L 1975 Classification and nomenclature of morphological defects. Lancet 1: 513

Heinonen O P, Slone D, Shapiro S 1977 Complete listing of malformations found in the offspring of 50,282 women (Appendix 2). In: Heinonen O P, Slone D, Shapiro S (eds) Birth defects and drugs in pregnancy. PSG Publishing Company, Littleton, pp 446–455

Shokeir M H K 1979 Managing the family of the abnormal newborn. Birth Defects 15: 199–222

Skinner R 1983 Genetic counselling. In: Emery A E H, Rimoin D L (eds) Principles and practice of medical genetics. Churchill Livingstone, Edinburgh, vol 2, pp 1427–1436

Wilson J G 1977 Current status of teratology: general principles and mechanisms derived from animal studies. In: Wilson J G, Fraser F C (eds) Handbook of teratology. Plenum Press, New York, vol 1, p 47

Index